Stem Cells in Reproductive Medicine

Basic Science and Therapeutic Potential
Third edition

Stem Cells in Reproductive Medicine

Basic Science and Therapeutic Potential
Third edition

Edited by

Carlos Simón MD PhD
Instituto Valenciano de Infertilidad [IVI], Valencia, Spain

Antonio Pellicer MD PhD
Instituto Valenciano de Infertilidad [IVI], Valencia, Spain

Renee Reijo Pera PhD
Department of Obstetrics and Gynecology, Stanford University
School of Medicine, Palo Alto, CA, USA

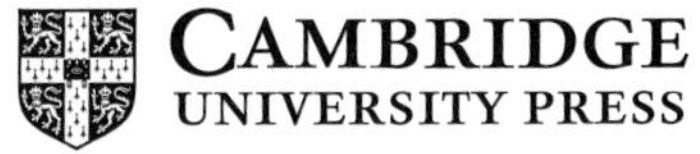

CAMBRIDGE
UNIVERSITY PRESS

CAMBRIDGE UNIVERSITY PRESS
Cambridge, New York, Melbourne, Madrid, Cape Town,
Singapore, São Paulo, Delhi, Mexico City

Cambridge University Press
The Edinburgh Building, Cambridge CB2 8RU, UK

Published in the United States of America by Cambridge University Press,
New York

www.cambridge.org
Information on this title: www.cambridge.org/9781107034471

This edition published 2013

Printed and bound in the United Kingdom by Bell and Bain Ltd

A catalogue record for this publication is available from the British Library

Library of Congress Cataloguing in Publication data
Stem cells in reproductive medicine : basic science and therapeutic potential
/ edited by Carlos Simón, Antonio Pellicer, Renee Reijo Pera. – 3rd ed.
     p.   ;   cm.
Rev. ed. of: Stem cells in human reproduction / edited by Carlos Simón,
Antonio Pellicer. 2009.
Includes bibliographical references and index.
ISBN 978-1-107-03447-1 (hbk.)
I. Simón, Carlos.   II. Pellicer, Antonio.   III. Reijo Pera, Renee.
IV. Stem cells in human reproduction.
[DNLM: 1. Adult Stem Cells.   2. Embryonic Stem Cells.
3. Genitalia – cytology.   4. Reproductive Medicine – methods.
5. Reproductive Techniques, Assisted.   QU 325]
QP277
616.02′774 – dc23   2013017143

ISBN 978-1-107-03447-1 Hardback

Contents

See color plates between pages 110 and 111.

Contributors

Anthony Atala
Wake Forest Institute for Regenerative Medicine, Wake Forest University Health Sciences, Winston-Salem, NC, USA

Karl W. Broman
Department of Biostatistics and Medical Informatics, University of Wisconsin-Madison, Madison, WI, USA

Irene Cervelló
CIPF & Fundación Instituto Valenciano de Infertilidad (FIVI), Valencia University, INCLIVA, Valencia, Spain

David K. Gardner
Department of Zoology, University of Melbourne, Parkville, Victoria, Australia

Caroline E. Gargett
The Ritchie Centre, Monash Institute of Medical Research and Monash University Department of Obstetrics and Gynaecology, Clayton, Victoria, Australia

Nicolás Garrido
Instituto Universitario IVI and FIVI, (Fundación IVI), Valencia, Spain

Ellen Goossens
Research Group Biology of the Testis, Department of Embryology and Genetics, Vrije Universiteit Brussel, Brussels, Belgium

Jennifer R. Gruhn
School of Molecular Biosciences and the Center for Reproductive Biology, Washington State University, Pullman, WA, USA

Alexandra J. Harvey
Department of Zoology, University of Melbourne, Parkville, Victoria, Australia

Terry J. Hassold
School of Molecular Biosciences and the Center for Reproductive Biology, Washington State University, Pullman, WA, USA

Patricia A. Hunt
School of Molecular Biosciences and the Center for Reproductive Biology, Washington State University, Pullman, WA, USA

Orkan Ilbay
Department of Obstetrics, Gynecology, and Reproductive Sciences, Yale University School of Medicine, New Haven, CT, USA

Irina Klimanskaya
Advanced Cell Technology, Inc., Marlborough, MA, USA

Tippi C. MacKenzie
Eli and Edythe Broad Center of Regeneration Medicine and Stem Cell Research and the Department of Surgery, University of California, San Francisco, CA, USA

Ana M. Martínez-Arroyo
CIPF & Fundación Instituto Valenciano de Infertilidad (FIVI), Valencia University, INCLIVA, Valencia, Spain

Jose V. Medrano
CIPF & Fundación Instituto Valenciano de Infertilidad (FIVI), Valencia University, INCLIVA, Valencia, Spain

Heidi Mertes
Bioethics Institute Ghent, Ghent, Belgium

Marcos Meseguer
Instituto Universitario IVI and FIVI, (Fundación IVI), Valencia, Spain

Sergio Mora
Control of Stem Cell Potency Group, Institute for Bioengineering of Catalonia (IBEC) and Center for Networked Biomedical Research on Bioengineering, Biomaterials, and Nanomedicine (CIBER-BBN), Barcelona, Spain

Sean V. Murphy
Wake Forest Institute for Regenerative Medicine, Wake Forest University Health Sciences, Winston-Salem, NC, USA

Hong P.T. Nguyen
The Ritchie Centre, Monash Institute of Medical Research and Monash University Department of Obstetrics and Gynaecology, Clayton, Victoria, Australia

Amar Nijagal
Eli and Edythe Broad Center of Regeneration Medicine and Stem Cell Research and the Department of Surgery, University of California, San Francisco, CA, USA

Takehiko Ogawa
Department of Urology, Yokohama City University, Yokohama, Japan

Guido Pennings
Bioethics Institute Ghent, Ghent, Belgium

Joy Rathjen
Department of Zoology, University of Melbourne, Parkville, Victoria, and Menzies Research Institute, University of Tasmania, Hobart, Tasmania, Australia

Angel Raya
Control of Stem Cell Potency Group, Institute for Bioengineering of Catalonia (IBEC); Center for Networked Biomedical Research on Bioengineering, Biomaterials, and Nanomedicine (CIBER-BBN); and Institució Catalana de Recerca i Estudis Avançats (ICREA), Barcelona, Spain

Renee A. Reijo Pera
Institute for Stem Cell Biology & Regenerative Medicine, Department of Obstetrics and Gynecology, Stanford University School of Medicine, Stanford University, Palo Alto, CA, USA

Rocío Rivera
Instituto Universitario IVI and FIVI, (Fundación IVI), Valencia, Spain

Emre Seli
Department of Obstetrics, Gynecology, and Reproductive Sciences, Yale University School of Medicine, New Haven, CT, USA

Carlos Simón
CIPF & Fundación Instituto Valenciano de Infertilidad (FIVI), Valencia University, INCLIVA, Valencia, Spain

Herman Tournaye
Centre for Reproductive Medicine, UZ Brussel, Brussels, Belgium

Agustín G. Zapata
Department of Cell Biology, Faculty of Biology, Complutense University, Madrid, Spain

Preface

Stem Cells in Reproductive Medicine: Basic Science and Therapeutic Potential, Third edition completes the trilogy devoted to this topic. It was initiated in 2007 with the publication of the first book that became a bestseller, continued in 2009 and the third book now sees the light in 2013.

This trilogy has witnessed an extraordinary evolution of the advances in stem-cell science that have impacted human reproductive medicine. There is no effort without error and shortcomings, therefore some of the topics initially presented have been consolidated, others have vanished, while a few have served as the initial step for actual breakthroughs.

Since the successful derivation of human embryonic stem cells (hESCs) from the inner cell mass (ICM) of a human blastocyst by the Thomson group in 1998, the mechanisms controlling pluripotency have started to be unraveled. As a result, in 2006 Yamanaka's group identified the factors responsible for reprogramming somatic cells toward a pluripotent phenotype. Initially, 24 factors were selected as candidates based on their functions, and after various combinations, the above authors demonstrated that only four were required to produce induced pluripotent stem cells (iPSCs) from fibroblasts, these being Oct3/4, Sox2, c-Myc, and Klf4. Despite the reprogramming process requiring subsequent modifications and improvements, this finding proved to be the milestone in the pluripotency road map, and was recognized by the Nobel Laureate of Medicine 2012. A large number of somatic cells has been reprogrammed by applying different approaches, including direct transdifferentiation from one lineage to another, and disease-/patient-specific reprogrammed cells produced, which represent an invaluable possibility for generating cell types of interest to be applied to autologous cell replacement therapies, e.g., the development of specific disease models and, in our discipline, artificial gamete generation. However, their clinical application is presently limited due to serious obstacles in biosafety terms. These general concepts in regenerative medicine can also be applied to our field.

Part I of this composition is devoted to the female gamete. Emre Seli introduces the genetics of germline formation, which is nicely followed by germ-cell differentiation from pluripotent cells by the groups of Rene Reijo and Carlos Simón. *Part II* focuses on the male gamete. Nicolas Garrido and Marcos Meseguer introduce the state of the art in this topic, and Takehiko Ogawa presents his data on in-vitro manipulation and differentiation of spermatogonial stem cells (SSCs), namely in vitro spermatogenesis that due to his work recently became possible in animal models. Finally, Herman Tournaye translates these perspectives to humans, exploring hopes and hypes. *Part III* starts with an outstanding chapter on meiotic recombination in human oocytes by the well-reputed group of Terry Hassold, which opens the gate for the understanding of the gene expression dynamics during human embryonic development by the co-editors' groups, followed by the concept of the human blastomere as the physiological unit of the embryo for the derivation of hESC, maintaining embryo viability, by the group of Irina Kliminskaya, that has a Phase I clinical trial underway on retinal degeneration using retinal pigment epithelial cells derived from hESCs. The ethical concerns of gamete generation from stem cells to avoid gamete donation, and customized hESC from blastomeres as the cellular insurance for the newborn are masterly treated by Guido Pennings. In *Part IV*, the amniotic fluid as an unexpected source of highly multipotent cells is presented by the group of Antony Atala who pioneered this discovery. Achievements in the research and translation of the stem-cell population in the human endometrium is presented by the groups of Caroline Gargett and Carlos Simón, and the new revolutionary concept of in-utero hematopoietic cell transplantation by the group of MacKenzie. The relevance of bone- marrow stroma as a source of mesenchymal stem cells for cell therapy is covered by Agustín Zapata.

Finally, *Part V* is dedicated to the state of the art in amazing, cutting-edge technologies such as reprogramming and transdifferentiation presented by Angel Raya and the metabolic framework of pluripotent stem cells and potential mechanisms of regulation from the experience of one of the most prominent embryologists in the field, David Gardner.

We would like to highlight the masterwork performed by our international colleagues who have generously contributed to this publication; to them we express our gratitude for the time and effort they have devoted. We do hope that the readers will find the contents of this third book useful as a reference, and as a valuable tool for the continued advancement of reproductive medicine.

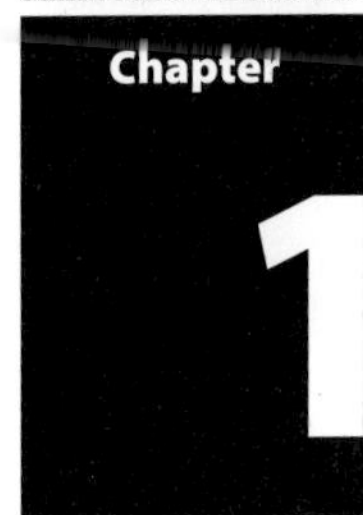

Genetics of germline formation

Orkan Ilbay and Emre Seli

Introduction

Survival of sexually reproducing organisms in the course of evolution depends on their success in producing gametes. The male gamete, or sperm, and the female gamete, the egg or oocyte, and their precursors are referred to as germ cells. Gametes develop from primordial germ cells (PGCs) that are set-aside during early embryogenesis [1]. In most metazoans, PGCs have an extragonadal origin and migrate to reach the somatic gonad where they proliferate by mitosis to form oocytes or spermatoza [1]. Specification, migration, proliferation, and differentiation of PGCs are tightly regulated and share common features among evolutionarily distant species.

In this chapter, we will review molecular mechanisms that control germline formation through a complex cascade of gene activation (Figure 1.1). These mechanisms have significant implications for our understanding of reproductive disorders and for ongoing efforts in using stem cells to generate functional gametes.

Primordial germ-cell specification

In mammals, primordial germ cells (PGCs) are derived from the proximal epiblast during early embryogenesis. In humans, the first PGCs are detected in the yolk sac on day 24 of embryo development [2]. In mice embryos, at day E7.25, PGCs are distinguished as alkaline phosphatase-positive cells in the extra-embryonic mesoderm posterior to the primitive streak [3,4]. Specification of PGCs from pluripotent epiblast cells requires induction by extracellular signals, which results in the activation of PGC-specific genes and the suppression of somatic genes (Table 1.1).

BMP4

One of the signals that induce PGC precursors is bone morphogenetic protein 4 (BMP4), which belongs to the transforming growth factor-β (TGF-β) superfamily [5]. BMP4 is expressed by extra-embryonic ectoderm in pre-implantation mouse embryos at around E6.0. BMP4 diffuses into the epiblast, setting up a gradient, and induces expression of genes involved in PGC specification in epiblast cells that are adjacent to the extra-embryonic ectoderm. *Bmp4*-null mice embryos are devoid of PGCs [5]. They also lack allantois, which, like PGCs, is derived from precursor cells in the proximal epiblast.

BMP8B

Another protein that belongs to the BMP and TGF-β families and is required for PGC formation is bone morphogenetic protein 8B (BMP8B) [6]. *In situ* hybridization of embryo sections shows *Bmp8b* expression in the extra-embryonic ectoderm of pre-gastrula- and gastrula-stage embryos. Similar to *Bmp4*, *Bmp8b*-null mice lack PGCs. Further studies on BMP4/BMP8B signaling shows that the number of PGCs formed during in vitro culture of proximal epiblast cells obtained from E6.0–E6.25 mouse embryos markedly increases upon addition of BMP4- and BMP8B-expressing feeder cells [7]. Although other unidentified signals may be required for acquiring PCG competence before BMP4/BMP8B signaling, current data suggest that these proteins are necessary and sufficient for PGC formation from epiblast cells on day E6.0.

Stem Cells in Reproductive Medicine 3rd edition, ed. Carlos Simón, Antonio Pellicer and Renee Reijo Pera.
Published by Cambridge University Press. © Cambridge University Press 2013.

Table 1.1 Regulatory proteins involved in primordial germ-cell specification.

Protein	Common Alias	Protein Function	Mutant Phenotype	Reference
BMP4		A TGF-Beta/Bmp family cytokine. Induces PGC formation.	Lack of PGCs and allantois.	Lawson *et al.* 1999 [5]
BMP8B		A TGF-Beta/Bmp family cytokine. Induces PGC formation.	Lack of PGCs (43%) or severe reduction in PGC number on a mixed genetic background. Lack PGCs on C57BL/6 background. Short or no allantois on both genetic backgrounds.	Ying *et al.* 2000 [6]
BMP2		A TGF-Beta/Bmp family cytokine. Structurally highly similar to Bmp4.	Reduced number of founding PGC. Short allantois. Additive effect with Bmp4 on PGC generation.	Ying *et al.* 2001 [9]
IFITM3	FRAGILIS	A trans-membrane protein implicated in cellular innate immunity to human pathogens (IFITM3). A PGC marker.	No effects on PGC formation and have no detectable effects on development of the germline.	Lange *et al.* 2008 [12]
DPPA3	STELLA	May play a role in maintaining cell pluripotentiality. A PGC marker.	No effect on PGC formation, but oocytes from mutant mice fail to develop normally beyond the four-cell stage.	Bortvin *et al.* 2004 [14]
PRDM1	BLIMP1	A PR domain-containing transcriptional repressor. Acts as a repressor of beta-interferon gene expression.	PGC-like cells at E7.5 that do not proliferate or migrate. Inconsistent repression of Hoxa1 and Hoxb1 genes.	Ohinata *et al.* 2005 [16]
PRDM14		A PR domain-containing transcriptional regulator. Necessary for PGC specification.	Lack of germ cells in adult ovaries and testes. Male and female infertility.	Yamaji *et al.* 2008 [18]

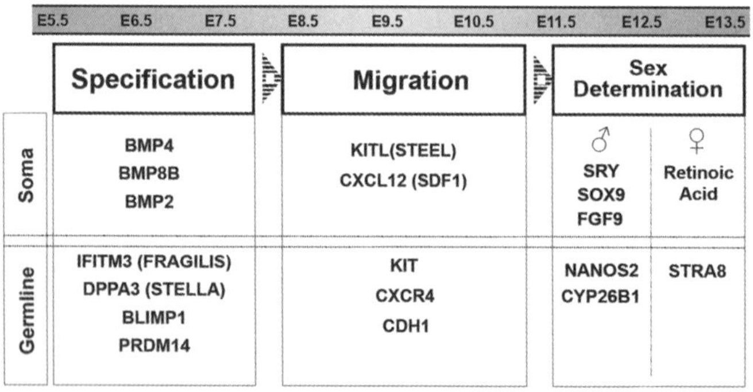

Figure 1.1 Germline formation: Bone morphogenetic proteins BMP4, BMP8B, and BMP2 induce PGC specification from the epiblast. BLIMP1 and PRDM14 are necessary for PGC specification. Nascent PGCs express FRAGILIS and STELLA, but these proteins are not necessary for PGC specification or germline formation. PGC specification is followed by migration. During migration PGCs express KIT while surrounding somatic cells express KITL. KITL is necessary for PGC motility as well as survival and proliferation of PGCs. CXCL12 is secreted from gonadal ridges and acts as a chemoattractant for PGCs. CXCR4 is a CXCL2 receptor expressed on the membranes of PGCs. E-CADHERIN expression on PGC membrane allows PGCs to interact with each other and migrate as a compact cluster. Migration ends when PGCs colonize the gonadal ridges and is followed by sex determination. FGF9 and retinoic acid (RA) from somatic cells regulate germ-cell sex determination in males and females, respectively. RA induces STRA8 expression and meiotic entry. CYP26B1 degrades RA protecting XY gonads from premature meiosis. FGF9 induces NANOS2 expression in germ cells, which in turn suppresses STRA8 expression.

BMP2

In addition to BMP4 and BMP8B expressed in the extra-embryonic ectoderm, expression of a third bone morphogenetic protein, BMP2, is detected in visceral endoderm at E6.0–E6.5 [8,9]. The highest BMP2 expression is observed in endoderm surrounding the posterior proximal epiblast, where BMP4/BMP8B signals act on PGC precursors. In *Bmp2*-null mice, the size of the PGC founding population is markedly reduced. BMP2 has >90% amino acid sequence homology to BMP4, and PGC numbers in double heterozygous mutants show BMP2 and BMP4 have an additive effect on PGC generation [9].

FRAGILIS and STELLA

Once specified, PGCs are characterized by expression of specific genes. Comparison of single-cell gene expression profiles of nascent PGCs and their somatic neighbors reveals up-regulation of an interferon-inducible trans-membrane protein, FRAGILIS/IFITM3 in PGCs [10]. Expression of FRAGILIS is induced by BMP signaling from extra-embryonic ectoderm in a dose-dependent manner. FRAGILIS expression is absent in *Bmp4*-null mouse embryos, while it is significantly reduced in *Bmp4*-heterozygous mutants. Moreover, intimate contact with extra-embryonic ectoderm is sufficient to induce FRAGILIS expression in distal epiblast. Expression of two more members of the Fragilis family, FRAGILIS2 and FRAGILIS3, has also been detected in nascent PGCs [11]. Among FRAGILIS-positive cells, only the ones with the highest expression become committed to germ-cell fate. These committed cells start expressing STELLA (DPPA3) during PGC specification, and STELLA expression remains restricted to developing PGCs [10]. Interestingly, although both FRAGILIS and STELLA are differentially expressed in PGCs, neither appears to be essential for PGC specification [12–14].

BLIMP1/PRDM1

Homeobox (Hox) genes are turned on sequentially throughout the embryo during embryonic pattern formation and play an important role in metazoan embryonic development. However, PGC specification, which requires an escape from somatic cell fate, is marked by down-regulation of *Hox* genes. There are several findings suggesting that BLIMP1/PRDM1, a PR domain-containing transcriptional repressor, which has been shown to regulate plasma cell differentiation, plays a role in the suppression of the somatic program in PGC precursors (or nascent PGCs) [15,16]. In mice, four to eight BLIMP1-positive cells are observed among E6.25 epiblast cells that are always directly in contact with extra-embryonic ectoderm. At E6.5 BLIMP1 expression is observed in approximately 20 cells in the epiblast

that are defined as lineage-restricted PGCs [16,17]. In *Blimp1*-deficient mice embryos at E7.5, the number of alkaline phosphatase-positive cells is markedly reduced. More importantly, although these PGC-like cells are alkaline phosphatase-positive, they do not proliferate or migrate as wild-type PGCs do. Comparison of transcripts from single PGC-like cells in *Blimp1*-deficient embryos with wild-type PGCs shows inconsistent repression of HOXA1 and HOXB1 [16].

PRDM14

More recently, expression of another PR-domain-containing transcriptional regulator, PRDM14, has been detected in BLIMP1/PRDM1-positive PGCs starting on E6.75 [18]. When both BLIMP1/PRDM1 and PRDM14 expression are examined in whole embryos, PRDM14 expression is more restricted to PGCs than BLIMP1/PRDM1. Germline-specific expression of PRDM14 is supported by the *Prdm14*-null phenotype. When crossed, $Prdm14^{+/-}$ mice deliver $Prdm14^{-/-}$ mice in the expected Mendelian ratio and with no apparent defects, suggesting that PRDM14 is not critical for embryonic development. However, adult *Prdm14*-null females and males are sterile and they lack germ cells, indicating that PRDM14 is essential for germ-cell development.

PGC migration

Once specified in the proximal epiblast, at around E7.5, PGCs start moving through the primitive streak into the adjacent endoderm [19] (Figure 1.1). At E8.0 PGCs migrate along the endoderm, while the endoderm gives rise to hindgut. PGCs then become incorporated into the hindgut and move along with the hindgut epithelium. Between E9.0–E9.5, PGCs exit from the hindgut, split into two populations, and migrate towards the dorsal body wall. PGCs reach and colonize the nascent gonadal ridges between E11.5 and E12.5 [20]. In humans, PGC migration and colonization of gonads take place between the 4th and 6th weeks of gestation [21].

In general, migration of PGCs from primitive streak to genital ridges is believed to be governed by chemotactic cytokines, cell surface receptors, and cell adhesion factors. In addition, PGCs seem to migrate passively during embryonic morphogenetic

Table 1.2 Regulatory proteins involved in primordial germ-cell migration.

Protein	Common Alias	Protein Function	Mutant Phenotype	Reference
KITLG *Kitl* *(mouse)*	*STEEL, STEEL FACTOR*	A cytokine that binds to the Kit receptor. Can exist both as a trans-membrane protein and a soluble protein. Facilitates PGC motility and essential for survival and proliferation of PGCs.	Marked decrease in PGC motility from the site of specification till they colonize the genital ridges.	Mahakali Zama *et al.* 2005 [23] Gu *et al.* 2009 [25]
KIT	*C-KIT*	Trans-membrane receptor for Kitl. Facilitates PGC motility and essential for survival and proliferation of PGCs.	Severe defects in PGC migration, number of PGC colonize gonadal ridges severely reduced.	Buehr *et al.* 1993 [88]
CXCL12		A cytokine secreted by genital ridges and acts as a chemoattractant for PGCs. Also produced by activated monocytes and neutrophils and expressed at sites of inflammation.	Reduced number of PGCs in the gonads.	Ara *et al.* 2003 [27]
CXCR4		A G-protein-coupled receptor, specific for Cxcl12.	Defects in PGC migration and survival; number of PGCs in the gonads is reduced.	Molyneaux *et al.* 2003 [26]
CDH1	*CD324*	(E-cadherin) a calcium-dependent cell–cell adhesion glycoprotein.	Chd1-null embryos die around the time of implantation. Perturbed PGC compaction in gonads when E-cadherin is blocked in embryo slice cultures.	Larue *et al.* 1994 [89] Bendel-Stenzel *et al.* 2000 [28]

movements and expansion of the hindgut endoderm. Although molecular mechanisms behind PGC migration are not well established there are several proteins that seem to be involved in this process (Table 1.2).

Expression of FRAGILIS and STELLA persist in PGCs during migration. Together with other interferon-induced trans-membrane (IFTM) family proteins, IFTM1 was thought to regulate initiation of PGC migration in mice [22]. However, targeted deletion of the *Iftm* gene cluster including *Iftm1* did not disturb initiation or completion of PGC migration [12].

KITL and c-KIT

KITL (Steel Factor) and its receptor KIT (c-KIT) are implicated in the regulation of PGC migration in mice, especially during the migration along the endoderm for about two days starting on E7.5 [23–25]. As a surface receptor, c-KIT is expressed on PGCs throughout all stages of their migration, while all the somatic cells surrounding PGCs express KITL. KITL expression in the surrounding somatic cells seems to facilitate PGC motility rather than acting as a chemotactic stimulus. Hence, PGCs in *Kitl*-deficient mice embryos

move in the proper direction but at a reduced rate, which is described as 50% reduction in average velocity. In addition to facilitating migration, KITL emerges as a niche factor that is essential for survival and proliferation of PGCs.

CXCL12 (SDF1), CXCR4, and E-cadherin

A chemotactic cytokine and its receptor regulate homing of PGCs to gonadal ridges after they leave the hindgut at E9.5. Chemokine (C-X-C motif) ligand 12 (CXCL12, also called SDF1), secreted by genital ridges and the surrounding mesenchyme, acts as a chemoattractant for PGCs. A SDF1-specific receptor, chemokine (C-X-C motif) receptor 4 (CXCR4), expressed by migrating germ cells, responds to the SDF1 signal from genital ridges [26,27]. In both $Sdf1^{-/-}$ and $Cxcr4^{-/-}$ mice, PGC colonization of the gonads is impaired, while the number of PGCs reaching the mesentery of the hindgut at E9.5 is not affected. Moreover, ubiquitous expression of SDF1 in cultured embryo slices perturbs homing of PGCs to genital ridges, and ectopic SDF1 expression causes PGCs to migrate to designated locations [26]. In addition to homing by SDF1/CXCR4, migration of PGCs from

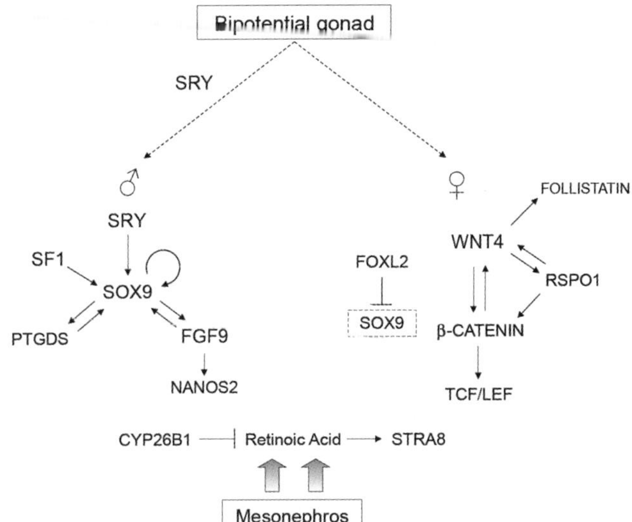

Figure 1.2 Sex determination: Sex determination in gonads precedes germ-cell sex determination. In XY gonads, transient SRY expression up-regulates SOX9 expression. SOX9 induces up-regulation of PTDGS and FGF9 expression. SOX9 itself, FGF9, and PGD2 (which is produced by PTGDS) induce SOX9 expression. Therefore, once induced by SRY, SOX9 expression is maintained. SF1 plays a role in synergistic activation of SOX9 by SRY and SOX9 itself. FGF9 up-regulates NANOS2 expression in germ cells. Together with CYP26B1, which degrades retinoic acid (RA), NANOS2 plays a role in preventing premature meiotic entry in XY germ cells. In XX gonads, RSPO1 up-regulates WNT4 expression and β-CATENIN activity. WNT4 up-regulates RSPO1, Follistatin, and β-catenin activity. β-CATENIN signaling, in turn, up-regulates WNT4 expression and regulates TCF/LEF-mediated transcriptional activation. FOXL2 suppresses SOX9 expression, hence male sex differentiation. RA signaling induces STRA8 transcription in germ cells, which leads to meiosis.

the hindgut to genital ridges is accompanied by up-regulation of a cell–cell adhesion glycoprotein, E-cadherin, which allows PGCs to interact or recognize each other to form a compact cluster and condense into the genital ridges [28].

Sex determination

Until the colonization of the genital ridges, XX and XY PGCs are indistinguishable in terms of morphology and behavior [29]. At the end of their migratory pathway, at around E12.0 in mice, PGCs colonize the genital ridges and are thereafter referred to as germ cells (GCs) or gonocytes. After entry into the gonadal ridges, expression of germline-specific gene products GCNA1 (germ cell nuclear antigen 1), DDX4 (DEAD (Asp-Glu-Ala-Asp) box polypeptide 4), DAZL (deleted in azoospermia-like) commences in both XX and XY germ cells [30–32]. Germ-cell sex determination starts in gonadal ridges and is largely regulated by the niche. Both XX and XY germ cells have the potential to be committed to spermatogenesis or oogenesis, when/if exposed to the somatic cells of a developing testis or ovary, respectively. In mice, male germ cells become committed to spermatogenesis between E11.5 and E12.5 and female germ cells become committed to oogenesis between E12.5 and E13.5 [33].

In mammals, genital ridges, or gonadal primordia, are derived from the coelomic epithelium of the mesonephros, and become visible at E10.0 in mice and at day 32 of pregnancy in humans. Proliferation and differentiation of epithelial cells give rise to gonadal primordia, which express the same gonadal-specific gene products (SF1, WT1, M33/CBX12, EMX2) in both XX and XY tissues [34]. Hence, early gonadal ridges are bipotential, which means they can follow either a testicular or an ovarian fate (Figure 1.2). At this point, the expression of sex-determining region Y (SRY) encoded by a gene on the Y chromosome, triggers a cascade of molecular events that strongly dictate initiation of differentiation of bipotential genital ridges into testes [35,36]. Female sex determination and development of gonadal ridges into ovaries also requires the onset of female-specific gene expression. However, molecular mechanisms establishing the female fate can be superseded by SRY expression in XX mice, which results in testes formation [37]. Moreover, absence of a functional *Sry* gene is enough for XY genital ridges to develop into ovaries and XY GCs to develop as oocytes [38]. In brief, mammalian sex determination seems to require a precise switch mechanism between ovary and testis formation, which is regulated by a single gene on the Y chromosome. SRY, and other genes involved in sex determination are listed in Table 1.3.

Male germline formation

In mice, male germ cells become committed to spermatogenesis between E11.5 and E12.5 [33]. Germ cells develop into spermatogonia and enter mitotic arrest, which takes place between E12.5 and E14.5 in mice. Mitotic arrest lasts until a few days after birth in mice

Table 1.3 Regulatory proteins involved in male and female germline formation.

Protein	Common Alias	Protein Function	Mutant Phenotype	Reference
SRY		A HMG-box-containing transcription factor that initiates male sex determination.	XY-to-female sex reversal.	Lovell-Badge *et al.* 1990 [38]
SOX9		A HMG-box-containing transcription factor activated by Sry.	Complete XY-to-female sex reversal.	Chaboissier *et al.* 2004 [46] Barrionuevo *et al.* 2006 [47]
FGF9		A fibroblast growth factor family protein. Involved in maintenance of Sox9 and germ line sex determination in males.	Disturbed Sertoli cell differentiation. Male-to-female sex reversal.	Colvin *et al.* 2001 [51]
PTGDS		Catalyzes the conversion of prostaglandin H_2 (PGH_2) to prostaglandin D_2 (PGD_2). PGD_2 is involved in regulation of Sox9 expression.	Reduced Sox9 expression in XY gonads but normal testis formation.	Moniot *et al.* 2009 [55]
NANOS2		Plays a role in suppression of meiosis, promotes male fate in germ cells.	Premature meiosis in XY germ cells.	Suzuki *et al.* 2008 [59]
CYP26B1		Involved in specific inactivation of retinoic acid.	Increased retinoic acid level in fetal testis. Premature meiotic entry in XY germ cells (at E13.5) and increased apoptosis after E13.5. Lack of germ cells in male neonates.	MacLean *et al.* 2007 [61]
WNT4		A secreted signaling protein involved in female fetal genital development and suppression of male fate. Involved in activation of β-catenin.	Formation of coelomic vessel and presence of steroidogenic cells in XX gonads.	Vainio *et al.* 1999 [65]
FST		Binds to activin and functions as an activin antagonist. Specifically inhibits follicle-stimulating hormone release. Co-expressed with Wnt4 in female gonads.	Coelomic vessel formation and presence of steroidogenic cells in XX gonads. Increased germ-cell apoptosis, almost no germ cells at birth. No defect in XY testes formation.	Yao *et al.* 2004 [67]
RSPO1		A secreted activator protein of R-spondin family. Activator of the beta-catenin signaling cascade, leading to TCF-dependent gene activation	Differentiation of seminiferous tubules and coelomic vessel formation in XX gonads.	Chassot *et al.* 2008 [70]
CTNNB1		(β-catenin) a key component of the canonical Wnt signaling pathway. Regulates TCF/LEF-mediated transcriptional activation.	Partial sex reversal in females. Formation of steroidogenic cells and a coelomic vessel in XX gonads. Down-regulated Wnt4 expression.	Liu *et al.* 2009 [72]
FOXL2		A fork-head DNA-binding domain-containing transcriptional regulator. Critical factor essential for ovary differentiation and maintenance, and repression of the genetic program for somatic testis determination.	Post-natal sex reversal in XX gonads. Transdifferentiation of granulosa cells into Sertoli-like cells.	Uhlenhaut *et al.* 2009 [77] Ottolenghi *et al.* 2005 [78]
NR0B1	DAX1, AHCH	A transcriptional regulator. Functions as an anti-testis gene by acting antagonistically to Sry.	No effect on female development. XY-to-female sex reversal depending on the mouse strain.	Yu *et al.* 1998 [84] Meeks *et al.* 2003 [85] Bouma *et al.* 2005 [86]
STRA8		A retinoic acid-responsive protein involved in the regulation of meiotic initiation in both spermatogenesis and oogenesis.	Failure in undergoing pre-meiotic DNA replication in germ cells. No oocytes or follicles in ovaries of 8-week-old mice.	Baltus *et al.* 2006 [90]

and until puberty in men. During adult life, spermatogonial cells proliferate while maintaining their identity, hence producing a pluripotent spermatogonia population. They also differentiate into spermatocytes. Spermatocytes enter meiosis to give rise to spermatids, which will mature into spermatozoa. Mitotic arrest in fetal testes, and each step in spermatogenesis in adult life, is regulated by signals from the somatic environment.

SRY

Mammalian male sex determination is initiated by SRY (sex-determining region Y) expression in XY genital ridges, which triggers Sertoli cell differentiation in supporting cell precursors. SRY is encoded by a single exon gene located on the Y chromosome and is the founding member of the SOX (SRY-like box) gene family, which comprises 20 genes in mice and humans. SRY protein (204 amino acids) is a chromatin-remodeling transcription factor and a member of the high mobility group (HMG)-box family of DNA-binding proteins. SRY, through its HMG domain, binds DNA sequences that contain the (A/T)ACAA(T/A) motif and bends the DNA [39]. SRY expression in mouse XY genital ridges starts at E10.5, reaches a peak at E11.5, and ceases by E12.5 [35]. Although it has a transient pattern, any delay (even 6 hours) in initiation of SRY expression results in a failure in testis development, suggesting that SRY expression must start or reach a threshold in a specific time window [40,41]. This transient expression of SRY acts as a trigger and initiates the cascade of molecular events that induce Sertoli cell differentiation and testis formation. A crucial part of the downstream events is activation of SOX9 expression.

SOX9

SOX9 (SRY-like box 9) is a HMG-box-containing transcription factor encoded by a member of the *SOX* gene family. In mice, low levels of SOX9 expression is observed in both XX and XY genital ridges at E10. However, in females, SOX9 expression is repressed and becomes undetectable in genital ridges by E11.5, whereas in XY genital ridges SOX9 expression is up-regulated soon after the onset of SRY expression [42,43]. Up-regulated SOX9 expression is restricted to Sertoli cell lineage and persists after E12.5 [42]. In humans, heterozygous *SOX9* mutations can result in partial or complete male-to-female sex reversal [44],

and duplication of *SOX9* gene has been reported in a female-to-male sex reversed case [45]. Mice lacking *SOX9* fail to perform male-specific differentiation and undergo complete male-to-female sex reversal [46,47]. Conversely, transgenic XX mice failing to repress SOX9 expression undergo sex reversal [48]. Therefore, current evidences suggest that while SRY expression in a specific time window is necessary for the onset of up-regulation of SOX9, SOX9 is necessary and sufficient for male sex determination.

SRY directly binds to TESCO (testis-specific enhancer of *SOX9* core), which is an enhancer element located upstream of SOX9, and activates SOX9 expression [49]. SOX9 itself binds to the TESCO element and creates a positive-feedback loop, which provides an insight to continuous SOX9 expression in Sertoli cell lineage. In both cases, together with SRY or SOX9, a transcriptional activator SF1 (steroidogenic factor 1), also called NR5A1, binds to and is involved in the synergistic activation of TESCO [49].

FGF9 and retinoic acid

In addition to the auto-regulatory positive-feedback loop involving SOX9 described above, FGF9 (fibroblast growth factor 9) seems to be required for maintenance of SOX9 expression and a positive feed-forward loop between FGF9 and SOX9 has been postulated [50]. FGF9 is a signaling molecule secreted by the Sertoli cells and induces differentiation in supporting cell precursors by up-regulating SOX9 expression. Targeted deletion of *Fgf9* or its receptor *Fgfr2* (fibroblast growth factor receptor 2) in mice disrupts Sertoli cell differentiation and leads to male-to-female sex reversal [51,52]. Prostaglandin D_2 (PGD_2) is another paracrine factor implicated in regulation of SOX9 expression [53]. SOX9, in turn, activates the expression of prostaglandin D synthase (PTGDS), which is the enzyme that produces PGD_2, forming a positive-feedback loop [54]. PGD_2 is able to induce SOX9 transcription in XX gonads in culture. In *Ptgds*-null mice, the SOX9 transcript level in XY gonads is reduced, but sex determination or testis formation is not affected [55].

FGF9 and retinoic acid (RA) are expressed at the gonadal niche and act as key determinants of sexual fate in XY and XX germ cells, respectively. Evidence suggests that FGF9 and RA have opposing effects on germ cells in terms of meiotic entry decision and sex determination. First, FGF9 promotes germ-cell survival specifically in XY gonads [56]. In *Fgf9*-null male mice, but not in females, the number of germ cells declines after E11.5 [57]. More importantly, FGF9 alone can markedly increase the survival of purified E11.5 XY germ cells in culture, proving that its effect is direct. Second, it has been shown that FGF9 acts to inhibit meiosis in XY germ cells, and also in XX germ cells [57,58]. The effect of RA on cultured E11.5 germ cells, which is determined by the expression level of an RA-activated gene (STRA8), is attenuated when FGF9 is included in the media [57]. In control of meiotic fate decision, FGF9 up-regulates NANOS2 (nanos homolog 2 (Drosophila)) expression in germ cells, which in turn prevents STRA8 expression [58]. NANOS2 expression is restricted to germ cells in male gonads and in *Nanos2*-null mice fetal germ cells enter meiosis and undergo apoptosis at around E15.5 [59]. Lastly, a P450 enzyme, CYP26B1, is expressed in somatic cells of the embryonic testes by E12.5, which effectively degrades pro-meiotic RA [60]. In *Cyp26b1-null* mice RA levels are increased in E12.5 testes and germ cells prematurely enter meiosis at E13.5, which is followed by apoptosis [61].

Female germline formation

In mice, female germ cells become committed to oogenesis between E12.5 and E13.5 [33]. Unlike the mitotically arrested spermatogonia in male fetal testis, female germ cells in fetal ovaries (oogonia) initiate meiosis and give rise to primary oocytes by E13.5 in mice, and between the 8th and the 13th week of gestation in humans [62]. Primary oocytes become arrested in the prophase of the first meiotic division and remain arrested until puberty. After puberty, with each menstrual cycle a number of primary oocytes are released from the prophase I arrest, continue meiosis and become arrested again in the metaphase of the second meiotic division; this second meiotic arrest is maintained until fertilization. As a crucial step in female germ-cell sex determination, cues to initiate meiosis are provided by female fetal ovaries.

Due to the fact that the presence or absence of male sex-determining factor, SRY, can greatly affect sex determination in mammalian gonads, differentiation of XX gonadal ridges into ovaries is often described as the "passive" or the "default" developmental path. In addition, molecular mechanisms establishing the female fate may be redundant, as implied by the fact that SRY-negative female-to-male sex reversal is very rare in humans and even in transgenic mice. Nevertheless, identification of SRY-negative female-to-male sex reversal cases in two siblings in three families, has led researchers to postulate that there is a recessive gene (termed the Z gene) that is responsible for repressing male development and/or activating female development [63]. While the Z gene is yet to be discovered, transcriptome analysis of mouse gonads during sex determination (between E10.5 and E13.5) shows that 1223 genes in females (and 1083 genes in males) are up-regulated [64]. Some of these genes have well-studied implications in female sex determination.

WNT4

WNT (wingless-related MMTV integration site) genes play key roles as intercellular signaling molecules in development that are conserved between *C. elegans* and vertebrates. In the canonical WNT signaling pathway, WNT ligands bind to cell surface receptors of the FRIZZLED family, leading to stabilization of cytoplasmic β-catenin. In turn, β-catenin transduces the signals to the nucleus and activates TCF/LEF (T-cell factor/lymphoid enhancer factor) family transcription factors to promote specific gene expression. There are 19 WNT and 10 FRIZZLED genes in mouse and human genomes.

WNT4 (wingless-related MMTV integration site 4) is a secreted signaling protein, which is implicated in control of female sexual development and the prevention of testes formation. During embryogenesis, between E9.5 and E10.5, WNT4 is expressed in both males and females, in the mesenchyme of the mesonephros and müllerian duct, and is essential for müllerian duct formation [65]. As sex-specific differentiation commences, WNT4 expression is repressed in the male gonad, while it is maintained in the female gonad. *Wnt4* deficiency has no effect in male sexual development, whereas it results in the presence of steroidogenic cells and formation of coelomic vessels in XX gonads. A loss-of-function mutation in human *WNT4* resulting in a phenotype similar to that observed in *Wnt4*-null mice, including regression of müllerian ducts, has been reported [66]. Downstream of WNT4, an activin-binding protein encoded by *Fst* gene, FOLLISTATIN, is employed [67]. FOLLISTATIN expression co-localizes with WNT4 in the female gonad, whereas it is absent in *Wnt4*-null mice. Moreover, *Fst*-deficient female mice fail to repress coelomic vessel formation and greatly mimic the *Wnt4*-null phenotype.

RSPO1

RSPO1 (R-sponsin 1) mutations have been associated with complete female-to-male sex reversal in humans [68]. In mouse embryos, RSPO1 expression is observed in the urogenital ridge, starting by E10.5, and in various other tissues, including the dorsal neural tube (E10–12), developing dermis (E12.5) and kidneys (E11.5) [68,69]. The sex-specific expression pattern is observed at E12.5 as a marked increase in RSPO1 expression in XX gonads. By E14.5, RSPO1 expression in XX gonads is fivefold higher than XY gonads [68]. Ablation of *Rspo1* in mice induces differentiation of seminiferous tubules in XX gonads but does not result in sex reversal as expected [70]. In addition, WNT4 expression is down-regulated in *Rspo1*-null gonads at E11.5 and E12.5, implying that RSPO1 is required for activation of WNT4 expression. Moreover, RSPO1 is a potent activator of WNT/β-catenin signaling and has been shown to inhibit internalization of LRP6 (low density lipoprotein receptor 6), which acts as a co-receptor with FRIZZLED in WNT signaling [71]. Hence, *Rspo1* deficiency results in a marked reduction in β-catenin activity [70].

β-catenin

As the key intracellular component of WNT signaling, β-catenin (CTNNB1) is required during female development. Binding of extracellular WNT ligands to FRIZZLED cell surface receptors leads to stabilization of cytoplasmic β-catenin, which is otherwise subject to phosphorylation and degradation. Ultimately, β-catenin accumulates and translocates to the nucleus to regulate TCF/LEF-mediated transcriptional activation. Employing a *LacZ*/target-gene fusion reporter, the active β-catenin-signaling pathway is detected in somatic cells of XX gonads starting by E12.5, but not in XY gonads [70]. Both WNT4 and RSPO1 contribute to stabilization of β-catenin in female gonads. *Wnt4*-null and *Rspo1*-null mice show only partial XX sex reversal and have similar ovarian phenotypes. Conditional ablation of *Ctnnb1* in SF1-positive somatic cells in female gonads results in a phenotype very similar to *Wnt4*-null and *Rspo1*-null mice [72]. Moreover, WNT4 expression is down-regulated in β-catenin-deficient female gonads, while RSPO1 expression is not affected. This may suggest a positive-feedback loop between WNT4 and β-catenin, while RSPO1 functions upstream of β-catenin. Interestingly, while overexpression of WNT4 has not been successful in causing male-to-female sex reversal [73,74], ectopic expression of a stable β-catenin in XY gonads has been sufficient to disrupt the male pathway and promote ovarian development [75].

FOXL2

Forkhead box L2 (FOXL2) is a transcriptional regulator containing a fork-head DNA-binding domain. In mice, FOXL2 expression is activated in XX gonads at around E12.5. FOXL2 is required for granulosa cell differentiation and ovary maintenance [76]. Moreover, it has been shown that FOXL2 can bind and repress TESCO (an enhancer element of SOX9) [77]. Hence, FOXL2 deficiency results in SOX9 up-regulation in XX ovaries, but only in perinatal and adult mice [77, 78]. In addition, conditional deletion of *Foxl2* in 8-week-old mice results in transdifferentiation of granulosa cells into Sertoli-like cells, which is described as post-natal sex reversal in the XX gonad [77]. A similar phenotype, transdifferentiation and post-natal sex reversal, is reported in mice lacking both *Esr1* (estrogen receptor 1) and *Esr2* (estrogen receptor 2) [79].

DAX1

DAX1, also called NR0B1 (nuclear receptor subfamily 0, group B, member 1), is encoded by an X-linked gene and has the potential to interfere with sex determination in a dose-dependent manner. DAX1 is first expressed in the bipotential genital ridges of both XX and XY mice embryos at E11.5 [80]. Between E12 and E12.5 DAX1 expression ceases to exist in males while it persists at least until E15.5 in female gonads. Duplications of a *DAX1*-containing region of Xp21 in XY individuals are associated with male-to-female sex reversal [81,82]. Also in mice, extra copies of the *Dax1* gene can cause complete male-to-female sex reversal [83]. Unexpectedly, DAX1 deficiency does not affect sex determination in XX mice, which demonstrates that DAX1 is not required for female development [84]. Moreover, targeted deletion of *Dax1* can cause complete male-to-female sex reversal in some mouse strains in a *Sry*-dependent manner [85,86].

Retinoic acid

Sex determination in XX germ cells is regulated by retinoic acid (RA) signaling, which triggers meiosis to initiate oogenesis. RA is produced not by gonads but by mesonephros of both sexes by E10 [60]. In females, RA signal induces up-regulation of the premeiotic marker STRA8 (stimulated by retinoic acid gene 8) at around E12.5 [86], while it is degraded by CYP26B1 in developing male testes. Still, high levels of RA in fetal testis can induce STRA8 up-regulation and meiosis in XY germ cells, as in *Cyp26b1*-null mice [60,61].

Summary

In mammals, germline is established early in embryogenesis. Primordial germ cells (PGCs) are derived from the distal epiblast, under the control of extracellular signals. Specifically, BMP4 and BMP8B are essential for PGC formation. Critical regulators for PGC specification like BLIMP1 and PRDM14, as well as novel PGC markers like FRAGILIS and STELLA have been identified by comparison of single-cell gene expression profiles of early PGCs with surrounding somatic cells. PGC specification is followed by migration of PGCs to gonadal ridges. During migration, cell surface receptors on PGCs, secreted ligands from surrounding somatic cells, and chemotactic cues from gonadal ridges play important roles.

Germ-cell colonization of the gonads is followed by sex determination. Expression of sex-specific genes in somatic tissues initiates molecular events that lead to testis or ovary development. Particularly, expression of Y-linked SRY, which activates SOX9 expression promotes testis differentiation. As for female sex determination, although a major player has not been identified, WNT/β-catenin signaling seems to plays a key role. FGF9 and retinoic acid signaling from differentiated somatic cells to germ cells controls meiotic entry and germ-cell sex differentiation in developing testes and ovaries, respectively.

In recent years, elegant studies in a multitude of model organisms have improved our understanding of the genetic regulation of germline formation. Further studies will enable us to better understand the biology

of this complex yet extremely important process and reinforce the framework for studies directed at generation of gametes from stem cells.

References

1. Matova, N., Cooley, L. Comparative aspects of animal oogenesis. *Developmental Biology*. 2001; 231(2): 291–320.

2. Witschi, E. Migration of germ cells of human embryos from the yolk sac to the primitive gonadal folds. *Contributions to Embryology Carnegie Institution*. 1948; 32(32): 67–80.

3. Chiquoine, A.D. The identification, origin, and migration of the primordial germ cells in the mouse embryo. *The Anatomical Record*. 1954; 118(2): 135–146.

4. Ginsburg, M., Snow, M.H., McLaren, A. Primordial germ cells in the mouse embryo during gastrulation. *Development*. 1990; 110(2): 521–528.

5. Lawson, K.A., Dunn, N.R., Roelen, B.A., *et al.* Bmp4 is required for the generation of primordial germ cells in the mouse embryo. *Genes and Development*. 1999; 13(4): 424–436.

6. Ying, Y., Liu, X.M., Marble, A., Lawson, K.A., Zhao, G.Q. Requirement of Bmp8b for the generation of primordial germ cells in the mouse. *Molecular Endocrinology*. 2000; 14(7): 1053–1063.

7. Ying, Y., Qi, X., Zhao, G.Q. Induction of primordial germ cells from murine epiblasts by synergistic action of BMP4 and BMP8B signaling pathways. *Proceedings of the National Academy of Sciences of the United States of America*. 2001; 98(14): 7858–7862.

8. Coucouvanis, E., Martin, G.R. BMP signaling plays a role in visceral endoderm differentiation and cavitation in the early mouse embryo. *Development*. 1999; 126(3): 535–546.

9. Ying, Y., Zhao, G.Q. Cooperation of endoderm-derived BMP2 and extraembryonic ectoderm-derived BMP4 in primordial germ cell generation in the mouse. *Developmental Biology*. 2001; 232(2): 484–492.

10. Saitou, M., Barton, S.C., Surani, M.A. A molecular programme for the specification of germ cell fate in mice. *Nature*. 2002; 418(6895): 293–300.

11. Lange, U.C., Saitou, M., Western, P.S., Barton, S.C., Surani, M.A. The fragilis interferon-inducible gene family of transmembrane proteins is associated with germ cell specification in mice. *BMC Developmental Biology*. 2003; 3: 1.

12. Lange, U.C., Adams, D.J., Lee, C. *et al.* Normal germ line establishment in mice carrying a deletion of the Ifitm/Fragilis gene family cluster. *Molecular and Cellular Biology*. 2008; 28(15): 4688–4696.

13. Payer, B., Saitou, M., Barton, S.C. *et al.* Stella is a maternal effect gene required for normal early development in mice. *Current Biology.* 2003; 13(23): 2110–2117.

14. Bortvin, A., Goodheart, M., Liao, M., Page, D.C. Dppa3 / Pgc7 / stella is a maternal factor and is not required for germ cell specification in mice. *BMC Developmental Biology.* 2004; 4: 2.

15. Shaffer, A.L., Lin, K.I., Kuo, T.C. *et al.* Blimp-1 orchestrates plasma cell differentiation by extinguishing the mature B cell gene expression program. *Immunity.* 2002; 17(1): 51–62.

16. Ohinata, Y., Payer, B., O'Carroll, D. *et al.* Blimp1 is a critical determinant of the germ cell lineage in mice. *Nature.* 2005; 436(7048): 207–13.

17. Saitou, M., Payer, B., O'Carroll, D., Ohinata, Y., Surani, M.A. Blimp1 and the emergence of the germ line during development in the mouse. *Cell Cycle.* 2005; 4(12): 1736–1740.

18. Yamaji, M., Seki, Y., Kurimoto, K. *et al.* Critical function of Prdm14 for the establishment of the germ cell lineage in mice. *Nature Genetics.* 2008; 40(8): 1016–1022.

19. Anderson, R., Copeland, T.K., Scholer, H., Heasman, J., Wylie, C. The onset of germ cell migration in the mouse embryo. *Mechanisms of Development.* 2000; 91(1–2): 61–68.

20. Molyneaux, K.A., Stallock, J., Schaible, K., Wylie, C. Time-lapse analysis of living mouse germ cell migration. *Developmental Biology.* 2001; 240(2): 488–498.

21. Fujimoto, T., Miyayama, Y., Fuyuta, M. The origin, migration and fine morphology of human primordial germ cells. *The Anatomical Record.* 1977; 188(3): 315–330.

22. Tanaka, S.S., Yamaguchi, Y.L., Tsoi, B., Lickert, H., Tam, P.P. IFITM/Mil/fragilis family proteins IFITM1 and IFITM3 play distinct roles in mouse primordial germ cell homing and repulsion. *Developmental Cell.* 2005; 9(6): 745–756.

23. Mahakali Zama, A., Hudson, F.P. III, Bedell, M.A. Analysis of hypomorphic KitlSl mutants suggests different requirements for KITL in proliferation and migration of mouse primordial germ cells. *Biology of Reproduction.* 2005; 73(4): 639–647.

24. Runyan, C., Schaible, K., Molyneaux, K. *et al.* Steel factor controls midline cell death of primordial germ cells and is essential for their normal proliferation and migration. *Development.* 2006; 133(24): 4861–4869.

25. Gu, Y., Runyan, C., Shoemaker, A., Surani, A., Wylie, C. Steel factor controls primordial germ cell survival and motility from the time of their specification in the allantois, and provides a continuous niche throughout their migration. *Development.* 2009; 136(8): 1295–1303.

26. Molyneaux, K.A., Zinszner, H., Kunwar, P.S. *et al.* The chemokine SDF1/CXCL12 and its receptor CXCR4 regulate mouse germ cell migration and survival. *Development.* 2003; 130(18): 4279–4286.

27. Ara, T., Nakamura, Y., Egawa, T. *et al.* Impaired colonization of the gonads by primordial germ cells in mice lacking a chemokine, stromal cell-derived factor-1 (SDF-1). *Proceedings of the National Academy of Sciences of the United States of America.* 2003; 100(9): 5319–5323.

28. Bendel-Stenzel, M.R., Gomperts, M., Anderson, R., Heasman, J., Wylie, C. The role of cadherins during primordial germ cell migration and early gonad formation in the mouse. *Mechanisms of Development.* 2000; 91(1–2): 143–152.

29. Hilscher, B., Hilscher, W., Bulthoff-Ohnolz, B. *et al.* Kinetics of gametogenesis. I. Comparative histological and autoradiographic studies of oocytes and transitional prospermatogonia during oogenesis and prespermatogenesis. *Cell and Tissue Research.* 1974; 154(4): 443–470.

30. Enders, G.C., May, J.J. II. Developmentally regulated expression of a mouse germ cell nuclear antigen examined from embryonic day 11 to adult in male and female mice. *Developmental Biology.* 1994; 163(2): 331–340.

31. Toyooka, Y., Tsunekawa, N., Takahashi, Y. *et al.* Expression and intracellular localization of mouse Vasa-homologue protein during germ cell development. *Mechanisms of Development.* 2000; 93(1–2): 139–149.

32. Seligman, J., Page, D.C. The Dazh gene is expressed in male and female embryonic gonads before germ cell sex differentiation. *Biochemical and Biophysical Research Communications.* 1998; 245(3): 878–882.

33. Adams, I.R., McLaren, A. Sexually dimorphic development of mouse primordial germ cells: switching from oogenesis to spermatogenesis. *Development.* 2002; 129(5): 1155–1164.

34. Swain, A., Lovell-Badge, R. Mammalian sex determination: a molecular drama. *Genes and Development.* 1999; 13(7): 755–767.

35. Gubbay, J., Collignon, J., Koopman, P. *et al.* A gene mapping to the sex-determining region of the mouse Y chromosome is a member of a novel family of embryonically expressed genes. *Nature.* 1990; 346(6281): 245–250.

36. Sinclair, A.H., Berta, P., Palmer, M.S. *et al.* A gene from the human sex-determining region encodes a

protein with homology to a conserved DNA-binding motif. *Nature*. 1990; 346(6281): 240–244.

37. Koopman, P., Gubbay, J., Vivian, N., Goodfellow, P., Lovell-Badge, R. Male development of chromosomally female mice transgenic for Sry. *Nature*. 1991; 351(6322): 117–121.

38. Lovell-Badge, R., Robertson, E. XY female mice resulting from a heritable mutation in the primary testis-determining gene, Tdy. *Development*. 1990; 109(3): 635–646.

39. Harley, V.R., Goodfellow, P.N. The biochemical role of SRY in sex determination. *Molecular Reproduction and Development*. 1994; 39(2): 184–193.

40. Bullejos, M., Koopman, P. Delayed Sry and Sox9 expression in developing mouse gonads underlies B6-Y(DOM) sex reversal. *Developmental Biology*. 2005; 278(2): 473–481.

41. Hiramatsu, R., Matoba, S., Kanai-Azuma, M. *et al.* A critical time window of Sry action in gonadal sex determination in mice. *Development*. 2009; 136(1): 129–138.

42. Morais da Silva, S., Hacker, A., Harley, V. *et al.* Sox9 expression during gonadal development implies a conserved role for the gene in testis differentiation in mammals and birds. *Nature Genetics*. 1996; 14(1): 62–68.

43. Sekido, R., Bar, I., Narvaez, V., Penny, G., Lovell-Badge, R. SOX9 is up-regulated by the transient expression of SRY specifically in Sertoli cell precursors. *Developmental Biology*. 2004; 274(2): 271–279.

44. Mansour, S., Hall, C.M., Pembrey, M.E., Young, I.D. A clinical and genetic study of campomelic dysplasia. *Journal of Medical Genetics*. 1995; 32(6): 415–420.

45. Huang, B., Wang, S., Ning, Y., Lamb, A.N., Bartley, J. Autosomal XX sex reversal caused by duplication of SOX9. *American Journal of Medical Genetics*. 1999; 87(4): 349–353.

46. Chaboissier, M.C., Kobayashi, A., Vidal, V.I. *et al.* Functional analysis of Sox8 and Sox9 during sex determination in the mouse. *Development*. 2004; 131(9): 1891–1901.

47. Barrionuevo, F., Bagheri-Fam, S., Klattig, J. *et al.* Homozygous inactivation of Sox9 causes complete XY sex reversal in mice. *Biology of Reproduction*. 2006; 74(1): 195–201.

48. Bishop, C.E., Whitworth, D.J., Qin, Y. *et al.* A transgenic insertion upstream of sox9 is associated with dominant XX sex reversal in the mouse. *Nature Genetics*. 2000; 26(4): 490–494.

49. Sekido, R., Lovell-Badge, R. Sex determination involves synergistic action of SRY and SF1 on a specific Sox9 enhancer. *Nature*. 2008; 453(7197): 930–934.

50. Kim, Y., Kobayashi, A., Sekido, R. *et al.* Fgf9 and Wnt4 act as antagonistic signals to regulate mammalian sex determination. *PLoS Biology*. 2006; 4(6): e187.

51. Colvin, J.S., Green, R.P., Schmahl, J., Capel, B., Ornitz, D.M. Male-to-female sex reversal in mice lacking fibroblast growth factor 9. *Cell*. 2001; 104(6): 875–889.

52. Kim, Y., Bingham, N., Sekido, R. *et al.* Fibroblast growth factor receptor 2 regulates proliferation and Sertoli differentiation during male sex determination. *Proceedings of the National Academy of Sciences of the United States of America*. 2007; 104(42): 16558–16563.

53. Wilhelm, D., Martinson, F., Bradford, S. *et al.* Sertoli cell differentiation is induced both cell-autonomously and through prostaglandin signaling during mammalian sex determination. *Developmental Biology*. 2005; 287(1): 111–124.

54. Wilhelm, D., Hiramatsu, R., Mizusaki, H. *et al.* SOX9 regulates prostaglandin D synthase gene transcription in vivo to ensure testis development. *The Journal of Biological Chemistry*. 2007; 282(14): 10553–10560.

55. Moniot, B., Declosmenil, F., Barrionuevo, F. *et al.* The PGD2 pathway, independently of FGF9, amplifies SOX9 activity in Sertoli cells during male sexual differentiation. *Development*. 2009; 136(11): 1813–1821.

56. DiNapoli, L., Batchvarov, J., Capel, B. FGF9 promotes survival of germ cells in the fetal testis. *Development*. 2006; 133(8): 1519–1527.

57. Bowles, J., Feng, C.W., Spiller, C. *et al.* FGF9 suppresses meiosis and promotes male germ cell fate in mice. *Developmental Cell*. 2010; 19(3): 440–449.

58. Barrios, F., Filipponi, D., Pellegrini, M. *et al.* Opposing effects of retinoic acid and FGF9 on Nanos2 expression and meiotic entry of mouse germ cells. *Journal of Cell Science*. 2010; 123(6): 871–880.

59. Suzuki, A., Saga, Y. Nanos2 suppresses meiosis and promotes male germ cell differentiation. *Genes and Development*. 2008; 22(4): 430–435.

60. Bowles, J., Knight, D., Smith, C. *et al.* Retinoid signaling determines germ cell fate in mice. *Science*. 2006; 312(5773): 596–600.

61. MacLean, G., Li, H., Metzger, D., Chambon, P., Petkovich, M. Apoptotic extinction of germ cells in testes of Cyp26b1 knockout mice. *Endocrinology*. 2007; 148(10): 4560–4567.

62. Gondos, B., Westergaard, L., Byskov, A.G. Initiation of oogenesis in the human fetal ovary: ultrastructural and squash preparation study. *American Journal of Obstetrics and Gynecology.* 1986; 155(1): 189–195.

63. McElreavey, K., Vilain, E., Abbas, N., Herskowitz, I., Fellous, M. A regulatory cascade hypothesis for mammalian sex determination: SRY represses a negative regulator of male development. *Proceedings of the National Academy of Sciences of the United States of America.* 1993; 90(8): 3368–3372.

64. Nef, S., Schaad, O., Stallings, N.R. *et al.* Gene expression during sex determination reveals a robust female genetic program at the onset of ovarian development. *Developmental Biology.* 2005; 287(2): 361–377.

65. Vainio, S., Heikkila, M., Kispert, A., Chin, N., McMahon, A.P. Female development in mammals is regulated by Wnt-4 signalling. *Nature.* 1999; 397(6718): 405–409.

66. Biason-Lauber, A., Konrad, D., Navratil, F., Schoenle, E.J. A WNT4 mutation associated with Mullerian-duct regression and virilization in a 46,XX woman. *The New England Journal of Medicine.* 2004; 351(8): 792–798.

67. Yao, H.H., Matzuk, M.M., Jorgez, C.J. *et al.* Follistatin operates downstream of Wnt4 in mammalian ovary organogenesis. *Developmental Dynamics.* 2004; 230(2): 210–215.

68. Parma, P., Radi, O., Vidal, V. *et al.* R-spondin1 is essential in sex determination, skin differentiation and malignancy. *Nature Genetics.* 2006; 38(11): 1304–1309.

69. Kamata, T., Katsube, K., Michikawa, M. *et al.* R-spondin, a novel gene with thrombospondin type 1 domain, was expressed in the dorsal neural tube and affected in Wnts mutants. *Biochimica et Biophysica Acta.* 2004; 1676(1): 51–62.

70. Chassot, A.A., Ranc, F., Gregoire, E.P. *et al.* Activation of beta-catenin signaling by Rspo1 controls differentiation of the mammalian ovary. *Human Molecular Genetics.* 2008; 17(9): 1264–1277.

71. Binnerts, M.E., Kim, K.A., Bright, J.M. *et al.* R-Spondin1 regulates Wnt signaling by inhibiting internalization of LRP6. *Proceedings of the National Academy of Sciences of the United States of America.* 2007; 104(37): 14700–14705.

72. Liu, C.F., Bingham, N., Parker, K., Yao, H.H. Sex-specific roles of beta-catenin in mouse gonadal development. *Human Molecular Genetics.* 2009; 18(3): 405–417.

73. Jeays-Ward, K., Hoyle, C., Brennan, J. *et al.* Endothelial and steroidogenic cell migration are regulated by WNT4 in the developing mammalian gonad. *Development.* 2003; 130(16): 3663–3670.

74. Jordan, B.K., Shen, J.H., Olaso, R., Ingraham, H.A., Vilain, E. Wnt4 overexpression disrupts normal testicular vasculature and inhibits testosterone synthesis by repressing steroidogenic factor 1/beta-catenin synergy. *Proceedings of the National Academy of Sciences of the United States of America.* 2003; 100(19): 10866–10871.

75. Maatouk, D.M., DiNapoli, L., Alvers, A. *et al.* Stabilization of beta-catenin in XY gonads causes male-to-female sex-reversal. *Human Molecular Genetics.* 2008; 17(19): 2949–2955.

76. Schmidt, D., Ovitt, C.E., Anlag, K. *et al.* The murine winged-helix transcription factor Foxl2 is required for granulosa cell differentiation and ovary maintenance. *Development.* 2004; 131(4): 933–942.

77. Uhlenhaut, N.H., Jakob, S., Anlag, K. *et al.* Somatic sex reprogramming of adult ovaries to testes by FOXL2 ablation. *Cell.* 2009; 139(6): 1130–1142.

78. Ottolenghi, C., Omari, S., Garcia-Ortiz, J.E. *et al.* Foxl2 is required for commitment to ovary differentiation. *Human Molecular Genetics.* 2005; 14(14): 2053–2062.

79. Couse, J.F., Hewitt, S.C., Bunch, D.O. *et al.* Postnatal sex reversal of the ovaries in mice lacking estrogen receptors alpha and beta. *Science.* 1999; 286(5448): 2328–2331.

80. Swain, A., Zanaria, E., Hacker, A., Lovell-Badge, R., Camerino, G. Mouse Dax1 expression is consistent with a role in sex determination as well as in adrenal and hypothalamus function. *Nature Genetics.* 1996; 12(4): 404–409.

81. Bardoni, B., Zanaria, E., Guioli, S. *et al.* A dosage sensitive locus at chromosome Xp21 is involved in male to female sex reversal. *Nature genetics.* 1994; 7(4): 497–501.

82. Zanaria, E., Bardoni, B., Dabovic, B. *et al.* Xp duplications and sex reversal. *Philosophical Transactions of the Royal Society of London Series B, Biological Sciences.* 1995; 350(1333): 291–296.

83. Swain, A., Narvaez, V., Burgoyne, P., Camerino, G., Lovell-Badge, R. Dax1 antagonizes Sry action in mammalian sex determination. *Nature.* 1998; 391(6669): 761–767.

84. Yu, R.N., Ito, M., Saunders, T.L., Camper, S.A., Jameson, J.L. Role of Ahch in gonadal development and gametogenesis. *Nature Genetics.* 1998; 20(4): 353–357.

85. Meeks, J.J., Weiss, J., Jameson, J.L. Dax1 is required for testis determination. *Nature Genetics.* 2003; 34(1): 32–33.

86. Bouma, G.J., Albrecht, K.H., Washburn, L.L. *et al.* Gonadal sex reversal in mutant Dax1 XY mice: a failure to upregulate Sox9 in pre-Sertoli cells. *Development.* 2005; 132(13): 3045–3054.

87. Menke, D.B., Koubova, J., Page, D.C. Sexual differentiation of germ cells in XX mouse gonads occurs in an anterior-to-posterior wave. *Developmental Biology.* 2003; 262(2): 303–312.

88. Buehr, M., McLaren, A., Bartley, A., Darling, S. Proliferation and migration of primordial germ cells in We/We mouse embryos. *Developmental Dynamics.* 1993; 198(3): 182–189.

89. Larue, L., Ohsugi, M., Hirchenhain, J., Kemler, R. E-cadherin null mutant embryos fail to form a trophectoderm epithelium. *Proceedings of the National Academy of Sciences of the United States of America.* 1994; 91(17): 8263–8267.

90. Baltus, A.E., Menke, D.B., Hu, Y.C. *et al.* In germ cells of mouse embryonic ovaries, the decision to enter meiosis precedes premeiotic DNA replication. *Nature Genetics.* 2006; 38(12): 1430–1434.

Germ-cell differentiation from pluripotent cells

Jose V. Medrano, Ana M. Martínez-Arroyo, Carlos Simón, and Renee A. Reijo Pera

Introduction

Germ-cell development and meiotic division lead to the conversion of diploid cells to haploid gametes that transfer genetic information to the offspring in species with sexual reproduction, like mammals. Thus, only haploid functional gametes are able to combine and form a new organism during fertilization.

According to the World Health Organization (WHO), infertility affects up to 14% of couples of reproductive age. This percentage tends to be increased mainly due to toxic habits and the delay of motherhood in Western countries. Based on the 2005 American National Survey on Family Growth report, approximately 12% of American couples experienced impaired fertility in 2002, which implies a 20% increase from the 6.1 million couples who reported difficulties in having children in 1995.

Donation of sperm and eggs is one solution when fertility problems are due to the absence or bad quality of gametes. Around 32% of the overall assisted reproduction cycles performed in 2000 in 49 countries worldwide involved egg donation [1]. The US Department of Health and Human Services stated that in the United States alone in 2004, 12.5% of assisted reproduction cycles were carried out with donor eggs. On the other hand, in the sixth report on European results of assisted reproductive techniques (ART) from treatments initiated during 2002, published by the European Society of Human Reproduction and Embryology (ESHRE) in 2006 (European IVF-monitoring programme, EIM), the proportion of ART cycles with egg donation increased to 22.4%, with a 34.9% pregnancy rate per transfer. Despite the variety of results that different reports state, there is a clear consensus that poor quality gametes is one of the most important causes of infertility. However, donation of gametes raises ethical, legal, and personal concerns, and this is why there is an increasing scientific interest in the study of germline development.

Most of the information we have regarding human germ-cell development has been extrapolated from studies of mouse germ-cell development in vivo [2]. However, our knowledge of this process in humans is limited, mainly due to ethical and technical limitations that complicate the accessibility to early human development stages for molecular and genetic analysis of germ cells. In this sense, pluripotent stem cells can be used as an in vitro model for the study of human germ-cell development [2].

Embryonic stem cells (ESCs) are derived from the inner cell mass of human blastocysts and have the ability to self-renew and remain undifferentiated under proper culture conditions, but also to differentiate to all the cell types of the three embryonic germ layers, as well as germ cells in vitro [3]. On the other hand, induced pluripotent stem cells (iPSCs) obtained by reprogramming adult cells with the four transcription factors OCT4, SOX2, KLF4, and c-MYC, resemble and share most of their characteristics with ESCs, representing an alternative to the use of human ESCs (hESCs), without the ethical issues usually associated with them [4].

This work aims to review the knowledge we have at this time about germline development in mammals and update readers on recent significant advances in the study of germ cell differentiation from pluripotent stem cells, focusing on the main challenges that have been raised, such as meiotic regulation and epigenetic reprogramming of germ cells.

Stem Cells in Reproductive Medicine 3rd edition, ed. Carlos Simón, Antonio Pellicer and Renee Reijo Pera.
Published by Cambridge University Press. © Cambridge University Press 2013.

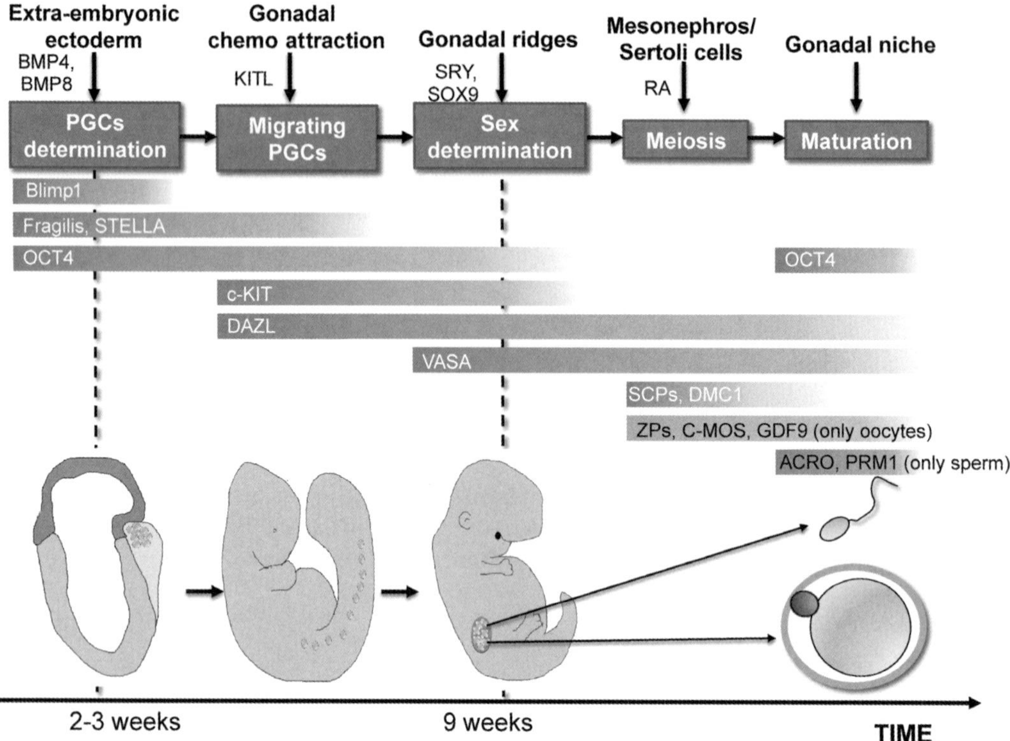

Figure 2.1 Schematic representation of the main developmental stages of human germline differentiation in vivo. Stages of germline differentiation are indicated within boxes. Tissue and/or cellular inducers with their signaling molecules are indicated above each differentiation stage and the specific molecular markers are indicated below. (See also color plate.)

Germline development in mammals

In order to understand the most recent advances in germline differentiation from human pluripotent stem-cell lines in vitro, it is necessary to give to the reader a brief introduction of the basics of germline development in mammals (Figures 2.1 and 2.2). Most of the data we present here comes from model organisms like the mouse. However, even though it is a common practice in biomedical sciences, it is possible that some of the events we discuss here differ in humans; thus the need to develop a human-genome-based system, such as human pluripotent stem cells to study specifically human germline development.

Pregonadal development: Specification, migration, and colonization of gonadal crests

In mammals, germ cells arise from a founder pluripotent cell population called primordial germ cells (PGCs) that segregates from the somatic lineage during gastrulation in response to the Bone Morphogenetic Proteins 4 and 8 (BMP4 and BMP8) secreted by adjacent extra-embryonic endoderm. As a consequence of this signaling, cells located in the proximal epiblast start to express Blimp1. BLIMP1 associates through its PR domain with the arginine methyltransferase PRMT5 to control global levels of histone H2A and H4 arginine-3 symmetrical dimethylation (H2A/H4R3me2s), which might be involved in the developmental transition from somatic to germ-cell fate [5]. At this stage, germ cells start to be subjected to large chromatin reorganization. During these first stages of germ-cell differentiation, genome-wide chromatin changes are similar in male and female germ cells and contribute to the suppression of somatic cell differentiation. In PGCs the genomes are clean of most of their DNA methylation and of other covalent chromatin modifications that are associated with somatic gene regulation, so that germ cells can acquire the capacity to support post-fertilization development [5]. In this way, the first detectable

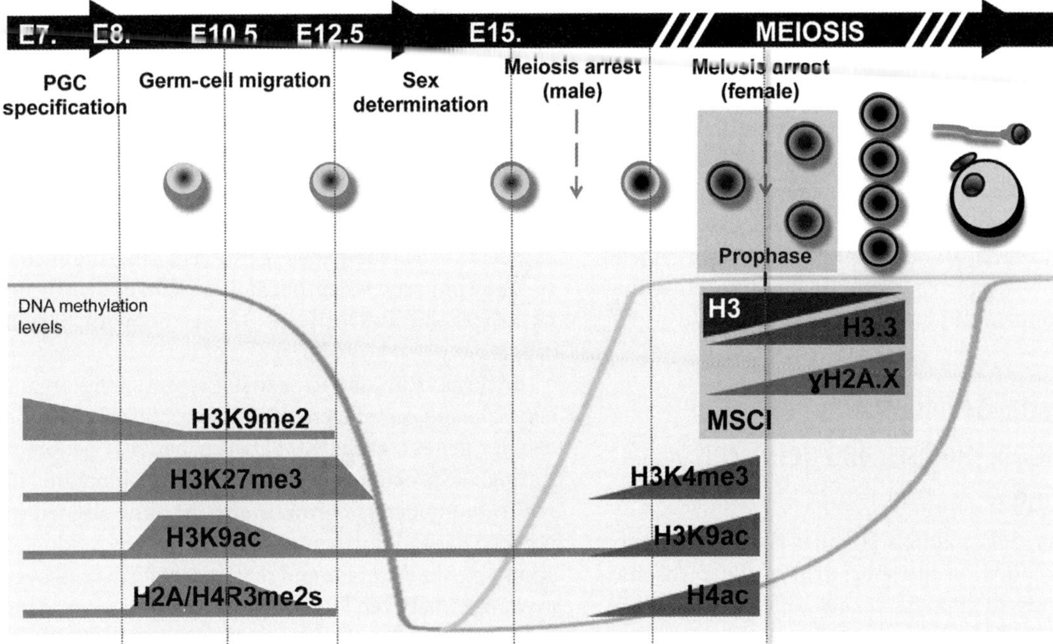

Figure 2.2 Major epigenetic changes during germ-cell differentiation in mice. DNA methylation changes decrease when germ cells start to migrate and there is a complete erasure of DNA methylation patterns once PGCs have entered the gonadal crests. In males (blue line) the DNA methylation pattern recovers before entering meiosis, while in females (pink) they are recovered during meiosis. Levels in histone modification change during germ-cell reprogramming from somatic cells (see text). Prophase I is the main checkpoint. During meiosis, there is a substitution of H3 by its variant H3.3, and the phosphorylation of H2AX is needed for correct meiotic progression, mainly in MSCI formation (see text). (See also color plate.)

population of PGCs appears out from the embryo, close to the yolk sac around the second or third week of pregnancy in humans. Among all the cells in the proximal epiblast that respond to the induction of extra-embryonic endoderm, only the subpopulation of commitent PGCs start to express Fragilis (also known as interferon-induced trans-membrane protein 1, Iftm1) and Stella (also known as developmental pluripotency-associated 3, Dppa3) and retain the expression of the pluripotency-associated transcription factors OCT4 (also known as POU class 5 homeobox 1, Pou5f1) and NANOG, as well as alkaline phosphatase activity after gastrulation (Figure 2.1).

Just after their specification, PGCs proliferate and migrate through subjacent endoderm to the genital ridges. This migration occurs between E8.5 and E12.5, and the fourth and sixth week of pregnancy in mice [6] and humans [7], respectively. During and after migration, PGCs undergo global epigenetic changes in chromatin organization, correlated with all the genetic changes that take place within these cells in response to extrinsic and intrinsic factors.

Once PGCs colonize genital ridges, they are termed gonocytes and are characterized by a rounded morphology, with a low cytoplasm: nucleus ratio. Also at this time, germ cells encounter a significant change in their genetic and epigenetic expression profiles and start to express some genes considered essential for their survival and maturation, such as *Deleted in azoospermia like (Dazl)* and *Vasa* [8]. Extensive changes in histone methylation have also been documented in murine PGCs, particularly gradual loss of H3 lysine-9 dimethylation (H3K9me2), together with DNA hipomethylation, two major repressive modifications for gene expression, from E7.5 onward. A global gain of H3 lysine-27 trimethylation (H3K27me3) occurs at E8.5–E9.0 and is maintained until at least E12.5. Thus, H3K4 methylation and H3K9 acetylation are modifications associated with transcriptionally permissive/active chromatin that are increased in germ cells upon their entry into the genital ridge [9]. On the other hand, a clear reduction in global DNA methylation in germ cells is observed between their specification and the arrival to the presumptive gonads at E10.5. Also, between E11.5 and E12.5 there is a marked demethylation of parentally imprinted genes, as well as other single-copy genes. It has been proposed that this orderly and extensive epigenetic reprogramming in pre-migratory and migratory germ cells might be necessary for their reacquisition of underlying totipotency, for subsequent specific epigenetic remodeling, including the resetting of parental imprints, and for the production of gametes with an appropriate epigenotype for supporting normal development [9].

Postgonadal development: Sex specification, meiosis, and germ-cell maturation

Once germ cells colonize gonadal ridges, expression of SRY, encoded on the short arm of the Y chromosome, drives their male sexual differentiation. SRY activates the expression of SOX9 in the supporting cells of the gonadal niche and induces its differentiation to Sertoli cells. In turn, Sertoli cells drive differentiation of the bipotential gonad into male testis by inducing the degeneration of the Müllerian duct in response to the anti-Müllerian hormone (AMH). Conversely, female gonad determination occurs when germ cells colonize the gonadal crest in the absence of SRY expression. Indeed, several reports suggest that ovarian development may occur independently of the germline and the somatic lineages (granulosa and theca cells) since germ cells that migrate outside of the ovary acquire oocyte-like morphology even if they are XX or XY cells [10]. Once sex determination has been initiated, DNA methylation patterns of germ cells are re-established progressively. Although precise timing remains unclear, this *de novo* methylation has been postulated as important for proper meiosis.

Once germ-cell sex is determined, male and female germ cells also differ in the time point to enter meiosis. In the female gonad, germ cells enter meiosis and stay arrested in the first meiotic prophase during embryonic development around E13.5 and week 12 in mice and humans, respectively, whereas in males, spermatogonia arrest in mitosis and do not enter meiosis until after birth, during puberty [11].

The ovary and testis have the same signaling systems to induce germ-cell meiosis, although at different times, as described above (Figure 2.3). Retinoic acid (RA) secreted by the mesonephros during development of both sexes or Sertoli cells during male adulthood is a key regulator responsible for the induction of germ-cell meiosis in the developing ovary by inducing the expression of the Stra8 gene [12]. However, in the fetal testis, SRY induces the degradation of RA by the activity of cytochrome P450 encoded by the Cyp26b1 gene in Sertoli cells. Thus RA degradation prevents male germ cells entering meiosis until puberty, when hormonal changes switch off its expression and activate RA secretion in Sertoli cells.

Meiosis is unique to sexually reproducing organisms. During gametogenesis, this exceptional cell cycle enables genetic exchange between parental genomes through a process called meiotic recombination, in which homologous chromosomes become aligned in pairs (synapsis) during prophase I, and DNA double-strand breaks are made and repaired, to form crossover exchanges between homologous chromosomes. This process is associated with specific chromatin changes. Also, chromosomes and chromosomal regions that are present in only one of the two homologous chromosomes cannot pair and are inactivated by a mechanism called meiotic silencing [13].

Once meiosis is initiated, synapsis is promoted by an evolutionarily conserved meiosis-specific protein structure, the synaptonemal complex, which is formed by synaptonemal complex proteins SCP1, SCP2, and SCP3, among others. These SCPs are meiosis-specific proteins essential for the synapses of homologous chromosomes since errors of synapses mean defects in homologous chromosome pairing and meiotic recombination, and these irregularities can contribute to meiotic arrest [14]. It has been suggested that SCP3 could be a target for DAZL-mediated translation in mammals. Then, azoospermia associated with a decrease in DAZ gene function in humans may in part be a consequence of failure at synapsis caused by reduced levels of SCP3 protein [15].

Major histone post-translational modifications also occur during meiosis. Levels of H3 lysine-4 mono-, di-, and trimethylation and H3K9me2 undergo global changes at meiotic prophase I and during chromosome pairing and recombination point formation and progression. The relevance of these epigenetic modifications is not known yet. However, several factors that control histone methylation are essential for meiotic transitions, particularly in the male germline [16].

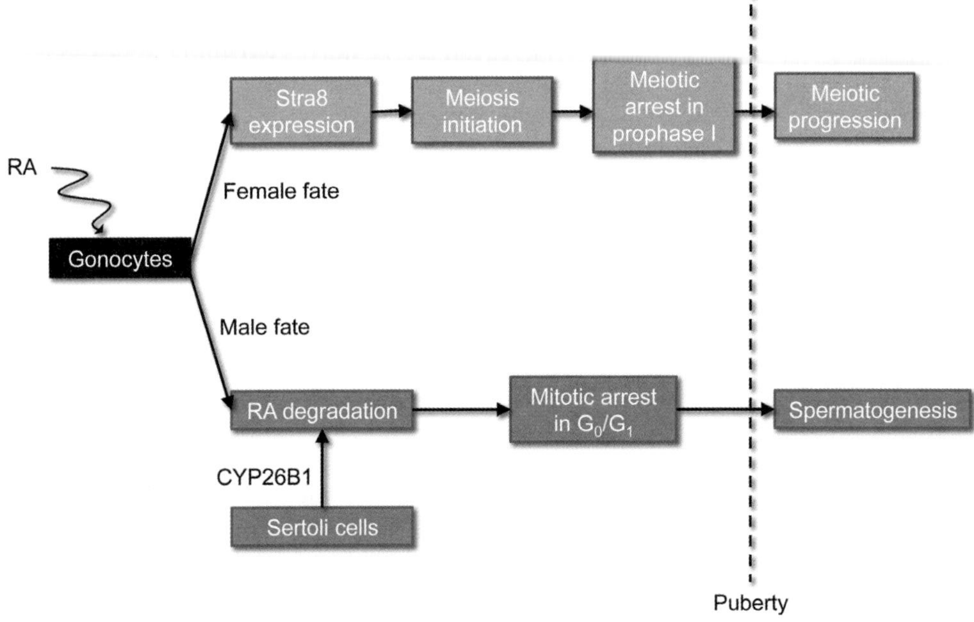

Figure 2.3 Model explanation of the divergent time point of meiotic initiation in males and females in response to the RA signaling from the adjacent mesonephros. (See also color plate.)

Besides specific DNA sequence motifs, histone modifications may contribute to synapsis formation and recombination, and enhance recombination at preferential regions called "hot spots of recombination" [16]. Recent studies in mice show that the initiation sites of recombination are enriched in H3K4me3 and in H3K9 acetylation (H3K9ac). This chromatin configuration could guide recombination initiation. Specific sequence elements are recognized during meiosis, leading to local H3K4 hypermethylation of the chromatin and thus specifying the recombination hotspots. Other histone modifications, including histone H4 acetylation, are also acquired. Some cases of male infertility are linked to loss of the lysine demethylase KDM5D (also called SMCY, JARID1D), a demethylase of H3K4me2/3. Its requirement could be linked to its observed association with MSH5, a meiosis-specific protein that controls synapsis and crossing over [17].

Chromosomes and chromosomal regions that do not become synapsed during meiosis undergo transcriptional silencing. This silencing mechanism called "meiotic silencing of unpaired chromatin" (MSUC) prevents illegitimate recombination and crossing over at unpaired sites and between non-homologous chromosomes. In mammals, the best-studied example of MSUC is the condensation and inactivation of the sex chromosomes during male meiosis, which is microscopically visible as the sex body. This process is referred to as meiotic sex chromosome inactivation (MSCI) and involves the exchange of histone H3 by the H3.3 variant, as well as the accumulation of phosphorylated H2AX [13,16].

Finally, gametic maturation in males occurs in a process called spermatogenesis that starts just after puberty. Spermatogenesis is initiated by asymmetric divisions of spermatogonia and is followed by their differentiation into meiotic spermatocytes I. Once meiosis occurs, haploid spermatocytes II start the second step of spermatogenesis, called spermiogenesis, that consists in significant morphological and epigenetic changes, including the replacement of histones by protamines, to form mature sperm [11].

Female gamete maturation in mammals occurs in waves following hormonal cycles that recruit pools of primordial follicles to progress through asymmetric meiosis. In each hormonal cycle, hundreds of follicles are recruited, but only one or two reach the metaphase II stage in which mature oocytes are ovulated in a selection process called atresia. Metaphase-II-ovulated oocytes only finish meiosis after their activation in fertilization [10].

Stem cells as a source of germ cells in vitro

Evidence of the in vitro generation of germ cells from pluripotent stem cells is now abundant, with several groups reporting the generation of cells expressing specific germline-related markers. In this section we briefly review the most important advances in the field during the last several years in order to illustrate the state of the art with the latest advances and main challenges (Figure 2.4).

State of the art in germ-cell differentiation from mESCs

In 2003, the scientific community was surprised by a report providing the first evidence of germline differentiation from mouse ESCs (mESCs) [18] (Figure 2.4A). In this study, mESC lines expressing GFP (green fluorescent protein) driven by a germ-cell-specific distal enhancer of OCT4 were spontaneously differentiated. Upon differentiation, GFP-positive cells were selected to continue their spontaneous differentiation. Surprisingly, authors observed that some follicle-like structures spontaneously started to detach from the monolayer and extrude oocyte-like cells (OLCs) that were parthenogenetically activated and formed pseudo-blastocysts. Interestingly, this phenomenon was observed in both male and female mESC cell lines, supporting previous findings that reported that in the absence of the expression of Sry from the gonadal niche, germ cells spontaneously differentiate to a female phenotype [10]. This fact brought a new breakthrough in regenerative medicine since it opened the possibility of obtaining germ cells in vitro to study genetics and development.

The same year, another group reported the differentiation of sperm-like cells from mouse ESCs. In a similar experimental design to that employed previously, the authors transfected mESCs with the post-migratory germ-cell marker Mvh (mouse VASA homologous), a promoter associated with GFP, and differentiated them in three-dimensional co-aggregates with a M15 cell line that secretes BMP4. Upon differentiation of the aggregates, the Mvh-GFP-positive cells were transplanted into host testes where they participated in spermatogenesis in vivo. However, this work reported no data about the fertilization capacity of these generated gametes [19].

Only one year later, the apparent functionality of germ cells derived in vitro was reported for the first time. In this report, mESCs were three-dimensionally differentiated in embryoid bodies (EBs) and spontaneously formed putative germ cells. SSEA1+/OCT4+ were isolated by flow cytometry and further cultured in the presence of retinoic acid (RA) to induce their meiotic entrance. The resulting haploid cells showed an epigenetic pattern of the imprinted genes, Igf2r and H19, similar to mature male gametes and their functionality was assessed by the formation of blastocysts after their injection into mouse oocytes by ICSI (intracytoplasmatic sperm injection) [20].

Despite several reports that have claimed the derivation of germ cells from mESCs by employing different approaches, the correct meiotic progression of these germ cells is still a controversy in the scientific community, as highlighted by another report that presented the difficulties related to the correct meiosis accomplishment in the mESCs-derived oocytes and the related aneuploidies [21]. In this study, the authors obtained follicular structures from mouse ESCs through EB formation, and analyzed oocyte-like cells to detect evidence of meiosis. Despite the presence of the meiotic marker SCP3, they found no expression of other important molecules implicated in meiosis, such as SCP1, SCP2, REC8, STAG3, and SMC1-β. Moreover, the chromosomal arrangement in these oocyte-like structures was aberrant compared with the synaptic disposition found in oocytes in vivo.

To date there is only one report of live offspring obtained from in-vitro-derived gametes [22]. In this work, the authors established spermatogonial stem-cell lines from mouse ESCs, selecting them by the expression of two fluorescent reporter genes linked to the late male germ-cell markers Stra8 and Prmt1. After the purification of spermatogonial cells, RA was added to the culture media to induce meiosis and EBs were formed. The authors observed the in vitro formation of sperm-like cells that expressed several meiotic and post-meiotic markers after RA. Moreover, these cells were able to form haploid sperm with limited motility when transplanted into the testes of previously sterilized recipient mice. Functionality of the in-vitro-derived male germ cells was finally demonstrated by their ability to produce live offspring after oocyte fertilization by ICSI. However, all pups showed phenotypic alterations, such as growth retardation, and died prematurely due to abnormal methylation patterns

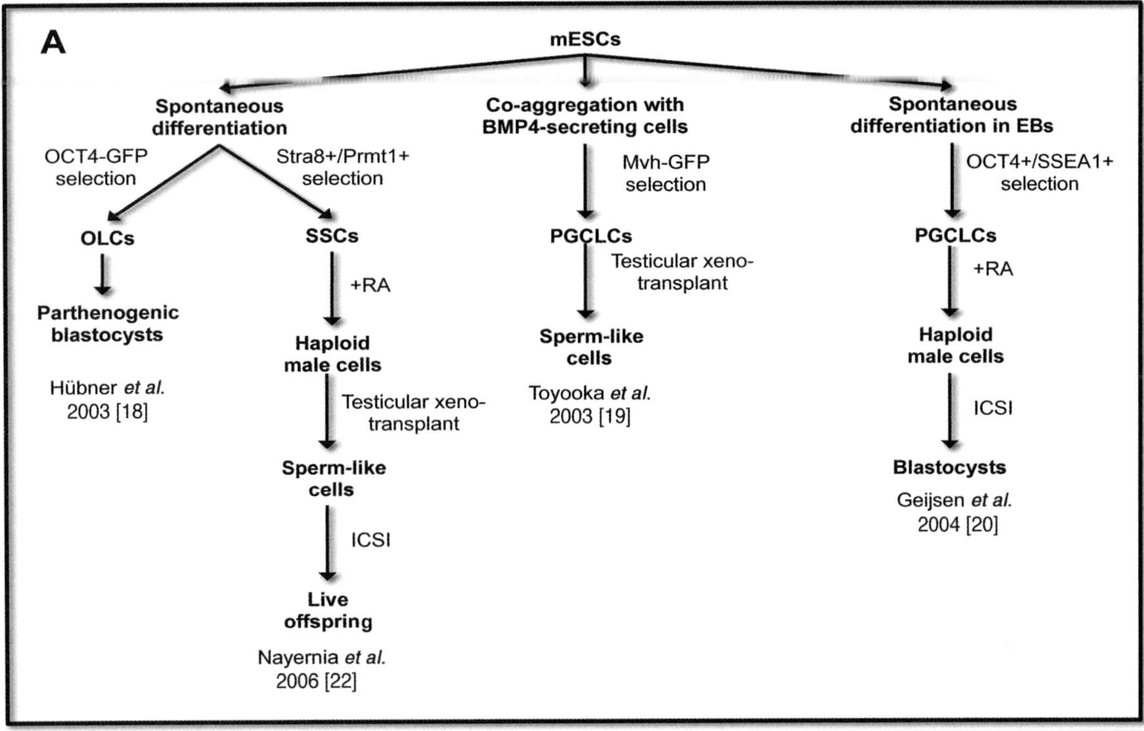

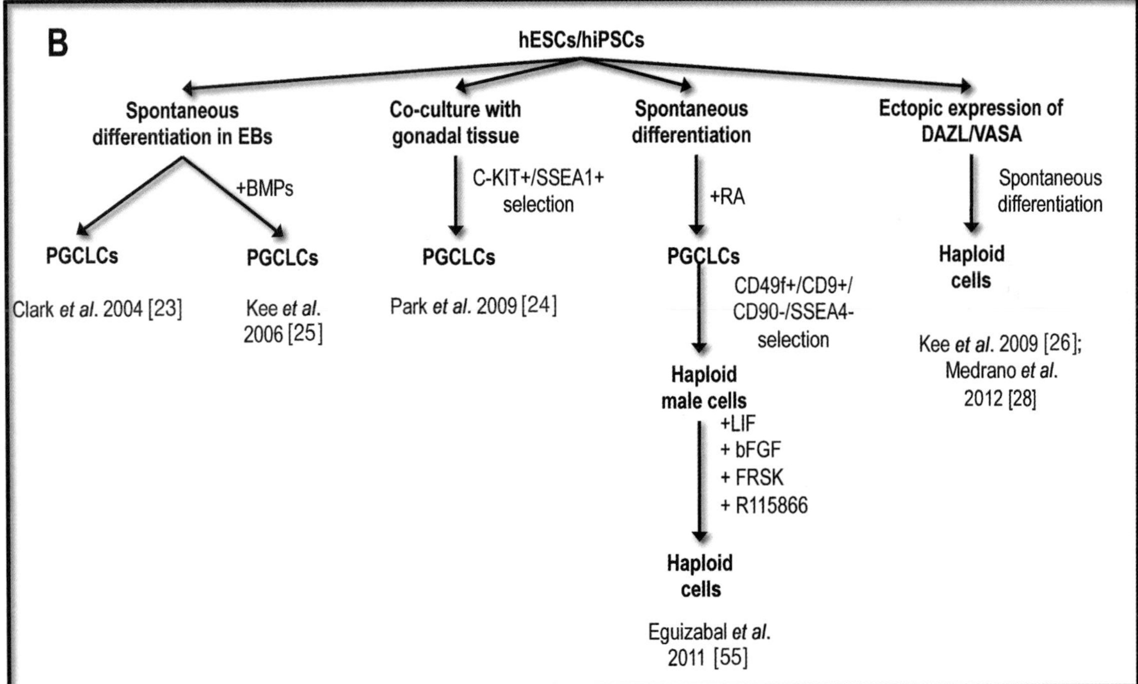

Figure 2.4 Strategies employed by different groups to accomplish germline differentiation from (A) mouse ESCs and (B) human ESCs and iPSCs.

because of a failure in establishing germline imprinting in the ESC-derived gametes.

State of the art in germ-cell differentiation from hESCs and hiPSCs

Concurrent with studies of mouse ESC differentiation, studies of differentiation of human pluripotent stem cells have progressed. The current state of research into germline differentiation processes from human pluripotent cells is very different from that achieved with mice ESCs, given the different limitations. First, ethical limitations make it difficult to carry out functional assays with the germ cells obtained from human pluripotent cells. Second, it seems that in vitro germline differentiation from hESCs and human iPSCs (hiPSCs) is a process more complex than that from mESCs, since in-vitro-derived germ cells usually show arrest in early pre-meiotic stages of germline formation (Figure 2.4B).

The first evidence of germline formation from human ESCs (hESCs) in vitro was reported in 2004 by EB spontaneous differentiation [23]. This study consisted in an exhaustive characterization of the stage-specific expression of different germ-cell markers in both undifferentiated and spontaneously differentiated hESC lines and established a reference model for the germline in vitro differentiation from hESCs. Among their findings, the authors showed that undifferentiated hESCs expressed some early germ-cell markers, such as c-KIT and DAZL, but not late markers such as VASA or SCP3, and hypothesized that hESCs could actually be a heterogeneous pluripotent population in which some cells have a predisposition to a germ-cell fate.

Following this work, several groups have reported the in vitro formation of human germ cells by employing different techniques. Briefly, the main approaches used to date to achieve germ-cell differentiation from human pluripotent stem cells can be classified as purification of germ cells obtained by spontaneous differentiation, in vitro co-culture models with gonadal tissue [24], and/or addition of growth factors to the culture media [25] (Figure 2.4B). However, problems to accomplish the maturation of germ cells derived in vitro and the initiation of meiosis were showed in most of these reports.

Recently, it has been reported that the ectopic expression of the DAZ gene family members DAZ2, DAZL, and BOULE in both hESC and hiPSC lines subjected to spontaneous differentiation can drive the complete meiotic progression of in-vitro-derived germ cells [26,27]. These studies described how the genetic modification of the expression of highly conserved RNA-binding proteins can lead to the correct meiotic progression of germ cells in vitro in the absence of a gonadal niche, and showed the important regulatory role that intrinsic factors related to post-transcriptional regulation can play in this process. Supporting these results, more recently meiosis induction in in-vitro-derived germ cells by the ectopic expression of another highly conserved RNA-binding protein in the germ line of all metazoans such as VASA [28] has been reported. All this evidence provides examples of how the establishment of models for in vitro germline differentiation from pluripotent stem cells can help us to understand insights of germline regulation and open new lines to study post-translational regulation mechanisms in germ cells.

On the other hand, another group recently reported complete meiosis from in–vitro-derived germ cells based on the purification of spontaneously differentiated germ cells and subsequent culture with the addition of a cocktail of growth factors, without any genetic manipulation [29]. However, the efficiency of formation of haploid cells in all these reports is far from anecdotic and further research is needed in order to understand the insights of gamete meiotic maturation.

Main challenges in germ-cell differentiation from pluripotent cells

Here we review two of the most exciting challenges that have been raised recently in the study of germ-cell differentiation from pluripotent stem cells.

Meiosis and its molecular regulation

Although there are several reports that have demonstrated the in vitro derivation of germ cells from mouse and human pluripotent cell lines, the correct meiotic progression in vitro represents one of the most important challenges for regenerative medicine. Here, we will give a concise review of our knowledge of meiotic regulation in mammals and the challenges we must overcome in order to improve the maturation efficiency of germ cells derived in vitro from pluripotent stem cells.

Meiosis in mammals is a complicated process consisting in two consecutive cell divisions without DNA replication to generate haploid cells. Among the different checkpoints that regulate the meiotic process, the prophase I has been described as one of the most important since the alignment of homologous chromosomes occurs during this stage. Prophase I of meiosis has been classically divided into four consecutive stages called leptotene, zigotene, pachytene, and diplotene.

In leptotene, homolog chromosomes are aligned but not yet paired. This process is driven by the formation of a chromosomal scaffold called a synaptonemal complex, formed by cohesins REC8, STAG3, and SMC1β, and axial elements SCP3 and SCP2. In zygotene, toposiomerase SPO11 mediates programmed double-strand breaks of DNA that allow recombination. These breaks are recognized by the recombination repair machinery. Phosphorylation of H2AX to form γH2AX is necessary to recruit the recombinase-related RECA, DMC1, and RAD51, among others, to repair breaks by homolog recombination. At this stage, pairing of chromosomes is completed and axial elements become lateral elements of the synaptonemal complex along the strands of the DNA being zipped. Chromosomal synapsis is completed during pachytene driven by the structural function of SCP1 and the central elements SYCE1 and SYCE2. Pachytene is also characterized by the appearance of specific recombination sites (crossovers) while MLH1 and MLH3 mediate mismatch repair of DNA breaks by homolog recombination. Finally, after recombination events in pachytene, in diplotene chromosomes undergo desynapsis and start to condense. At this stage, recombination sites can be observed by the formation of chiasmata [30].

Following prophase I, the first reductional cell division occurs and homologous chromosomes are separated, followed by a second equational division where sister chromatids are separated to form haploid daughter cells. As commented above, these two consecutive cell divisions without DNA replication occur in a different time point in males and females. In males, these divisions occur subsequently and give rise to four phenotypically similar daughter cells that will continue their maturation process during spermiogenesis. However, in females the first division occurs during the follicular recruitment stage following hormonal cycles, whereas the second is completed at fertilization. Also in females, divisions are not symmetrical, giving rise to both polar bodies that will degenerate.

On the other hand, meiosis has several checkpoints at different stages. Most of these checkpoints are also present in mitosis. One of the most important checkpoints is the spindle assembly checkpoint (SAC). This SAC is formed by the Mad (mitotic arrest deficient) proteins MadI and MadII, the Bub (budding uninhibited by benzimidazole) proteins BubI, Bub3 and BubRI, and MpsI. It is a mechanism that detects unattached tubules or loss of tension in the kinetochores of chromosomes during metaphase to ensure the correct segregation of chromosomes. Also, there are several protein complexes such as the Ndc80 complex, the chromosomal passenger complex (CPC), the mitotic centromere-associated kinesis (MCAK), the kintochore null I (KNLI), and the MisI2 complexes that act as microtubule-kinetochore attachment regulators [31].

However, despite our knowledge of meiotic regulation and checkpoints, mechanisms of meiotic initiation in mammals remain currently unclear. Unlike events in yeast, where there exist two well-characterized proteins that initiate meiosis, NDT80 and IME2 [32], in mammals there are no clear orthologous genes that regulate meiosis. However, it has been postulated that germ-cell intrinsic factors, such as the RNA-binding protein Dazl, can act upstream of Stra8, being a master regulator of meiotic initiation in mammals in a process that the authors called *germ-cell licensing* [33]. Because of the lack of a conserved regulatory mechanism to enter meiosis between yeast and mammals, further studies are needed and it seems that post-transcriptional regulation by RNA-binding proteins and small non-coding RNAs could be the key to understanding.

Post-transcriptional regulation by RNA-binding proteins and small non-coding RNAs

Post-transcriptional gene regulation appears critical in several developmental processes, including germ-cell maturation and meiosis initiation. This regulation is essential in gametogenesis since germ cells are transcriptionally silenced periodically during their development. The increased levels of micro-RNA (miRNA) expression in germ cells compared with somatic cells, together with miRNA clusters on chromosomes 2 and X up-regulated in 14-day-old mouse neonatal testis and ovaries, is also indicative of their importance in germline development [34].

Briefly, small non-coding RNA are short single-stranded non-coding RNAs that bind specifically in conjunction with a protein complex to complementary 3′ untranslated regions (UTR) of target mRNAs and inhibit their translation or induce their degradation. Three major classes of functional small noncoding RNAs have been found in mammals: microRNAs (miRNAs), endogenous small interfering RNAs (endo-siRNAs), and Piwi-interacting RNAs (piRNAs); they differ from one another in their biogenesis and maturation to form the final active functional molecule [35].

Usually, miRNAs are transcribed by RNA polymerase II and cleaved by the RNase Drosha to form hairpin loops [36]. These hairpin loops are recognized by the cytoplasmic endonucelase Dicer and cleaved to form double-stranded mature miRNAs that are loaded into the miRNA-induced silencing complex (miRISC). Finally, the effector miRISC incorporates specific RNA-binding proteins such as Argonaute (AGO) that mediate the post-transcriptional regulation of target mRNAs. In contrast, siRNAs derived from long double-stranded RNAs (dsRNAs) or as long hairpins, are directly processed by Dicer consecutively along the dsRNA to produce multiple siRNAs [37]. From this point, both miRNA and siRNA act in a similar way. Therefore, post-transcriptional regulation efficiency depends on two main components: the complementarity of miRNAs and siRNAs with their target mRNAs, and the catalytic activity of their associated RNA-binding proteins [35].

The best-characterized miRNA pathway in mammalian germ cells is the repression of the miRNA Let7 by the RNA-binding protein Lin28 that allows Blimp1 translation during the first steps of mouse germ-cell determination [38]. Additionally, it seems that the roles of the reciprocal regulation pathway of Lin28 and Let7 extend also to later stages of spermatogenesis as pluripotency regulators in conjunction with the miRNAs miR-125a and miR-9 [39].

Apart from this, there are several examples of regulation of germ-cell development by miRNAs. The miRNA cluster miR-17–92 is thought to promote survival and proliferation of pre-meiotic germ cells, and its expression is down-regulated in female primordial oocytes following meiotic arrest [40]. Moreover, miR-125 is implicated in post-transcriptional repression of Oct4 during male meiotic silencing [41], whereas miR-181c targets Sox5 and Sox6. In the same way, miR-181c, together with miR-181b and miR-355 targets the post-meiotic marker Rsbn I [42], and miR-320 and miR-214 are predicted to target cell adhesion

and heat shock proteins in germ cells, respectively [43]. Interestingly, it has been shown that the overexpression of the miR-34 family, which targets several cell-cycle regulators, together with the RNA-binding protein Vasa in HeLa cells promotes the expression of germ-cell markers, suggesting a possible link between them [44]. Finally, there are studies that predict that miRNAs such as miR-34b and 34c can even post-transcriptionally regulate the expression of RNA-binding proteins such as Dazl [45].

However, most of the information we have about miRNA functions in germ cells has two important issues. First, because the germ-cell profile is different depending on the developmental stage, most of the studies conducted to date to elucidate miRNA functions in germ cells with whole gonadal tissue samples are not totally informative since they analyze heterogeneous populations of germ cells, so it is essential to design future studies with purified and homogeneous populations of germ cells. In this sense, improvement of in vitro germ-cell differentiation techniques could be a solution. Second, most of the reported miRNA targets are based in *in silico* bioinformatic prediction tools that must be experimentally validated. Also in this case, the in-vitro-derived germ cells can be a model to experimentally confirm these predictions.

The third class of small non-coding RNAs is the class of Piwi-interacting RNAs (piRNAs). Expression of piRNAs is specific to the germline in mammals, and differs from miRNAs and siRNAs in that they do not require Dicer for their processing. Instead, piRNAs are generated from long single-stranded RNA precursors that are often encoded by complex and repetitive intergenic sequences and are defined by their interaction with the Piwi proteins, a distinct family of Argonaute proteins (including Miwi, Miwi2, and Mili in mouse; also known as Piwil1, Piwil4, and Piwil2, respectively) [35,46]. One proposed model for the biogenesis of piRNAs is the "ping-pong mechanism" (Figure 2.5). In this model, Mili, an Argonaute protein, cleaves the primary piRNA to define the 5′ end, which is then recognized by Miwi2. Afterwards, Miwi2 cleaves the other strand of the precursor, thereby generating a 5′ end of the piRNA that can then bind to Mili, thus forming a positive amplification loop [35]. Many of the details of this model remain poorly characterized and the mechanism of action is not well understood. Moreover, the ping-pong model explains the biogenesis of the piRNAs that are derived from repetitive sequences,

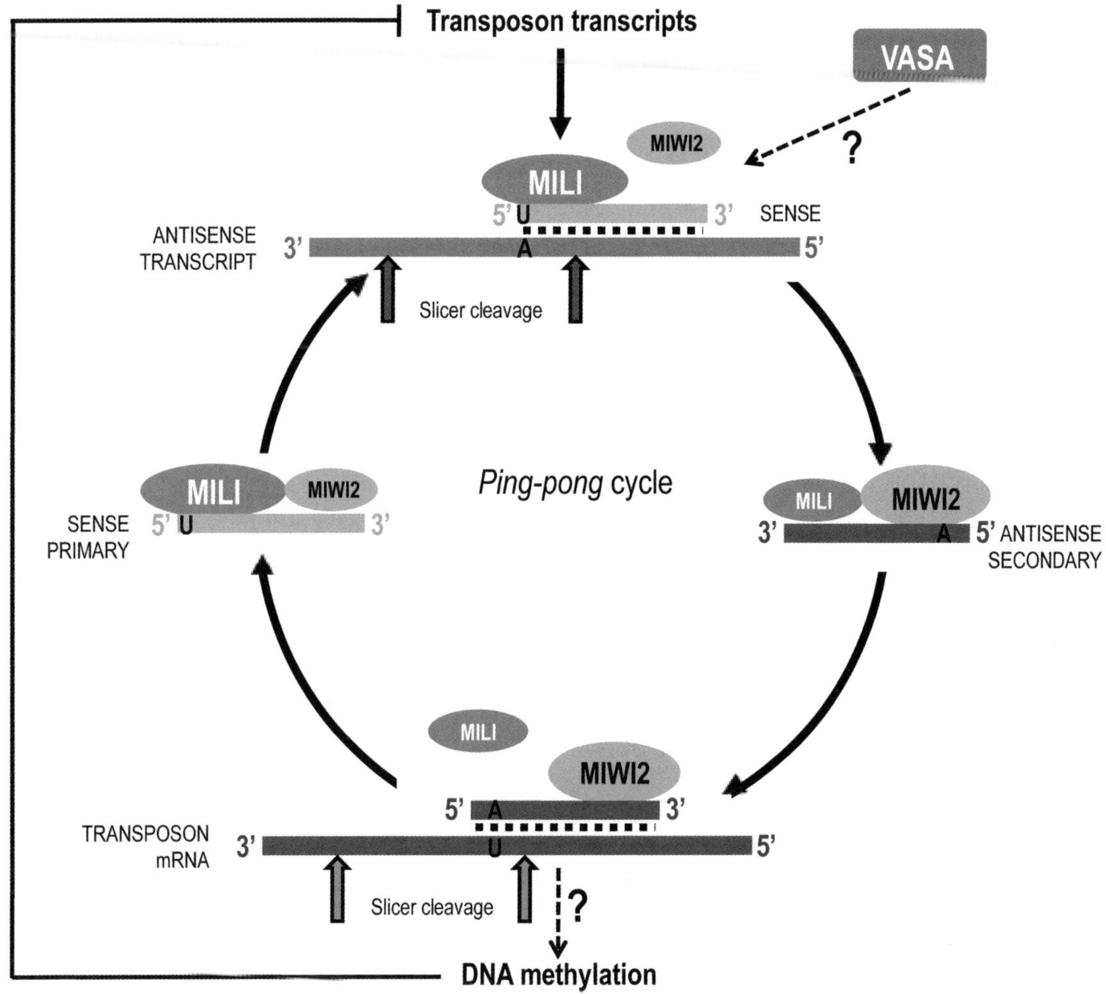

Figure 2.5 First class piRNA processing in mammals. Primary processing of mRNAs of active transposable elements are the source of sense piRNA that associate to MILI and enter a ping-pong cycle where MIWI2 binds secondary antisense piRNA. Antisense piRNA are the responsible of DNA methylation at transposable elements, even though this mechanism remains unclear. VASA may participate in promoting this cycle (see text), although the mechanism is not clear. (See also colour plate.)

such as transposons, characteristic of the early stages of spermatogenesis. The mechanism of biogenesis of the second class of piRNAs, derived from complex intergenic sequences and associated with the later stages of spermatogenesis, is unclear. It is thought that repetitive piRNA acts by promoting *de novo* demethylation of the transposons, thus repressing them and maintaining genomic stability during spermatogenesis. However the mechanism by which piRNA can direct the DNA methylation machinery is still unclear [35,37, 46].

Genetic studies imply that, like miRNAs, piRNAs are also essential for spermatogenesis. During this process, two kinds of piRNAs can be differentiated. The first class has a highly repetitive nature and is expressed before meiotic pachytene. This class of piRNA interacts with Mili and Miwi2 and consistent with this, deletion of Mili and Miwi2 results in early arrest in meiosis I at the primary spermatocyte stage. The second class of piRNA has a non-repetitive nature and becomes abundant during the pachytene stage, associated with Mili and Miwi proteins. Thus, deletion of Miwi results in arrest following meiosis II at the round spermatid stage [47,48].

On the other hand, there are several highly conserved RNA-binding proteins that have been described as essential for correct germline maturation in mammals. Among them, the DAZ gene family of RNA-binding proteins is one of the most important [49]. In humans, this family is composed of the autosomic genes *BOULE* and *DAZL* together with the cluster of *DAZ* genes on the Y chromosome. In mice, Dazl has a role as a master regulator of spermatogenesis, whereas Boule seems to be critical for meiosis, since knockout models show a clear increase in apoptosis of germ cells just before the moment of initiation of meiosis [49].

VASA is another RNA-binding protein that has been postulated as an essential factor in meiosis and germ-cell maturation. It is also highly conserved along the germ cells of all metazoans and is specifically located in an electron-dense perinuclear structure that is rich in RNAs and other RNA-binding proteins called germ plasm [8]. In humans and mice, it is encoded by the gene *DDX4*. This gene is a member of the DEAD-box gene family and transcribes an ATP-dependent RNA-helicase protein that is specifically expressed from the moment of gonadal crest in all peri-meiotic stages of mammalian germ cells. Knockout models for VASA in Drosophila show defects in polar bodies (also known as germ plasm) assembly and in oogenesis [50], whereas knockout mice for Mvh (Mouse VASA homolog) show infertility in males [51].

It has recently been suggested that there may be a need for Vasa for the correct ping-pong amplification cycle of the piRNAs. The authors based this suggestion on the shared phenotype of knockout mice for Mvh and for the mouse Argonaute-like Piwi homolog proteins Miwi, Mili, and Miwi2, which regulate piRNAs [47]. Since one of the functions of piRNAs is retrotransposon silencing by *de novo* methylation of DNA, this phenotype showed meiotic arrest as a consequence of the high expression of retrotansposons. Moreover, given their functions as retrotransposon silencers, it is possible that piRNAs are also implicated in the meiotic silencing of unpaired chromatin (MSUC) during male meiotic prophase I in mammals. Therefore, this fact could explain why only males are sterile in Mvh knockout mice. However, further basic studies are needed to understand the existing link between Lin28, Nanos, Dazl, Vasa, Piwi homologs and other RNA-binding proteins with meiotic progression (Figure 2.5).

Despite the lack of knowledge we have about these and other germline-related RNA-binding proteins, it has been suggested that they can work as chaperones that mediate the correct folding of target RNAs in order to facilitate their interaction with accessory proteins [52], as well as post-transcriptional regulators of meiosis-related proteins. Indeed, it has been recently suggested that Dazl is an upstream post-transcriptional regulator of Scp3 and Vasa [15,53] in mice. Additionally, it has also been suggested that Vasa can target mRNAs encoding another highly conserved proteins such as Nanos2, which maintains mitotic arrest in mice spermatogonia [54].

Concluding remarks and future applications

Here, we have provided a brief review of the main advances in germline differentiation from pluripotent stem cells, with special emphasis on the challenges that we must overcome in order to achieve the correct maturation of germ cells in vitro. Thus, derivation of germ cells in vitro is our optimal model to obtain insights into human germ-cell development.

Moreover, the divergent efficiency of derivation of germ cells in vitro between human and murine stem cells indicates the existence of interspecific differences in germline development, as shown by the low meiotic initiation rates in human experiments. Therefore, further studies are needed to describe these differences in both germline programs in order to achieve a better understanding.

Moreover, gametogenesis is a dynamic process of cross-talk between the gonadal niche and the germ cells in order to orchestrate germline maturation. Thus, it is essential to find suitable cell niches that provide the required environment for the proper development of gametes in vitro. Creation of defined culture media to enable complete differentiation process is also desirable, avoiding the use of serum containing unspecified components to improve reproducibility of experiments among groups.

Finally, epigenetics is an amazing and evolving field of knowledge that has made great advances in recent years. Due to the special epigenetic reprogramming of germ cells in vivo, further studies are needed to achieve the correct functionality for in-vitro-derived germ cells. In this sense, it is likely that fine tuning of meiotic regulation meiosis may be accomplished by RNA-binding proteins and small non-coding RNAs.

References

1. Adamson, G.D., de Mouzon, J., Lancaster, P. *et al*. World collaborative report on in vitro fertilization, 2000. *Fertility and Sterility*. 2006; 85(6): 1586–1622.

2. Marques-Mari, A.I., Lacham-Kaplan, O., Medrano, J.V. *et al*. Differentiation of germ cells and gametes from stem cells. *Human Reproduction Update*. 2009; 15(3): 379–390.

3. Thomson, J.A., Itskovitz-Eldor, J., Shapiro, S.S. *et al*. Embryonic stem cell lines derived from human blastocysts. *Science*. 1998; 282(5391): 1145–1147.

4. Takahashi, K., Yamanaka, S. Induction of pluripotent stem cells from mouse embryonic and adult fibroblast cultures by defined factors. *Cell*. 2006; 126(4): 663–676.

5. Ancelin, K., Lange, U.C., Hajkova, P. *et al*. Blimp1 associates with Prmt5 and directs histone arginine methylation in mouse germ cells. *Nature Cell Biology*. 2006; 8(6): 623–630.

6. Wylie, C.C., Stott, D., Donovan, P.J. Primordial germ cell migration. *Developmental Biology (New York 1985)*. 1986; 2: 433–448.

7. Fujimoto, T., Miyayama, Y., Fuyuta, M. The origin, migration and fine morphology of human primordial germ cells. *Anatomical Record*. 1977; 188(3): 315–330.

8. Castrillon, D.H., Quade, B.J., Wang, T.Y. *et al*. The human *VASA* gene is specifically expressed in the germ cell lineage. *Proceedings of the National Academy of Sciences of the United States of America*. 2000; 97: 9585–9590.

9. Seki, Y., Hayashi, K., Itoh, K. *et al*. Extensive and orderly reprogramming of genome-wide chromatin modifications associated with specification and early development of germ cells in mice. *Developmental Biology*. 2005; 278(2): 440–458.

10. McLaren, A. Germ cells and germ cell sex. *Philosophical Transactions of the Royal Society of London B, Biological Science*. 1995; 350(1333): 229–233.

11. McLaren, A. Meiosis and differentiation of mouse germ cells. *Symposia of the Society for Experimental Biology*. 1984; 38: 7–23.

12. Bowles, J., Knight, D., Smith, C. *et al*. Retinoid signaling determines germ cell fate in mice. *Science*. 2006; 312(5773): 596–600.

13. Kelly, W.G., Aramayo, R. Meiotic silencing and the epigenetics of sex. *Chromosome Research* 2007; 15(5): 633–51.

14. Pittman, D.L., Cobb, J., Schimenti, K.J. *et al*. Meiotic prophase arrest with failure of chromosome synapsis in mice deficient for Dmc1, a germline-specific RecA homolog. *Molecular Cell*. 1998; 1(5): 697–705.

15. Reynolds, N., Collier, B., Bingham, V. *et al*. Translation of the synaptonemal complex component Sycp3 is enhanced in vivo by the germ cell specific regulator Dazl. *RNA*. 2007; 13(7): 974–981.

16. Kota, S.K., Feil, R. Epigenetic transitions in germ cell development and meiosis. *Developmental Cell*. 2010; 19(5): 675–686.

17. Akimoto, C., Kitagawa, H., Matsumoto, T. *et al*. Spermatogenesis-specific association of SMCY and MSH5. *Genes to Cells*. 2008; 13(6): 623–633.

18. Hübner, K., Fuhrmann, G., Christenson, L.K. *et al*. Derivation of oocytes from mouse embryonic stem cells. *Science*. 2003; 300(5623): 1251–1256.

19. Toyooka, Y., Tsunekawa, N., Akasu, R. *et al*. Embryonic stem cells can form germ cells in vitro. *Proceedings of the National Academy of Sciences of the United States of America*. 2003; 100(20): 11457–11462.

20. Geijsen, N., Horoschak, M., Kim, K. *et al*. Derivation of embryonic germ cells and male gametes from embryonic stem cells. *Nature*. 2004; 427(6970): 148–154.

21. Novak, I., Lightfoot, D.A., Wang, H. *et al*. Mouse embryonic stem cells form follicle-like ovarian structures but do not progress through meiosis. *Stem Cells*. 2006; 24(8): 1931–1936.

22. Nayernia, K., Nolte, J., Michelmann, H.W. *et al*. In vitro-differentiated embryonic stem cells give rise to male gametes that can generate offspring mice. *Developmental Cell*. 2006; 11(1): 125–132.

23. Clark, A.T., Bodnar, M.S., Fox, M. *et al*. Spontaneous differentiation of germ cells from human embryonic stem cells in vitro. *Human Molecular Genetics*. 2004; 13: 727–739.

24. Park, T.S., Galic, Z., Conway, A.E. *et al*. Derivation of primordial germ cells from human embryonic and induced pluripotent stem cells is significantly improved by coculture with human fetal gonadal cells. *Stem Cells*. 2009; 27(4): 783–795.

25. Kee, K., Gonsalves, J.M., Clark, A.T. *et al*. Bone morphogenetic proteins induce germ cell differentiation from human embryonic stem cells. *Stem Cells and Development*. 2006; 15(6): 831–837.

26. Kee, K., Angeles, V., Flores, M. *et al*. Human DAZL, DAZ and BOULE genes modulate primordial germ cell and haploid gamete formation. *Nature*. 2009; 462: 222–225.

27. Panula, S., Medrano, J.V., Kee, K. *et al*. Human germ cell differentiation from fetal- and adult-derived induced pluripotent stem cells. *Human Molecular Genetics*. 2011; 20(4): 752–762.

28. Medrano, J.V., Ramathal, C., Nguyen, H.N. *et al.* Divergent RNA-binding proteins, DAZL and VASA, induce meiotic progression in human germ cells derived in vitro. *Stem Cells.* 2012; 30(3): 441–451.

29. Eguizabal, C., Montserrat, N., Vassena, R. *et al.* Complete meiosis from human induced pluripotent stem cells. *Stem Cells.* 2011; 29(8): 1186–1195.

30. Handel, M.A., Schimenti, J.C. Genetics of mammalian meiosis: regulation, dynamics and impact on fertility. *Nature Reviews Genetics.* 2010; 11(2): 124–136.

31. Sun, S.C., Kim, N.H. Spindle assembly checkpoint and its regulators in meiosis. *Human Reproduction Update.* 2012; 18(1): 60–72.

32. Kassir, Y., Adir, N., Boger-Nadjar, E. *et al.* Transcriptional regulation of meiosis in budding yeast. *International Review of Cytology.* 2003; 224: 111–171.

33. Gill, M.E., Hu, Y.C., Lin, Y. *et al.* Licensing of gametogenesis, dependent on RNA binding protein DAZL, as a gateway to sexual differentiation of fetal germ cells. *Proceedings of the National Academy of Sciences of the United States of America.* 2011; 108(18): 7443–7448.

34. Buchold, G.M., Coarfa, C., Kim, J. *et al.* Analysis of microRNA expression in the prepubertal testis. *PLoS One.* 2010; 5(12): e15317.

35. Suh, N., Blelloch, R. Small RNAs in early mammalian development: from gametes to gastrulation. *Development.* 2011; 138(9): 1653–1661.

36. Han, J., Pedersen, J.S., Kwon, S.C. *et al.* Posttranscriptional crossregulation between Drosha and DGCR8. *Cell.* 2009; 136(1): 75–84.

37. Fabian, M.R., Sonenberg, N., Filipowicz, W. Regulation of mRNA translation and stability by microRNAs. *Annual Review of Biochemistry.* 2010; 79: 351–379.

38. West, J.A., Viswanathan, S.R., Yabuuchi, A. *et al.* A role for Lin28 in primordial germ-cell development and germ-cell malignancy. *Nature.* 2009; 460(7257): 909–913.

39. Zhong, X., Li, N., Liang, S. *et al.* Identification of microRNAs regulating reprogramming factor LIN28 in embryonic stem cells and cancer cells. *Journal of Biological Chemistry.* 2010; 285(53): 41961–41971.

40. Hayashi, K., Chuva de Sousa Lopes, S.M., Kaneda, M. *et al.* MicroRNA biogenesis is required for mouse primordial germ cell development and spermatogenesis. *PLoS One* 2008; 3(3): e1738.

41. Western, P.S., van den Bergen, J.A., Miles, D.C. *et al.* Male fetal germ cell differentiation involves complex repression of the regulatory network controlling pluripotency. *FASEB Journal* 2010; 24(8): 3026–3035.

42. Yan, N., Lu, Y., Sun, H. *et al.* A microarray for microRNA profiling in mouse testis tissues. *Reproduction* 2007; 134(1): 73–79.

43. Marcon, E., Babak, T., Chua, G. *et al.* miRNA and piRNA localization in the male mammalian meiotic nucleus. *Chromosome Research.* 2008; 16(2): 243–260.

44. Bouhallier, F., Allioli, N., Lavial, F. *et al.* Role of miR-34c microRNA in the late steps of spermatogenesis. *RNAA Publication of the Rna Society.* 2010; 16(4): 720–31.

45. Luo, L., Ye, L., Liu, G. *et al.* Microarray-based approach identifies differentially expressed microRNAs in porcine sexually immature and mature testes. *PLoS One* 2010; 5(8): e11744.

46. Aravin, A.A., Sachidanandam, R., Bourc'his, D. *et al.* A piRNA pathway primed by individual transposons is linked to de novo DNA methylation in mice. *Molecular Cell.* 2008; 31(6): 785–799.

47. Kuramochi-Miyagawa, S., Watanabe, T., Gotoh, K. *et al.* MVH in piRNA processing and gene silencing of retrotransposons. *Genes Development.* 2010; 24(9): 887–892.

48. Carmell, M.A., Girard, A., van de Kant, H.J. *et al.* MIWI2 is essential for spermatogenesis and repression of transposons in the mouse male germline. *Development Cell.* 2007; 12(4): 503–514.

49. Ruggiu, M., Speed, R., Taggart, M. *et al.* The mouse Dazla gene encodes a cytoplasmic protein essential for gametogenesis. *Nature.* 1997; 389(6646): 73–77.

50. Lasko, P.F., Ashburner, M. The product of the Drosophila gene vasa is very similar to eukaryotic initiation factor-4A. *Nature.* 1988; 335(6191): 611–617.

51. Tanaka, S.S., Toyooka, Y., Akasu, R. *et al.* The mouse homolog of Drosophila Vasa is required for the development of male germ cells. *Genes Development.* 2000; 14(7): 841–853.

52. Mohr, S., Stryker, J.M., Lambowitz A.M. A DEAD-box protein functions as an ATP-dependent RNA chaperone in group I intron splicing. *Cell.* 2002; 109(6): 769–779.

53. Reynolds, N., Collier, B., Maratou, K. *et al.* Dazl binds in vivo to specific transcripts and can regulate the pre-meiotic translation of Mvh in germ cells. *Human Molecular Genetics*. 2005; 14(24): 3899–3909.

54. Becalska, A.N., Gavis E.R. Lighting up mRNA localization in Drosophila

oogenesis. *Development*. 2009; 136(15): 2493–2503.

55. Eguizabal, C., Montserrat, N., Vassena, R, *et al.* Complete meiosis from human induced pluripotent stem cells. *Stem Cells*. 2011; 29(8): 1186–1195.

The male gamete

Nicolás Garrido, Rocío Rivera, and Marcos Meseguer

Introduction

Men producing no spermatozoa are the main potential beneficiary of sperm cells created from stem cells. Up to now, these couples were directed to the use of donor sperm.

Sperm donation has been an effective way to achieve pregnancies and healthy newborns safely when no sperm cells are available within the ejaculate and testicular tissue, or the sperm cell count is dramatically decreased, until ICSI incorporation, and after several assisted reproduction failures when the male factor is suspected to be the main cause. Obviously, the main concern using donated sperm is the lack of biological paternity.

In these cases, the objective is to develop functional spermatozoa to be employed in assisted reproduction treatments, in order to achieve healthy newborns, containing the father's genetic traits. Initially, testicular stem cells can be identified in some males, but their use in creating sperm is dubious, given their origin: malfunctioning testis. The ideal situation is to achieve sperm creation by reprogramming the father's own adult stem cells obtained from other tissues, reaching this end in vitro.

Sperm production is defective in a significant proportion of males attempting fatherhood, leading to the creation of sperm cells without the optimal features to fertilize, produce embryos able to be implanted, develop, and result in a healthy newborn. The study of these situations enabled us to better define what a sperm cell needs to be successful.

Sperm-related defects can be divided into those leading to abnormally decreased sperm production, resulting from low to absent sperm in the ejaculate, and defects in sperm physiological characteristics, that may be independent from sperm count, but causing reproductive failure.

Moreover, several concerns must be taken into account in order to avoid genetic problems in the offspring once these cells are created. These include epigenetic deregulation and the high risk of chromosomal abnormalities when immature spermatogenic cells are employed in assisted reproduction.

Investigations are underway to create sperm from adult stem cells, but no clinical application in humans is available, and a long journey remains until it is.

In this chapter, our aim is to describe the existing knowledge regarding the ideal molecular profile of sperm cells, in order to define the model to be mimicked when stem cells are employed in order to create male gametes.

When sperm cells are absent or fail

Help wanted: Sperm donation in the era of ICSI

Sperm donation can solve with a reasonably high effectiveness those cases where sperm cells are absent, and also those cases where they are produced, and even found within the ejaculate in minimum or adequate amounts, but are physiologically ineffective.

Unfortunately, the latter case is only possible after repeated failures using different ART procedures have been done, given that predictive tools to forecast success, based on molecular sperm features, are not currently available.

Obviously, the main concern with the use of donated sperm is the lack of biological paternity, and thus genetic link with the offspring.

Stem Cells in Reproductive Medicine 3rd edition, ed. Carlos Simón, Antonio Pellicer and Renee Reijo Pera.
Published by Cambridge University Press. © Cambridge University Press 2013.

Over the last decade the clinical indication of sperm donation has been growing together with the rest of the assisted reproduction treatments in our unit, and several reasons can explain this phenomenon, such as open distribution of all new advances and new technologies related to assisted reproduction in the media (newspapers, radio, TV, etc.) enabling a better public understanding of the problems and therapeutic options, changing their minds, abolishing previously established taboos, and permitting a better acceptance of donated gametes.

We describe a higher use of sperm donation for artificial insemination than conventional IVF, and this difference is probably based on the favorable cost–benefit ratio that an AID cycle could offer to a patient, with acceptable pregnancy rates when the sperm bank is adequately managed. Artificial insemination with the use of semen from anonymous donors (AID) has been a low-complexity assisted reproduction technique widely used for many years in the treatment of women wishing to conceive in specific situations [1]. But ART also covers interventions like IVF and intracytoplasmic sperm injection (ICSI), which have the ultimate aim of assisting the infertile patient to become pregnant and deliver a live infant. In both situations the use of donor sperm could be mandatory although the indications for its employment could or should be different [2,3]. Actually, these are severe male factors, both in patients with very low or absent spermatogenesis but also in males with genetic disorders that might be transmissible to the progeny, as well as repeated ICSI failure (IF) and in homosexual women or women without a male partner. The introduction of ICSI to the assisted reproduction laboratory has notably decreased the number of AIDS over recent years, mainly in patients showing severe alterations in spermatogenesis. In other cases, we expect a reduction in the use of donor sperm as new techniques develop or when other techniques become firmly established, for instance, pre-implantation diagnosis of genetic diseases, as well as sperm washing for HIV serodiscordant couples [4]. Hence, it is essential to determine the relevant factors affecting the indications for donor sperm in AID and IVF/ICSI and how they influence the results of the programs, and in this way we can establish adequate criteria to counsel, estimate success prognosis, and improve success rates. Different studies have described the influence of different parameters, such as maternal age, male aetiology, female aetiology, ovarian stimulation protocol, and many

others, with controversial or rather divergent results. Nevertheless, some significant risk factors for low pregnancy and live birth rates have been identified of which female infertility, older maternal age, low number of previous births, and lack of ovulatory stimulation are those with clear effects [5,6]. A number of studies with adequate sample sizes were conducted from different clinics together with multicenter studies, where probably the selection criteria, control, and management of patients are slightly different, thus adding heterogeneity to the sample [7].

In AID procedures we have the highest pregnancy rates in patients without sperm production compared with those having had IVF/ICSI failures and single women. This marked difference could be explained because azoospermic female partners are fertile and have never been in contact with a male gamete when attempting pregnancy. Moreover, those coming from IVF failure could have some associated female factors, often linked to bad oocyte quality, and regarding single women, frequently also advanced maternal age.

In IVF procedures we found similar pregnancy rates in those patients coming from IVF failure or unsuccessful sperm retrieval, and always higher than single women.

Despite the use of sperm banks for assisted reproduction increasing in recent years, we have observed a significant reduction in the number of cycles related to IVF failure. The cause seems to be quite evident: new procedures in clinical embryology have been developed and others improved, and this has been reflected in successful treatments and less IVF/ICSI fertilization or transference failures.

Clinical indications and reproductive outcome

From our experience, spanning more than eight years, with almost 3000 AID and IVF non-selected consecutive cycles, we investigated the distribution of the clinical indications to use donated sperm, comparing AID and IVF, and studying their evolution during the period analyzed. Approximately 57% of ART cycles using donor sperm were AID and 42.8% were IVF.

We compared the indications for sperm donation between patients undergoing IUI and IVF/ICSI. There were significant differences between them, while women without a partner had the same proportions

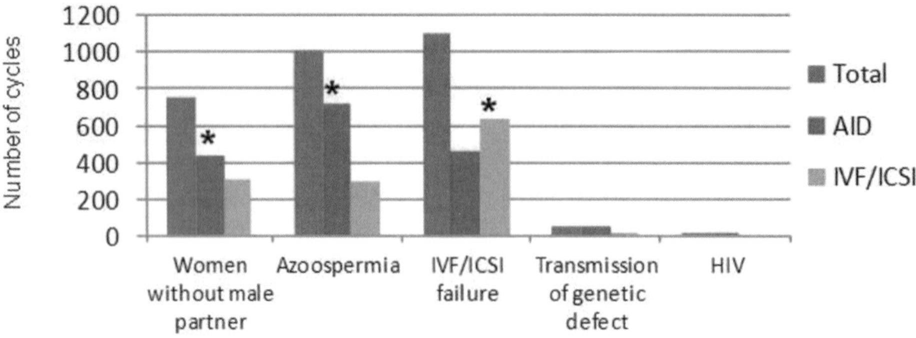

Figure 3.1 Number of cycles with donor sperm depending on the ART procedure (AID vs. IVF/ICSI) and clinical indications for donor sperm. The distribution of the proportions were compared by chi-square analysis. * denotes a statistically significant difference between proportions presented in AID vs. IVF $p < 0.0001$. (See also color plate.)

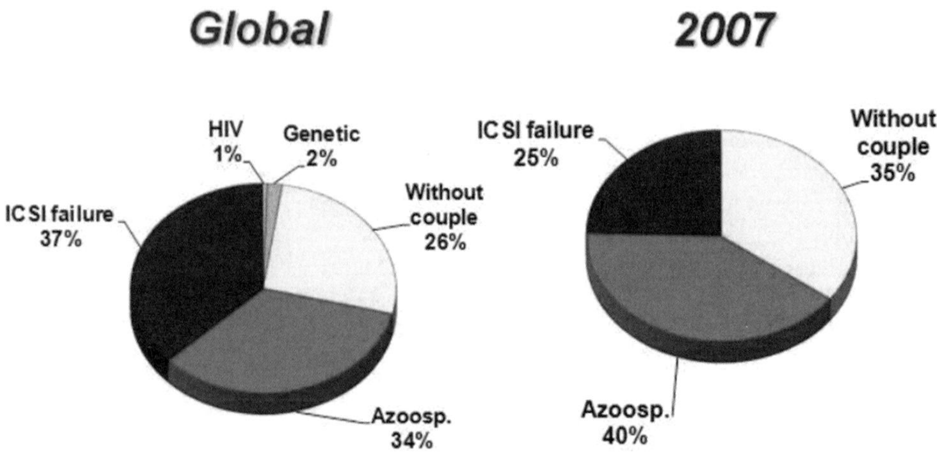

Figure 3.2 Distribution of the clinical indications for sperm donation. In the left graph the global proportion of each indication is represented (from 1999 to 2007). In the right graph the proportions observed in the last year are represented. The distribution of the proportions was compared by chi-square analysis. A statistically significant difference in the proportions presented in the two distributions was observed. $p < 0.0001$. (See also color plate.)

in both groups. We also observed an increased number of patients coming from ICSI failure in IVF and a decreased percentage with a previous diagnosis of non-obstructive azoospermia (Figure 3.1).

We studied the evolution in the indications for the use of donor sperm in recent years, comparing global distributions with the indications in the last year (2007), and there are significant increases in women without a heterosexual partner (from 26.4% to 34.9%) and azoospermia (from 33.9% to 40.1%), and a decrease in IVF/ICSI failure (from 37.2% to 25.0%), with indications to replace male gametes because of a genetic disorder or the presence of a sexually transmitted disease almost disappearing (Figure 3.2). We also represented the evolution in the number of

cycles and the different indications from 2000 to 2007 in AID and IVF cycles (Figure 3.3). We observed that whilst in AID the indications kept the same proportions, in IVF the proportions tended to invert from the original distribution.

Regarding pregnancy rates (AID), non-obstructive azoospermia patients presented the highest (29.1%) in comparison with ICSI failure and single women (27.6% and 22.6%, respectively). Couples with previous ICSI failures presented the highest pregnancy rates in IVF cycles (48.7%) compared with azoospermia and single women (42.0% and 38.2%, respectively).

All this information may help to describe the niche of patients that would potentially benefit from the development of the laboratory procedures to

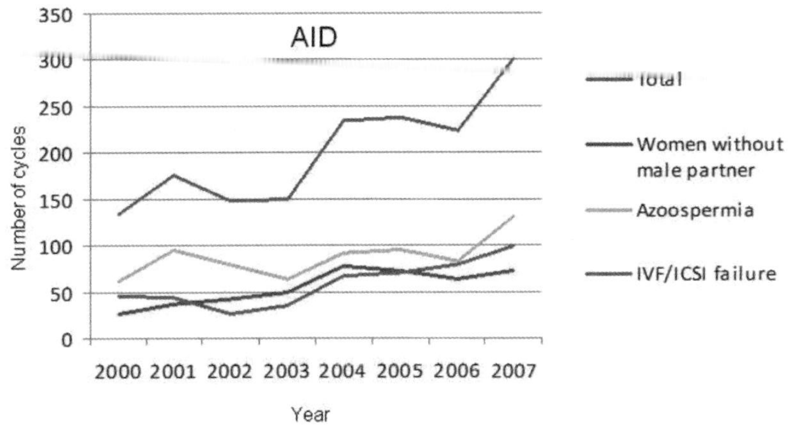

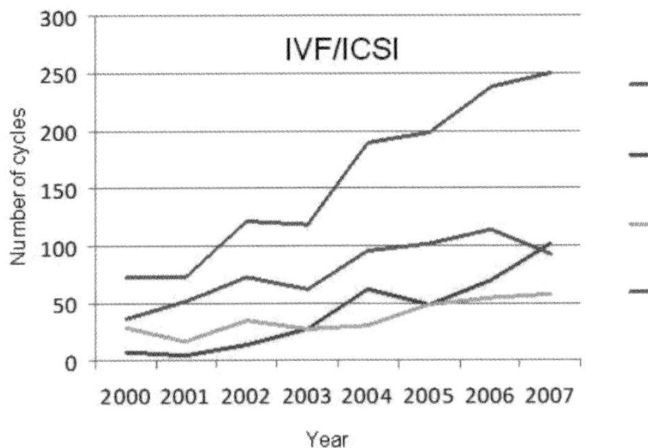

Figure 3.3 Number of cycles with donor sperm depending on the clinical indication in the ART procedure. These values are presented in a linear fashion for the years from 2000 to 2007. The upper panel represents the AID cycles and the lower panel the IVF/ICSI cycles. (See also color plate.)

obtain valid and physiologically competent spermatozoa from adult stem cells.

What we learned from infertile male sperm

To date, several research works have attempted to describe the physiology of sperm cells, aiming to determine the molecular features needed for a sperm to succeed. To reach this goal, and complete their function, sperm cells need to be able to adequately surpass a series of steps towards fertilization, correct embryo development, implantation, and the maintenance of a healthy pregnancy to finally deliver a child. Moreover, to increase the ejaculate's chances, it seems that numbers matter.

A myriad of molecules and processes have been related to one or more of these pathways, in a positive or negative manner. An in-depth knowledge of this "combination lock" is essential in order to establish what the ideal sperm created in a laboratory should look like.

Male infertility and defective sperm production

Sperm production is defective in a significant proportion of males aiming at fatherhood.

These defects can be divided into those leading to abnormally decreased sperm production, resulting from low or absent sperm in the ejaculate, or defects in sperm physiological characteristics, independent of sperm count, but causing reproductive failure.

Sperm defects related to sperm counts

In the last two years we have seen the publication of reports that suggest a global decline in semen quality [8]. Within Western Europe, a four-center study of fertile couples [9] has shown substantial variations in semen parameters. However, the data on trends in semen quality are conflicting and sensitive to geographical variations [10]. It has also been difficult to prove an association between deterioration in semen quality and male infertility, and the quality of existing studies has been questioned on the basis of population and selection biases, variations in laboratory standards, and statistical methodologies used for the analysis. The public impact and the "fear factor" of their conclusions (the modern's man apocalypse?) increase the public awareness of these studies.

There are little published data regarding the seminal patterns of the male partners of infertile couples referred to infertility units for assisted reproduction [11].

From our results we have observed that 15% of our patients had normal sperm parameters following WHO criteria, while 85% had abnormal semen analysis, with morphologic alterations (teratozoospermia) being the most common (27.8%) of the disorders observed, although there is no link between teratozoospermia and total reproductive failure [12].

Azoospermia, defined as the absence of spermatozoa in the ejaculate after assessment of centrifuged semen on at least two ejaculates, is observed in 1% of the general population and in 10–15% of infertile men [13]. The introduction of intracytoplasmic sperm injection (ICSI) offered a novel opportunity for parenthood to these couples. The first pregnancies reported after fertilization by ICSI with frozen testicular sperm in men with obstructive azoospermia (OA) were published by our group in 1995 [14]. The use of testicular sperm extraction (TESE) in non-obstructive azoospermia (NOA) was first reported by Tournaye [15]. This problem affects 10% of infertile men and is diagnosed in 60% of azoospermic men [16]. Aetiologies for testicular failure include genetic disorders such as sexual chromosomal abnormalities, translocations and microdeletions of the Y chromosome, cryptorchidism, testicular torsion, radiation, and toxins [17]. Testicular spermatozoa can be retrieved in some NOA men despite the absence of ejaculated spermatozoa in their semen, because of the existence of isolated foci of active spermatogenesis. However, lower recovery rates (around 50%) were observed in large series [18].

Current recommendations on the diagnosis of NOA dictate that it should only be based on histopathological findings, since clinical and endocrine parameters cannot accurately distinguish between OA and NOA [19]. The former represents an important issue, since sperm can be retrieved in almost all cases of OA, but only in 50% of NOA, when no preliminary selection of patients on the basis of histopathology has been performed [18].

Given the close relationship between genetic problems and very low sperm counts, this factor needs to be considered when using these individuals' testicular stem cells aiming to build sperm.

Sperm defects unrelated to sperm counts

Highly differentiated spermatozoa are generated through multiple cellular and molecular processes maintained by Sertoli cells. The cellular events associated with germ cells include proliferation, protein folding, and transportation, as well as sequential changes in chromatin and cell organelles.

These processes are strictly controlled by the expression of specific genes, and defects could induce structural and ultrastructural faults. These may affect function and could be closely related to male infertility and could compromise all the sections of the sperm cells, as has been widely described in multiple works.

Instead of a "big" molecular defect causing, or being 100% responsible for reproductive failure, it seems a lot of "small" physiological obstacles could be potentially guilty of the lack of success of sperm cells, in an additive manner. Hence, diagnostic tools aiming to predict success when analyzing semen should consider several aspects of sperm function.

Changes have been described in the morphology of the acrosome membrane and head of infertile sperm. The acrosome of infertiles can represent a bigger proportion of the sperm head than in the fertile males. The acrosome membrane in infertile men can also be less intact and less smooth than in fertile men. More droplets are attached to the acrosome membrane in infertile than fertile men [20].

The morphological analysis of spermatozoa from fertile and infertile men using light and electron microscopy can clarify the relationship between sperm morphology and fertility. Abnormalities in the spermatozoa can be classified into three types for the tails, two for the midsections, and six for the heads, according to the criteria adapted from WHO (World Health Organization) guidelines, as stated in the WHO Laboratory Manual for the Examination of Human Semen And Semen–Cervical Mucus Interaction (4th edition) in 1999. Approximately 14% of the spermatozoa from fertile men have abnormal tails at the light micro-scopic level, while approximately 44% have abnormal heads. Most abnormal cell types are encountered in semen from fertile men too, although the incidence of abnormalities is low [21].

Asthenozoospermia is a frequent cause of male infertility and can be explained by alterations in flagellum structure. These alterations may be non-specific and acquired, affecting a variable number of spermatozoa, or primary and specific, observed in most spermatozoa [22]. Numerous abnormalities of the axoneme and of the peri-axonemal structures are known in humans. An absence of both dynein arms revealed that these structures are essential to flagellar motion. Several other axonemal abnormalities have been found in infertile men, which could involve any of the axonemal components [23]. Abnormalities in the fibrous sheath, the mitochondrial sheath, and the attachment of the flagellum to the nucleus have also been found to be responsible for male infertility [24].

ICSI is considered an efficient treatment to overcome male infertility. Initially proposed in severe oligozoospermia [25], ICSI has been applied with ejaculated spermatozoa in the presence of oligoasthenoteratozoospermia, and with epididymal and testicular spermatozoa in azoospermia, with fresh or frozen–thawed samples [26]. Furthermore, fertilization and delivery were also obtained with ICSI using immotile but viable spermatozoa [27].

Until now, ICSI outcomes have only been reported in rare cases of specific flagellar abnormalities responsible for immotile spermatozoa, such as absent dynein arms [28], absent central microtubules [29] or dysplasia of the fibrous sheath [24]. Most of these infertile patients with ultrastructural defects of their sperm flagella also exhibited clinical features suggesting abnormalities of their respiratory cilia, i.e., Kartagener's syndrome, or chronic airway infections [28].

Globozoospermia is a very rare condition observed in <1% of infertile patients, where the major morphological anomaly is the absence of an acrosomal cap in sperm (Figure 3.4). The sperm head appears small and round due to the failure of the acrosome to develop [30]. The pathogenesis of globozoospermia most probably originates in spermatogenesis, more specifically in acrosome formation and sperm head elongation. The absence of the acrosome renders globozoospermic

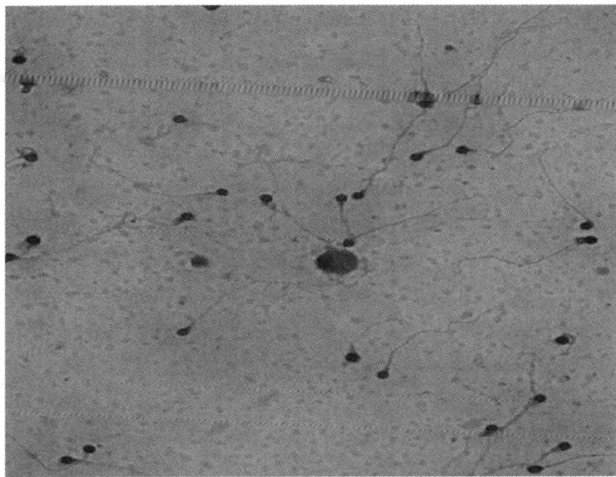

Figure 3.4 Hematoxylin-eosin staining of ejaculated spermatozoa from a patient suffering globozoospermia. Magnification 400×. (See also color plate.)

spermatozoa unable to bind to the zona pellucida (ZP) or fuse with the oocyte oolemma. Therefore, men affected by globozoospermia are infertile and untreatable by artificial insemination or conventional IVF. But when globozoospermic spermatozoa bypass the ZP and oocyte oolemma with ICSI, normal fertilization, embryo development, and pregnancy may occur. However, globozoospermia reduced ICSI fertilization rates compared with other forms of teratozoospermia. Fertilization failures have been attributed to a deficiency in oocyte activation capacity. Pregnancy and live birth can be achieved with chemical activation in a globozoospermic patient with a low fertilization rate in the previous cycle. Our group detected an improvement in the fertilization rate, development, and quality of the embryos generated with assisted oocyte activation [30].

Spermatogonial stem cells to restore male fertility

The introduction of intracytoplasmic sperm injection (ICSI) has played a significant role in the treatment of many severe male infertility problems [31]. However, in extreme cases of male infertility there is a complete absence of spermatozoa within the ejaculate due to absence of sperm production, or the obstruction or absence of some conduits. In these cases, testicular biopsy and ICSI is mandatory for proper diagnosis and treatment [32]. Moreover, in approximately one half of the non-obstructive azoospermia cases, it is almost impossible to recover the sperm from the testis [33]. Therefore, at the present time the only solution is sperm donation, resignation, or adoption [34].

Recently, the new avenue of research identifying testicular stem cells has arisen as a potential new field to be explored to treat these men. Spermatogonial stem cells (SSCs) are the adult stem cells of the testis [35]. They are located at the periphery of the seminiferous tubules flanked by the Sertoli cells, their niche cells. Like any other stem cell in the body, SSCs can either self-renew to maintain the SSC population, or differentiate and give rise to cells from the germ-cell line. The SSCs start to differentiate and will eventually produce mature spermatozoa in the continuous spermatogenesis process. This process of spermatogenesis occurs throughout a man's entire adult reproductive life and is preserved by the self-renewing capacity of the SSCs. Both proliferation and differentiation are well-regulated mechanisms, which are mainly directed by the Sertoli cells [36].

The importance of the testicular stem cells is reflected in a variety of research fields. The study of fundamental aspects of germ-cell development has become possible thanks to the introduction of the testicular stem-cell transplantation technique [37,38] and germ-cell culture [39]. In the future, these techniques may also have clinical applications. Indeed, the preservation of spermatogonial stem cells may be an important strategy in preserving fertility in young cancer patients [40].

These SSCs possess the capacity to repopulate nude mice treated with busulphan and to produce spermatozoa *de novo* [41]. Currently, a typical assay for the presence of spermatogonial stem cells in a cell suspension is the spermatogonial stem-cell transplantation technique; in the future this technique is intended to be used to restore fertility in patients with azoospermia. In experimental animals, azoospermia has been treated by the repopulation of the testes with SSCs obtained from different animals [42]. However, in humans, the main clinical objective is to obtain SSCs from a subject to repopulate the same testis [43] after a sterilizing treatment (such as chemotherapy on pre-pubertal boys because spermatogenesis has not been started in these patients). This presents the problem of reimplanting SSCs into destructured testis, and this problem led to an alternative option: to develop in vitro spermatogenesis and subsequent cryopreservation of the generated mature spermatozoa. Then, these in-vitro-derived spermatozoa could be used in assisted

reproduction techniques to obtain live offspring. This issue will be useful, for instance, in patients with maturation arrest [44] where the testicular niches are unable to produce the factors needed to support spermatogenesis.

On the other hand, the embryonic stem cells are pluripotent cells able to undergo meiosis, and generate functional haploid male gametes in vitro [45], as shown by Nayernia *et al.* [46], who achieved fertilization after intracytoplasmic injection into mouse oocytes. The resulting two-cell embryos were transferred into oviducts and live mice were born. However, the pups born were either too small or too large and died prematurely [46]. Due to this, this method cannot be employed in the treatment of infertility in humans.

Maintaining the genetic integrity of testicular stem cells is important in order to preserve the quality and function of the differentiated cells, but also to guarantee the correct transmission of genetic information from one generation to the next [45]. Adult testicular stem cells are thus essential for both the production of gametes and the continuation of the species.

Recent studies showed that murine SSCs have the ability to generate pluripotent cells and to differentiate spontaneously into derivates of the three embryonic germ layers [47]. This is an important alternative to the use of embryonic stem cells for cell-based regenerative medicine therapy [36].

In conclusion, several research lines are underway to create sperm cells from different origins, but we must keep in mind that spermatozoa are more than mere "DNA bags," and they should be structurally and physiologically competent to succeed, as we will discuss in the next section.

This rationale can explain why stem cells coming from non-functional testes could be a problematic cell type to start developing lab sperm.

Molecular features of the functional spermatozoa

To develop sperm from reprogrammed or undifferentiated cells, there are some aspects that need to be considered before assisted reproduction with laboratory-created gametes is conducted.

Until now, the only analysis to estimate the male potential to become a father is the spermiogram following World Health Organization criteria [34], where sperm volume, concentration, and the percentage of spermatozoa with progressive motility and normal shape are the main parameters considered. When men's fertility is analyzed, these values have been considered the best indicators for decades.

Interestingly, there are a significant proportion of infertile males presenting normal sperm counts, thus diagnosed as having idiopathic infertility [48]. This fact is clearly pointing to some underlying defects within their spermatozoa, confirming that male fertility is something other than having a high sperm output.

Several recent studies have suggested molecular factors implicated in sperm biology, which need to be considered when "creating" successful spermatozoa in the laboratory.

Chromosomal content and genetic status

Obviously, sperm chromosomal content is a key issue to consider when deriving sperm cells from stem cells, mainly taking into account that a correct chromosomal content obtained from an adequate meiotic division from diploid cells is necessary.

Actually, except for chromosomal aneuploidies [49,50], or Y chromosome microdeletion investigations [51], both linked to severe alterations in sperm count, no molecular features of sperm complementing the basic sperm analysis are available as a diagnostic tool.

The presence of chromosomal abnormalities in infertile males' ejaculates is relatively frequent, as the severity of the male factor increases, reaching almost 40% of males with sperm counts lower than 2–4 million [52], while the presence of microedeletions is confirmed in 14% of azoospermic males [51].

This clearly indicates a close relationship between testicular function and genetic problems that should be seriously considered when creating spermatozoa from stem cells.

Nevertheless, fluorescent *in situ* hybridization techniques to confirm the absence of chromosomal aneuploidies in created sperm are widely employed and available in research laboratories, and these tests are mandatory before these sperm cells are employed, although the presence of microdeletions caused by the methodology of gamete creation is unlikely.

Imprinting

Epigenetic mechanisms, including DNA methylation, covalent histone modification, and chromatine remodeling acting on mRNA transcription, and post-transcriptional modifications by non-coding mRNAs, genetically regulate the expression of one allelic copy, depending on their parental origin.

These genes present a highly relevant role in embryo development.

Given that epigenetic regulation is done during gametogenesis, this is a fundamental issue that needs to be tackled when aiming to create sperm from stem cells.

In the germline, epigenetic reprogramming begins with the complete deletion of all genes, starting with *de novo* methylation and chromatin remodeling of all the genome [53]. This reprogramming provides the gametes with the molecular programs required to activate the oocyte, the zygote, and embryo development.

Given that genetic imprinting is established during gametogenesis, it has been postulated that this process can be affected as a consequence of assisted reproduction treatments, mainly caused when immature sperm cells are employed, as a consequence of ovarian hyperstimulation protocols, in vitro oocyte maturation, germ-cell cryopreservation, and the stressful mechanisms caused by IVF micromanipulation procedures [54].

This fact is especially relevant when we consider their consequences. Several diseases have been related to imprinting defects, such as neurological and developmental diseases (Beckwith–Wiedemann, Prader-Willi, and Angelman syndromes), metabolic diseases (neonatal transitory diabetes mellitus), psychiatric and behavioral diseases (autism, schizophrenia, and bipolar disease), and cancer (retinoblastoma, Wilm's tumor, osteosarcoma, and rhabdomyosarcoma).

Moreover, some authors found data from newborns obtained by means of assisted reproduction supporting these affirmations, although it is still a controversial issue.

The same happens with imprinting-derived infertility: several authors found in their work results supporting a close link between imprinting defects and infertility, but this needs to be further confirmed [53,54].

Sperm DNA integrity

To date, there are a lot of studies concerning DNA analysis of human spermatozoa suggesting that the determination of DNA fragmentation levels can be a parameter of semen quality, directly implicated in male fertility [55,56].

The sperm chromatin structure assay (SCSA) from the work of Evenson *et al.* [57] has been the initial methodology to determine sperm DNA alterations, and several studies have found a negative predictive value in pregnancy outcome in ART [58,59]. A strong correlation between the SCD and SCSA tests has been found [60], as expected, since both of these tests determine susceptibility of sperm DNA to acid denaturation in vitro.

Nevertheless, among all the studies presented, highly controversial results have been reported [61]. A high percentage of the works are unable to find a significant relationship between sperm DNA fragmentation and the incapacity to reach pregnancy. Furthermore, among all the research work finding a positive relationship, different thresholds and cut-off values have been settled, thus limiting the clinical application of the test.

Moreover, some works are openly against the value of the measurement of the DNA fragmentation extent to predict fertility potential [62,65].

When we compared the results of sperm DNA fragmentation on the same samples employed in IUI cycles achieving a pregnancy with those who failed, in a total number of 100 samples, there were no statistical differences [64].

In IVF procedures, we can obtain further data to determine the influence of sperm DNA fragmentation in male fertility, due to the close follow-up of embryo development [63]. In this work, a negative correlation with fertilization, an increased proportion of zygotes showing asynchrony between the nucleolar precursor bodies of zygote pronuclei (73.8 vs. 28.8%, $p = 0.001$), implantation rate, and slower embryo development, together with worse morphology on day 6, was correlated with higher sperm DNA fragmentation sperm samples. It was also found that the situation does not compromise pregnancy chances, probably as a consequence of the embryo selection before transfer [63].

Oxidative stress defence in sperm

Reactive oxygen species (ROS) are by-products of the physiological metabolism of O_2 in cells under aerobic conditions, necessary for the normal cell function in organs or tissues, but controlled by the antioxidant content [66,67].

In sperm, ROS in controlled levels are required to achieve fertilization [68], fusion with the oocyte, and capacitation [69,70].

Under some circumstances, ROS are highly reactive against cellular structures and molecules, interfering with their biological functions and properties [71].

Therefore, oxidative stress (OS) in sperm is defined as the disequilibrium between pro-oxidative and anti-oxidative molecules in a complex biological system, where the oxidants prevail over the defensive systems, causing damage to DNA molecules, deregulating the acrosome reaction and impeding sperm/oocyte recognition and fusion [71].

It is known that human spermatozoa are extremely sensitive to ROS-induced damage due to their special plasma membrane composition [72]. This sensitivity is related to the high content of polyunsaturated fatty acids. This results in sperm–egg fusion, acrosome reaction, and motility being compromised in OS situations.

Free radical overload has been correlated with diminished fertilization rates and also with bad embryo quality [73].

GPX4 and GPX1 are differentially expressed in fertile and infertile males, and the protein formed from these mRNAs exhibited altered parameters, thus suggesting a role for these enzymes in male fertility [74–75].

Moreover, when day-3 embryo parameters were evaluated, GPX4 mRNA expression in sperm cells was significantly lower when asymmetric embryos were observed, and poorer embryo development and morphology on day 5 was statistically related to lower sperm GPX1 activity [75].

The appropriate control of these systems by the molecular content of sperm cells is essential for reproductive function.

Other molecular keys in sperm physiology

Other molecules have been described as relevant in sperm function, and thus they should be considered to be important in "artificially created" sperm.

Some of them are involved in the apoptosis process. For instance, when selecting non-apoptotic sperm cells via immunomagnetic separation after cell labeling against annexin-V-positive cells [76], sperm fertilization potential was shown to be higher, as assessed using the hamster oocyte penetration assay and hamster oocyte-intracytoplasmic sperm injection (ICSI)

Another example is platelet-activating factor (PAF), a signaling phospholipid found in sperm that has been studied and related to fertilizing potential [77].

Also heat shock protein2A (Hsp2A) has been detected in sperm and present in higher levels in infertile males [78]. The same group tested whether or not low sperm HspA2 ratios and CK activity were predictive of IVF pregnancies, showing excellent results, and the selection of sperm to bind HA-coated slides causes a significant decrease in sperm chromosomal anomalies, therefore providing better results in ICSI treatments.

Ubiquitin forms covalently linked polyubiquitin chains on substrate proteins and targets "ubiquitinated" substrates for degradation to assist in the removal of defective sperm and debris.

Increased levels of sperm ubiquitination in men with idiopathic infertility were found [79]. This could reveal the presence of a fault in defective sperm removal, thus increasing the chances of fertilization by a malfunctioning sperm cell. Moreover, there are negative correlations between sperm ubiquitin and several parameters reflective of embryo development after assisted fertilization [80].

In a recent study, we looked at the implications of mucin MUC-1 [81] in sperm-function infertile patients showing fewer stained spermatozoa than fertile sperm donors.

Oxygen consumption ability

Oxygen uptake is considered a good indicator of cellular metabolic activity, and it is directly related to viability and motility in sperm cells. To date, the only available system to measure oxygen diminution due to metabolic activity in spermatozoa needs the previous extraction of intracellular contents [82], and complex reagents, complex equipment like microspectrophotometry, ultramicrofluorescence, electrochemical methods, automatic tracking with electrodes, and electrochemical microscopic tracking [82,84], difficult to implement in assisted reproduction laboratories.

This is because most of these techniques are invasive, technically underdeveloped, take a long time, and require the use of UV light, radioactive proofs, or fluorescence markers; thus tests are unfeasible to

study sperm viability prior to assisted reproduction treatment.

The Microrespiration System is a technology based on the use of oxygen microsensors able to instantly measure O_2 concentration (OC) while maintaining sperm viability, enabling an easy and inexpensive way to measure OC dynamics in either ejaculates or prepared sperm samples.

This is the demonstration that many molecular features of sperm need to be considered before tagging spermatozoa as functional or not, once produced in vitro. Several quality-control checkpoints need to be implemented before their employment in human assisted reproduction procedures.

Information obtained from the application of massive analysis techniques to sperm

Finally, the massive analysis of sperm, by means of proteomics or genomics technologies, reveals huge differences between the molecular features of sperm able to yield a healthy pregnancy, or not.

The development of microarray technology, derived from the results of the human genome project, made it possible to determine cell or tissue expression profiles for the whole genome, enabling the comparison between two different biological conditions, which is expected to be essential in the development of research, diagnostic, and therapeutic tools [85].

Sperm mRNA was first described in the late 1980s in different animals and the mRNA detection as a potential infertility marker in human sperm was seriously considered several years later [86,87].

There is evidence of the need for adequate embryo formation of sperm-delivered mRNAs from experiments confirming the lack of success in the oocyte's parthenogenetic activation, the absence of certain mRNAs within the oocyte, and the implication of concrete sperm mRNAs in embryo development [88,90]. In these works, the bases for future research were established, since several known and unknown protein-coding mRNAs were described.

A comparison between ejaculates was obtained from idiopathically infertile males, with normal sperm counts and partners without evident infertility problems, in comparison with healthy and previously fertile sperm donors. Numerous genes were found to be differentially expressed in both directions, when a cut-off value of 2 was settled [91], expressed at least twice in fertile vs. infertile males, or vice versa. Only considering those genes expressed at least 10 times in one of the groups in comparison with the other, a total number of 116 genes were found. These results were confirmed by random quantitative PCR.

Among them, some were involved in spermatogenesis, such as microseminoprotein beta, t-complex-associated-testis-expressed-1 like-1, sperm-associated antigen 5 (SPAG5), and spermatogenesis-associated gene 7 (SPATA7), which are overexpressed in fertile males in comparison with infertile males without decreased sperm count and motility. Additionally, some genes with roles not yet described in spermatogenesis such as ornithine decarboxylase antizyme 3 (OAZ3), the suppressor of potassium transport defect (SKD), and ribosomal protein (RPS3A) were found with very different expression levels, being overexpressed in the fertile patient group [91].

Moreover, when applying functional analysis platforms to analyze genes grouped on the basis of their function blindly (the analyst not knowing the origin of the data), at different grouping levels of analysis, several processes implicated in gamete formation are found to be different between both groups. These analyses statistically test if the existence of a determined number of genes over- or underexpressed within each group is due to a real effect or chance.

As described in Figure 3.1, several groups reveal a significant disparity between the proportions of genes over- or underexpressed in infertile males and fertile sperm donors. At a different analysis level, different biochemical pathways or processes are implicated. Interestingly, when over- or underexpressed genes in infertile males were grouped by their function, those involving spermatozoa differentiation were present at all analysis levels. Also, a comparison between genes expressed in the sperm of fertile males, not found in infertile males, and inversely, detected in infertile males while they are not within sperm of fertile males, was performed.

We found 27 spermatogenesis- or testes-related genes expressed only in previously fertile sperm donors not expressed in infertile males with normal sperm count. Only one was expressed in infertile males, while it was not present in controls. Among those 27 genes we can remark on ODFP2 (outer dense fiber protein 2), which may have a modulating influence on sperm motility, and SPAT9 (spermatogenesis-associated protein 9), which is not expressed in testes of patients with Sertoli-cell-only syndrome and shows variable expression in patients with spermatogenic arrest. Meanwhile the unique gene in the infertile male group not present in fertile donors was H2BWT (H2B histone family member W testis-specific) an atypical histone H2B that does not recruit chromosome condensation factors and does not participate in the assembly of mitotic chromosomes, if present [92]. These findings are even more interesting when we consider that sperm samples did not differ in terms of sperm concentration and motility between fertile donors and infertile males, thus being focused on idiopathic male infertility.

Proteomic mapping of male infertility has also been recently attempted. This technology analyses a different aspect of the sperm physiology which could potentially be employed as an independent fertility predictor. The information contained in the sperm mRNA will be translated into proteins that will be later modified, and will result in the functional biomolecules of spermatozoa. Both human seminal plasma and sperm have been tested by means of this technology to determine their protein profile [93,94]. Lots of different spots can be found from the bidimensional electrophoresis analysis of a sperm protein profile, representing each a protein sequence.

A list of proteins present in human spermatozoa has been recently reported, from sperm lysates, in both soluble and insoluble fractions.

No report has yet considered the differences between fertile and infertile males, and this technology seems to be a step forward from the wide genomic analysis. Only the description of a case report of in vitro fertilization failure in comparison with fertile donors has been published [95].

Sperm lipidic profile

Sperm membrane lipid composition is of special interest, given their involvement in fertilization [96], capacitation, spermatozoa, and oocyte interaction [96,97]. Moreover, their particular lipidic composition, with very high levels of phospholipids, sterols, glycolipids, and saturated and polyunsaturated fatty acids, increases their sensitivity to oxidative attack and are positively correlated with sperm quality too, probably because these fatty acids provide higher fluidity of the plasma membrane [98].

Thus, an adequate sperm cell membrane lipidic composition seems essential to succeed.

Where are we now and where can we go: Conclusions

We can conclude that there are still several difficulties to confirm if derived sperm could be guaranteed to behave like sperm from fertile males, before undergoing assisted reproduction.

The future vision shows the possibility to create sperm cells from adult stem cells, with all the requirements to succeed fulfilled, thus guaranteeing a safe and successful use. The intermediate steps to reach it are the task that needs to be done by researchers.

Men with no sperm, and also men producing sperm cells with inappropriate characteristics will benefit from these developments.

References

1. Zuzuarregui, J.L., Meseguer, M., Garrido, N. *et al.* Parameters affecting the results in a program of artificial insemination with donor sperm. A 12-year retrospective review of more than 1800 cycles. *Journal of Assisted Reproduction and Genetics.* 2004; 21(4): 109–118.

2. Garrido, N., Zuzuarregui, J.L., Meseguer, M. Sperm and oocyte donor selection and management: experience of a 10 year follow-up of more than 2100 candidates. *Human Reproduction.* 2002; 17(12): 3142–3148.

3. Ferraretti, A.P., Pennings, G., Gianaroli, L. *et al.* Semen donor recruitment in an oocyte donation programme. *Human Reproduction.* 2006; 21(10): 2482–2485.

4. Meseguer, M., Garrido, N., Gimeno, C. *et al.* Comparison of polymerase chain reaction-dependent methods for determining the presence of human immunodeficiency virus and hepatitis C virus in washed sperm. *Fertility and Sterility.* 2002; 78(6): 1199–1202.

5. Freour, T., Jean, M., Mirallie, S. *et al.* Predictive value of CASA parameters in IUI with frozen donor sperm. *International Journal of Andrology.* 2008; 32: 498–504.

6. Allamaneni, S.S., Bandaranayake, I., Agarwal, A. *et al.* Use of semen quality scores to predict pregnancy rates in couples undergoing intrauterine insemination with donor sperm. *Fertility and Sterility.* 2004; 82(3): 606–611.

7. The European IVF-Monitoring Programme (EIM) for the European Society of Human Reproduction and Embryology (ESHRE), Andersen, A.N., Gianaroli, L., Felberbaum, R. *et al.* Assisted reproductive technology in Europe, 2002. Results generated from European registers by ESHRE. *Human Reproduction.* 2006; 21(7): 1680–1697.

8. Bilotta, P., Guglielmo, R., Steffe, M Analysis of decline in seminal fluid in the Italian population during the past 15 years. *Minerva Ginecologica.* 1999; 51(6): 223–231.

9. Jensen, T.K., Slama, R., Ducot, B. *et al.* Regional differences in waiting time to pregnancy among fertile couples from four European cities. *Human Reproduction.* 2001; 16(12): 2697–2704.

10. Pal, P.C., Rajalakshmi, M., Manocha, M. *et al.* Semen quality and sperm functional parameters in fertile Indian men. *Andrologia.* 2006; 38(1): 20–25.

11. Adeniji, R.A., Olayemi, O., Okunlola, M.A. *et al.* Pattern of semen analysis of male partners of infertile couples at the University College Hospital, Ibadan. *West African Journal of Medicine* 2003; 22(3): 243–245.

12. Garrido, N., Meseguer, M., Pellicer, A. Interpretation of sperm morphology analysis in gynecological practice for infertility. *Expert Reviews in Obstetrics and Gynecology.* 2006; 1: 7–8.

13. Jarow, J.P., Espeland, M.A., Lipshultz, L.I. Evaluation of the azoospermic patient. *Journal of Urology.* 1989; 142(1): 62–65.

14. Gil-Salom, M., Minguez, Y., Rubio, C. *et al.* Efficacy of intracytoplasmic sperm injection using testicular spermatozoa. *Human Reproduction.* 1995; 10(12): 3166–3170.

15. Tournaye, H., Camus, M., Goossens, A. *et al.* Recent concepts in the management of infertility because of non-obstructive azoospermia. *Human Reproduction.* 1995; 10 Suppl 1: 115–119.

16. Matsumiya, K., Namiki, M., Kondoh, N. *et al.* New indication of testis biopsy for azoospermia: a clinical study in Japanese patients. *International Journal of Urology.* 1994; 1(2): 177–180.

17. Raman, J.D., Schlegel, P.N. Testicular sperm extraction with intracytoplasmic sperm injection is successful for the treatment of nonobstructive azoospermia associated with cryptorchidism. *Journal of Urology.* 2003; 170(4 Pt 1): 1287–1290.

18. Gil-Salom, M., Romero, J., Minguez, Y. *et al.* Testicular sperm extraction and intracytoplasmic sperm injection: a chance of fertility in nonobstructive azoospermia. *Journal of Urology.* 1998; 160(6 Pt 1): 2063–2067.

19. McLachlan, R.I., Rajpert-De Meyts, E., Hoei-Hansen, C.E. *et al.* Histological evaluation of the human testis – approaches to optimizing the clinical value of the assessment: mini review. *Human Reproduction.* 2007; 22(1): 2–16.

20. Yu, J.J., Xu, Y.M. Ultrastructural defects of acrosome in infertile men. *Archives of Andrology*. 2004; 50(6): 405–409.

21. Kubo-Irie, M., Matsumiya, K., Iwamoto, T. *et al.* Morphological abnormalities in the spermatozoa of fertile and infertile men. *Molecular Reproduction and Development*. 2005; 70(1): 70–81.

22. Chemes, H.E., Olmedo, S.B., Carrere, C. *et al.* Ultrastructural pathology of the sperm flagellum: association between flagellar pathology and fertility prognosis in severely asthenozoospermic men. *Human Reproduction*. 1998; 13(9): 2521–2526.

23. Baccetti, B., Capitani, S., Collodel, G. *et al.* Recent advances in human sperm pathology. *Contraception*. 2002; 65(4): 283–287.

24. Chemes, E.H., Rawe, Y.V. Sperm pathology: a step beyond descriptive morphology. Origin, characterization and fertility potential of abnormal sperm phenotypes in infertile men. *Human Reproduction Update*. 2003; 9(5): 405–428.

25. Hamberger, L., Lundin, K., Sjogren, A. *et al.* Indications for intracytoplasmic sperm injection. *Human Reproduction*. 1998; 13 Suppl 1: 128–133.

26. Devroey, P., Van Steirteghem, A. A review of ten years experience of ICSI. *Human Reproduction Update*. 2004; 10(1): 19–28.

27. von Zumbusch, A., Fiedler, K., Mayerhofer, A. *et al.* Birth of healthy children after intracytoplasmic sperm injection in two couples with male Kartagener's syndrome. *Fertility and Sterility* 1998; 70(4): 643–646.

28. Peeraer, K., Nijs, M., Raick, D. *et al.* Pregnancy after ICSI with ejaculated immotile spermatozoa from a patient with immotile cilia syndrome: a case report and review of the literature. *Reproductive Biomedicine Online*. 2004; 9(6): 659–663.

29. Okada, H., Fujioka, H., Tatsumi, N. *et al.* Assisted reproduction for infertile patients with 9 + 0 immotile spermatozoa associated with autosomal dominant polycystic kidney disease. *Human Reproduction*. 1999; 14(1): 110–113.

30 Tejera, A., Molla, M., Muriel, L. *et al.* Successful pregnancy and childbirth after intracytoplasmic sperm injection with calcium ionophore oocyte activation in a globozoospermic patient. *Fertility and Sterility*. 2008; 90(4): 1202.e1–1202.e5.

31. Palermo, G., Joris, H., Devroey, P. *et al.* Pregnancies after intracytoplasmic injection of single spermatozoon into an oocyte. *Lancet*. 1992; 340: 17–18.

32. Meseguer, M., Garrido, N., Remohi, J. *et al.* Testicular sperm extraction (TESE) and ICSI in patients with permanent azoospermia after chemotherapy. *Human Reproduction*. 2003; 18: 1281–1285.

33. Gil-Salom, M., Romero, J., Minguez, Y. *et al.* Testicular sperm extraction and intracytoplasmic sperm injection: a chance of fertility in nonobstructive azoospermia. *Journal of Urology*. 1998; 160: 2063–2067.

34 World Health Organization. Towards more objectivity in diagnosis and management of male infertility. Results of a World Health Organisation Multicentre Study. *International Journal of Andrology*. 1987; 7 Suppl.: 1.

35 McLaren, A. Germ and somatic cell lineages in the developing gonad. *Molecular and Cellular Endocrinology*. 2000; 163: 3–9.

36 Ellen, G., Herman, T. Is there a clinical future for spermatogonial stem cells? *Current Stem Cell Research and Therapy*. 2007; 2: 189–195.

37. Brinster, R.L., Zimmermann, J.W. Spermatogenesis following male germ-cell transplantation. *Proceedings of the National Academy of Sciences of the United States of America*. 1994; 91: 11298–11302.

38. Brinster, R.L., Avarbock, M.R. Germline transmission of donor haplotype following spermatogonial transplantation. *Proceedings of the National Academy of Sciences of the United States of America*. 1994; 91: 11303–11307.

39. Falciatori, I., Lillard-Wetherell, K., Wu, Z. *et al.* Deriving mouse spermatogonial stem cell lines. *Methods in Molecular Biology*. 2008; 450: 181–192.

40. Tournaye, H., Goossens, E., Verheyen, G. *et al.* Preserving the reproductive potential of men and boys with cancer: current concepts and future prospects. *Human Reproduction Update*. 2004; 10: 525–532.

41. Kanatsu-Shinohara, M., Ogonuki, N., Inoue, K. *et al.* Restoration of fertility in infertile mice by transplantation of cryopreserved male germline stem cells. *Human Reproduction*. 2003; 18: 2660–2667.

42. Kanatsu-Shinohara, M., Miki, H., Inoue, K. *et al.* Germline niche transplantation restores fertility in infertile mice. *Human Reproduction*. 2005; 20: 2376–2382.

43. Ogawa, T., Ohmura, M., Yumura, Y. *et al.* Expansion of murine spermatogonial stem cells through serial transplantation. *Biology of Reproduction*. 2003; 68: 316–322.

44. Lee, D.R., Kim, K.S., Yang, Y.H. *et al.* Isolation of male germ stem cell-like cells from testicular tissue of non-obstructive azoospermic patients and differentiation into haploid male germ cells in vitro. *Human Reproduction*. 2006; 21: 471–476.

45. Geijsen, N., Horoschak, M., Kim, K. *et al.* Derivation of embryonic germ cells and male

gametes from embryonic stem cells. *Nature*. 2004; 427: 118–154.

46. Nayernia, K., Nolte, J., Michelmann, H.W. *et al.* In vitro-differentiated embryonic stem cells give rise to male gametes that can generate offspring mice. *Developmental Cell*. 2006; 11: 125–132.

47. Guan, K., Nayernia, K., Maier, L.S. *et al.* Pluripotency of spermatogonial stem cells from adult mouse testis. *Nature*. 2006; 440: 1199–1203.

48. Kumar, R., Gautam, G., Gupta, N.P. Drug therapy for idiopathic male infertility: rationale versus evidence. *Journal of Urology*. 2006; 176: 1307–1312.

49. Bernardini, L.M., Calogero, A.E., Bottazzi, C. *et al.* Low total normal motile count values are associated with increased sperm disomy and diploidy rates in infertile patients. *International Journal of Andrology*. 2005; 28: 328–336.

50. Rubio, C., Gil-Salom, M., Simón, C. *et al.* Incidence of sperm chromosomal abnormalities in a risk population: relationship with sperm quality and ICSI outcome. *Human Reproduction*. 2001; 16: 2084–2092.

51. Martinez, M.C., Bernabe, M.J., Gomez, E. *et al.* Screening for AZF deletion in a large series of severely impaired spermatogenesis patients. *Journal of Andrology*. 2000; 21: 651–655.

52. Rodrigo, L., Rubio, C., Mateu, E. *et al.* Analysis of chromosomal abnormalities in testicular and epididymal spermatozoa from azoospermic ICSI patients by fluorescence in-situ hybridization. *Human Reproduction*. 2004; 19(1): 118–123.

53. Allen, C., Reardon, W. Assisted reproduction technology and defects of genomic imprinting. *British Journal of Obstetrics and Gynecology*. 2005; 112(12): 1589–1594.

54. Trasler, J.M. Gamete imprinting: setting epigenetic patterns for the next generation. *Reproduction, Fertility and Development*. 2006; 18(1–2): 63–69.

55. Agarwal, A., Said, T.M. Role of sperm chromatin abnormalities and DNA damage in male infertility. *Human Reproduction Update*. 2003; 9: 331–345.

56. Ozmen, B., Caglar, G.S., Koster, F. *et al.* Relationship between sperm DNA damage, induced acrosome reaction and viability in ICSI patients. *Reproductive Biomedicine Online*. 2007; 15: 208–214.

57. Evenson, D.P., Jost, L.K., Marshall, D. *et al.* Utility of the sperm chromatin structure assay as a diagnostic and prognostic tool in the human fertility clinic. *Human Reproduction*. 1999; 14: 1039–1049.

58. Larson-Cook, K.L., Brannian, J.D., Hansen, K.A. *et al.* Relationship between the outcomes of assisted reproductive techniques and sperm DNA fragmentation as measured by the sperm chromatin structure assay. *Fertility and Sterility*. 2003; 80: 895–902.

59. Virro, M.R., Larson-Cook, K.L., Evenson, D.P. Sperm chromatin structure assay (SCSA) parameters are related to fertilization, blastocyst development, and ongoing pregnancy in in vitro fertilization and intracytoplasmic sperm injection cycles. *Fertility and Sterility*. 2004; 81: 1289–1295.

60. Chohan, K.R., Griffin, J.T., Lafromboise, M. *et al.* Comparison of chromatin assays for DNA fragmentation evaluation in human sperm. *Journal of Andrology*. 2006; 27: 53–59.

61. Evenson, D., Wixon, R. Meta-analysis of sperm DNA fragmentation using the sperm chromatin structure assay. *Reproductive Biomedicine Online*. 2006; 12: 466–472.

62. Payne, J.F., Raburn, D.J., Couchman, G.M. *et al.* Redefining the relationship between sperm deoxyribonucleic acid fragmentation as measured by the sperm chromatin structure assay and outcomes of assisted reproductive techniques. *Fertility and Sterility*. 2005; 84: 356–364.

63. Muriel, L., Garrido, N., Fernandez, J.L. *et al.* Value of the sperm deoxyribonucleic acid fragmentation level, as measured by the sperm chromatin dispersion test, in the outcome of in vitro fertilization and intracytoplasmic sperm injection. *Fertility and Sterility*. 2006; 85: 371–383.

64. Muriel, L., Meseguer, M., Fernández, J.L. *et al.* Value of the sperm chromatin dispersion test in predicting pregnancy outcome in intrauterine insemination: a blind prospective study. *Human Reproduction*. 2006; 21(3): 738–744.

65. Practice Committee of the American Society for Reproductive Medicine. The clinical utility of sperm DNA integrity testing. *Fertility and Sterility*. 2006; 86: S35–S37.

66. Garrido, N., Meseguer, M., Simón, C. *et al.* Pro-oxidative and anti-oxidative imbalance in human semen and its relation with male fertility. *Asian Journal of Andrology*. 2004; 6: 59–65.

67. Saleh, R.A., Agarwal, A. Oxidative stress and male infertility: from research bench to clinical practice. *Journal of Andrology*. 2002; 23: 737–752.

68. Aitken, R.J. The Amoroso Lecture. The human spermatozoon – a cell in crisis? *Journal of Reproduction and Fertility*. 1999; 115: 1–7.

69. O'Flaherty, C., de Lamirande, E., Gagnon, C. Positive role of reactive oxygen species in mammalian sperm capacitation: triggering and modulation of

phosphorylation events. *Free Radical Biology and Medicine.* 2006; 41: 528–540.

70. O'Flaherty, C., de Lamirande, E., Gagnon, C. Reactive oxygen species modulate independent protein phosphorylation pathways during human sperm capacitation. *Free Radical Biology and Medicine.* 2006; 40: 1045–1055.

71. Agarwal, A., Saleh, R.A., Bedawy, M.A. Role of reactive oxygen species in the pathophisiology of human reproduction. *Fertility and Sterility.* 2003; 79: 829–843.

72. Padron, O.F., Brackett, N.L., Sharma, R.K. *et al.* Seminal reactive oxygen species and sperm motility and morphology in men with spinal cord injury. *Fertility and Sterility.* 1997; 67: 1115–1120.

73. Zorn, B., Vidmar, G., Meden-Vrtovec, H. Seminal reactive oxygen species as predictors of fertilization, embryo quality and pregnancy rates after conventional in vitro fertilization and intracytoplasmic sperm injection. *International Journal of Andrology.* 2003; 26: 279–285.

74. Garrido, N., Meseguer, M., Alvarez, J. *et al.* Relationship among standard semen parameters, glutathione peroxidase/glutathione reductase activity, and mRNA expression and reduced glutathione content in ejaculated spermatozoa from fertile and infertile men. *Fertility and Sterility.* 2004; 82 Suppl 3: 1059–1066.

75. Meseguer, M., de los Santos, M.J., Simon, C. *et al.* Effect of sperm glutathione peroxidases 1 and 4 on embryo asymmetry and blastocyst quality in oocyte donation cycles. *Fertility and Sterility.* 2006; 86: 1376–1385.

76. Said, T.M., Grunewald, S., Paasch, U. *et al.* Effects of magnetic-activated cell sorting on sperm motility and cryosurvival rates. *Fertility and Sterility.* 2005; 83: 1442–1446.

77. Toledo, A.A., Mitchell-Leef, D., Elsner, C.W. *et al.* Fertilization potential of human sperm is correlated with endogenous platelet-activating factor content. *Journal of Assisted Reproduction and Genetics.* 2003; 20: 192–195.

78. Ergur, A.R., Dokras, A., Giraldo, J.L. *et al.* Sperm maturity and treatment choice of in vitro fertilization (IVF) or intracytoplasmic sperm injection: diminished sperm HspA2 chaperone levels predict IVF failure. *Fertility and Sterility.* 2002; 77: 910–918.

79. Sutovsky, P., Hauser, R., Sutovsky, M. Increased levels of sperm ubiquitin correlate with semen quality in men from an andrology laboratory clinic population. *Human Reproduction.* 2004; 19: 628–638.

80. Ozanon, C., Chouteau, J., Sutovsky, P. Clinical adaptation of the sperm ubiquitin tag immunoassay (SUTI): relationship of sperm ubiquitylation with sperm quality in gradient-purified semen samples from 93 men from a general infertility clinic population. *Human Reproduction.* 2005; 20: 2271–2278.

81. Martinez-Conejero, J.A., Garrido, N., Remohi, J. *et al.* MUC1 in human testis and ejaculated spermatozoa and its relationship to male fertility status. *Fertility and Sterility.* 2008; 90(2): 450–452.

82. Ferramosca, A., Focarelli, R., Piomboni, P., Coppola, L., Zara, V. Oxygen uptake by mitochondria in demembranated human spermatozoa: a reliable tool for the evaluation of sperm respiratory efficiency. *International Journal of Andrology.* 2008; 31: 337–345.

83. Stendardi, A., Focarelli, R., Piomboni, P. *et al.* Evaluation of mitochondrial respiratory efficiency during in vitro capacitation of human spermatozoa. *International Journal of Andrology.* 2011; 34: 247–255.

84. Deutch, D.S., Katz, D.F., Overstreet, J.W. Increases in human sperm oxygen consumption at low cell concentrations. *Biology of Reproduction.* 1985; 32: 865–871.

85. Hoheisel, J.D. Microarray technology: beyond transcript profiling and genotype analysis. *Nature Reviews Genetics.* 2006; 7: 200–210.

86. Kramer, J.A., Krawetz, S.A. RNA in spermatozoa: implications for the alternative haploid genome. *Molecular Human Reproduction.* 1997; 3: 473–478.

87. Miller, D., Briggs, D., Snowden, H. *et al.* A complex population of RNAs exists in human ejaculate spermatozoa: implications for understanding molecular aspects of spermiogenesis. *Gene.* 1999; 237: 385–392.

88. Dix, D.J., Garges, J.B., Hong, R.L. Inhibition of hsp70–1 and hsp70–3 expression disrupts preimplantation embryogenesis and heightens embryo sensitivity to arsenic. *Molecular Reproduction and Development.* 1998; 51: 373–380.

89. Krawetz, S.A. Paternal contribution: new insights and future challenges. *Nature Reviews Genetics.* 2005; 6: 633–642.

90. Ostermeier, G.C., Dix, D.J., Miller, D. *et al.* Spermatozoal RNA profiles of normal fertile men. *Lancet.* 2002; 360: 772–777.

91. García-Herrero, S., Garrido, N., Martínez-Conejero, J.A. *et al.* Microarray analysis of infertile males in absence of abnormal sperm count reveals profound expression changes in spermatogenesis related gene products. *Abstracts of the 2nd International IVI Congress, Barcelona (Spain).* 2007.

92. García-Herrero, S., Meseguer, M., Martínez-Conejero, J.A. *et al.* Spermatogenic and testis related (str) genes "switched on/off" in fresh sperm from fertile donors vs. infertile patients. *Abstracts of the 33rd Annual Meeting of the American Society of Andrology, Alburquerque (USA).* 2007.

93. Martinez-Heredia, J., Estanyol, J.M., Ballesca, J.L. *et al.* Proteomic identification of human sperm proteins. *Proteomics.* 2006; 6: 4356–4369.

94. Pilch, B., Mann, M. Large-scale and high-confidence proteomic analysis of human seminal plasma. *Genome Biology.* 2006; 7: R40.

95. Pixton, K.L., Deeks, E.D., Flesch, F.M. *et al.* Sperm proteome mapping of a patient who experienced failed fertilization at IVF reveals altered expression of at least 20 proteins compared with fertile donors: case report. *Human Reproduction.* 2004; 19: 1438–1447.

96. Flesch, F.M., Gadella, B.M. Dynamics of the mammalian sperm plasma membrane in the process of fertilization. *Biochimica Biophysica Acta.* 2000; 1469: 197–235.

97. Kawano, N., Yoshida, K., Miyado, K. *et al.* Lipid rafts: keys to sperm maturation, fertilization, and early embryogenesis. *Journal of Lipids.* 2011; 264706.

98. Niu, D.M., Wang, J.J. Lipids in the sperm plasma membrane and their role in fertilization. *Zhonghua Nan Ke Xue.* 2009; 15: 651–655.

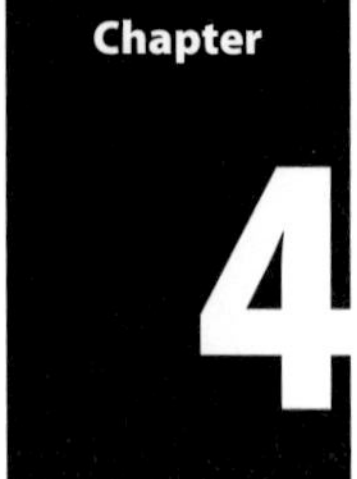

Chapter

4

In vitro production of functional sperm from neonatal mouse testes

Takehiko Ogawa

Introduction

Stem cells in the adult body are essential for the maintenance of tissues and organs. Spermatogonial stem cells (SSCs) enable continuous sperm production for almost the entire life of a male. Biological technologies and procedures for manipulating SSCs have progressed markedly over the last two decades. In particular, the in vitro manipulation of SSCs and their differentiation, namely in vitro spermatogenesis, recently became possible. These technological advances will contribute to a deeper understanding of the mechanism of spermatogenesis, and could be clinically applicable for male infertility in the future.

Development of spermatogonial transplantation technique

Historically, studies on SSCs were performed by morphological means to disclose their presence on the basement membrane inside the seminiferous tubules, and cell kinetics of SSCs and their daughter cells, including both undifferentiated and differentiating spermatogonia, were closely examined. Nonetheless, it has to be said that the nature of SSCs of mammals remained mysterious for a long time, because the exact identification of SSCs among other spermatogonia remained elusive. In 1994, a method to transplant SSCs from one mouse to another was developed to induce donor spermatogenesis in the testes of recipients [1]. This method, spermatogonial transplantation (SGT), modernized SSC research, because the functional evaluation of SSCs became possible. With SGT, it is feasible to enrich SSCs with a cell-separation technique like fluorescence-activated cell sorting (FACS). It was also shown that SSCs can be maintained in culture, at least for a while [2], and cryopreserved in

liquid nitrogen [3]. Besides, SGT allowed spermatogenesis of a certain species in xeno-recipients. A series of xeno-transplantation experiments showed that rat-to-mouse and reverse transplantation is possible to induce donor spermatogenesis in recipients [4,5]. In addition, the transplantation of hamster germ cells into mice was shown to work [6]. In other species, including humans as donors, however, when phylogenetic distances between the donor and recipient are larger than that mentioned above, the donor SSCs were observed to settle in the seminiferous tubules of recipient nude mice, but did not result in spermatogenesis [7].

SGT can also be used to treat infertility due to a spermatogenic defect. The spermatogenesis of a mutant sterile mouse was induced in a recipient mouse whose testicular microenvironment supported the donor SSCs' spermatogenesis, which never happened in the original testis [8].

In vitro multiplication of spermatogonial stem cells

As stated above, SGT was a revolutionary technique in the study of male germ-cell biology. The significance of SGT, however, might have not been well appreciated until it became possible to cultivate SSCs for multiplication in-vitro [9]. As SSCs can be identified only by their functional property, a functional assay system for SSCs was necessary before their manipulation became realistic. In this regard, SGT had to precede the culturing of SSCs. The culturing of stem cells of any origin is not easy. For instance, hematopoietic stem cells have yet to be propagated in-vitro, even though they are one of the most extensively studied stem cells. The culturing of SSCs remained reasonably difficult. In 2000, it was reported that GDNF was a key extrinsic factor for

Stem Cells in Reproductive Medicine 3rd edition, ed. Carlos Simón, Antonio Pellicer and Renee Reijo Pera.
Published by Cambridge University Press. © Cambridge University Press 2013.

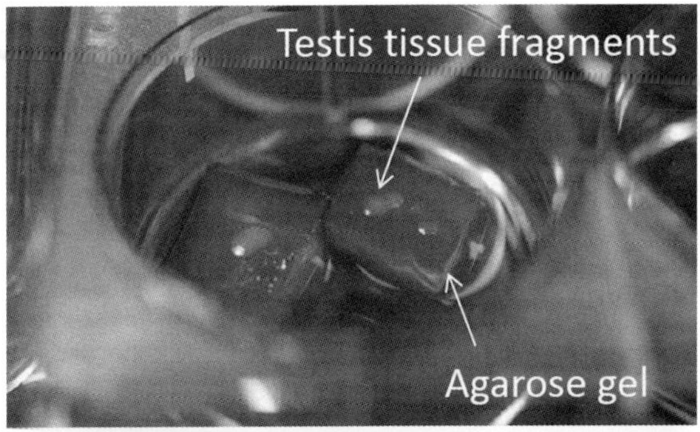

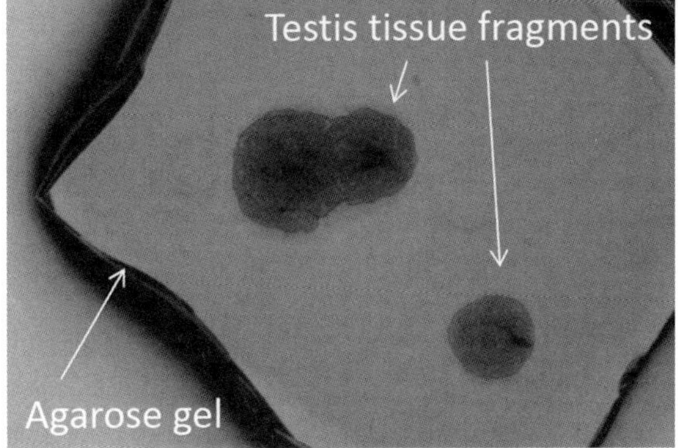

Figure 4.1 Testis tissue culture on agarose gel. (See also color plate.)

the propagation of SSCs [10]. Then, using GDNF and some other factors, a culture system that promotes in vitro propagation of SSCs was developed [9,11]. The SSCs propagated in vitro were named germline stem cells (GS cells) [9]. The GS cells increased their number in a logarithmic manner, while stably maintaining their genetic, karyotypic, and epigenetic characteristics. When GS cells were transplanted into a host testis, they settled in the seminiferous tubule to form colonies and initiated spermatogenesis, proving their identity as SSCs.

Facing the development of a culture system for SSCs, I thought it would soon become possible to develop an in vitro system of spermatogenesis using GS cells as experimental material, because a favorable amount of GS cells would be available for study. Even if the efficiency of in vitro spermatogenesis remained very low, sufficient numbers of GS cells as starting material could be harvested. Against such an optimistic prospect, spermatogenesis from GS cells in vitro did not show much progress. In our own experience, it appeared very difficult to induce meiosis from GS cells, let alone haploid production. These results made us

rethink the fact that in vivo spermatogenesis depends totally on the testicular microenvionment: complicated and not well clarified, but certainly orchestrated, support from testicular somatic cells. In particular, Sertoli cells were considered to play a pivotal role in spermatogenesis. Naturally, it appears that an organ culture method using a testis tissue fragment *en bloc* instead of a cell culture method would be a reasonable action to take first, even though it does not appear to be at the cutting edge of science.

Then, we embarked on a study of in vitro spermatogenesis by revisiting classic studies undertaken by Drs. Steinberger [12,13]. Our strategy was to repeat studies of testis tissue organ culture with a same gas–liquid interphase method [14]. Also, we tried to refine the method by adopting Miura's methods [15] and our own modifications. The final form of culturing is very simple and uses agarose gel, being half-soaked in the medium, on which small fragments of testis tissue are placed (Figure 4.1).

In vitro spermatogenesis with organ culture method

In order to make the evaluation of spermatogenesis simple and sensitive, we introduced two lines of transgenic mice (Tg) carrying GFP transgenes which are expressed in a meiosis- and haploid-specific manner. The germ cells of *Gsg2/Haspin*-GFP Tg express GFP strongly when they become round spermatids (haploids). Even though some weak expression of GFP starts at the end phase of meiosis in this Tg, the sharp and strong GFP expression is useful to identify the progress of in vitro spermatogenesis. The other Tg, *Acr*-GFP, shows GFP expression when germ cells have progressed into the mid-phase of meiosis. For further convenience, the GFP protein accumulates in the acrosome of the spermatids of *Acr*-GFP Tg, which could be a faithful marker of haploid production. These two Tg naturally do not express GFP when they are immature. The *Gsg2*-GFP starts expression around day 20 after birth, while *Acr*-GFP starts around day 15. Using immature testis tissues of these Tg, the culture experiment became facile, and evaluation can be made while leaving the culture experiment going.

Starting the experiment with these preparations, it soon appeared that cultured testis tissues expressed GFP at almost the same timing as in vivo. The optimal temperature for in vitro spermatogenesis was confirmed to be 34 °C. As for the culture media, alpha-MEM turned out the best among those tested. We also found that fetal bovine serum (FBS) was necessary for our culture system. With such optimal culture conditions, we observed the reliable induction of meiosis and occasional production of round spermatids [16]. However, we never found elongated spermatids or sperm, even in our best samples.

In the experiments until that time, we always added FBS to the media at 10% (v/v), because no sign of spermatogenesis developed without it. We tried to promote spermatogenesis further by incorporating additional factors, such as testosterone, FSH, and various growth factors, into the medium. However, none of those additional factors turned out to be beneficial, and we did not make any progress. It was thought that, although FBS is effective to induce spermatogenesis, it may have some adverse factors on spermatogenesis which, thus, inhibit the progression beyond the pachytene phase. We changed the strategy and abandoned FBS to adopt serum-free media. As the first step, we used commercially available serum replacements, including KSR. KSR is mostly used for the culture of ES and iPS cells to support their proliferation, while suppressing their differentiation. Thus, there is no reason to expect that KSR stimulates spermatogenesis. The addition of KSR to the culture media, however, surprisingly enhanced the expressions of both *Acr*- and *Gsg2*-GFP in our organ culture experiments. In addition, while the duration of these GFP expressions with FBS was about 1 month at the longest, it lasted for more than 2 months with KSR. Furthermore, KSR induced GFP expression even with testis tissues from neonates, 0.5 to 2.5 dpp, which was hardly accomplished with FBS.

Then, we examined whether those GFP expressions really reflected genuine meiosis and the production of haploid cells. Immunohistochemistry with antibodies to Sycp1 and Sycp3 demonstrated pachytene-specific chromosomal spreading in spermatocytes located at the center of seminiferous tubules. When *Acr*-GFP Tg tissues were used, we found GFP-expressing acrosomal cap structures on culture days 20 to 50, which were decisive markers of the production of round spermatids (haploids). In addition, we occasionally observed flagellated spermatids whose head was engulfed by Sertoli cells. Finally, even sperm were obtained.

We looked at Sertoli cells and checked their condition by immunostaining with antibody to the androgen receptor (AR). The Sertoli cells showed AR expression, which indicated their maturation during the cultivation. As the Sertoli cell is essential for spermatogenesis, its normal growth and maturation is necessary for proper spermatogenesis. Our culture system appeared to have supported both germ and somatic cell growth and differentiation.

Lastly, we tested the fertility of our in-vitro-produced sperm and spermatids by micro-insemination. With 23 round spermatids, we finally obtained 7 pups which grew normally to adults. On the other hand, with 35 sperms, 5 offspring were obtained, which also grew to healthy adults. When those progeny males and females were mated with each other, offspring were produced, which proved that all males and females were fertile. The probability of progeny production with micro-insemination was almost equivalent to using in-vivo-produced sperm or spermatids. Thus, it showed that the in-vitro-produced gametes with our organ culture method could be as normal as those produced in vivo [17].

In vitro transplantation and culture method (IVTC method)

We developed a new system of in vitro spermatogenesis with an organ culture technique. However, we were not really sure if the spermatogenesis started from SSCs. To address this question, we planned our next study. In fact, a goal we set initially in the study of in vitro spermatogenesis was to use GS cells as a starting sample. Then, we devised a new technique, which was a combination of SSC transplantation and organ culture. First, we transplanted mouse GS cells, which express GFP in a ubiquitous manner, into the seminiferous tubules of pup mice, either busulfan-treated wild-type or *W* mutant. These mice were chosen because they lack spermatogenic cells of their own; thus, they can provide donor cells with space for colonization. The host testes, having received donor cells, were removed from the recipient mouse and cut into pieces for culturing. The main concern then was whether the donor cells would settle in the niche as they do when the host testes are kept in the body of recipient mice. We observed the donor cell behavior closely over the course of culturing, and found that the donor cells showed signs of migration into their niche, namely on the basement membrane inside the seminiferous tubule, as early as several hours after transplantation.

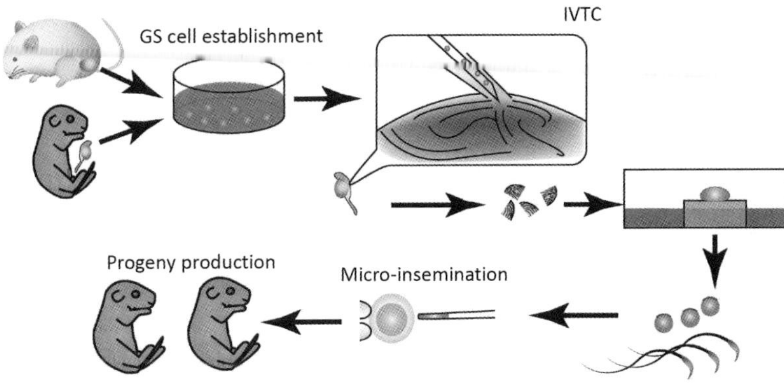

Figure 4.2 Experimental scheme of in-vitro transplantation and culture method. (See also color plate.)

In 3 days, the donor GS cells had finished migration and they were all on the peripheral inside, on the basement membrane, of the seminiferous tubules. Although these precise observations were not undertaken when the testis was in the body, their migration to niches in vitro must be comparable to what happens in vivo. The settled GS cells immediately started to proliferate to expand their colonies, which is also the same as in vivo. Naturally, spermatogenesis followed, and spermatocytes and even spermatids appeared. We finally found sperm, although not many, which were derived from GS cells. These haploid cells were applied for micro-insemination, and resulted in progeny production. These were healthy and grew normally and gave rise to the next generation by natural mating. Thus, our new experimental system, the in vitro transplantation and culture method (IVTC), induced GS cell differentiation up to sperm totally in vitro [18] (Figure 4.2).

Cryopreservation of SSCs and testis tissues

As cancer treatments have advanced, the number of cancer survivors is increasing. They undergo cyto-abrasive cancer treatments, namely chemo- and/or radiotherapies. Some survivors who are at or before reproductive age at the time of treatment may suffer toxic side effects of chemo- or radiotherapies on their gonads, resulting in permanent infertility. At present, one of the most promising measures to preserve their fertility is the cryopreservation of semen before these therapies. In fact, semen cryopreservation of young male cancer patients is becoming common in clinical practice.

On the other hand, in cases of pediatric cancer patients, semen cryopreservation is not applicable. Fertility protection or preservation of such pre-pubertal boys is as yet impractical. When the spermatogonial transplantation technique was introduced, people may have thought to cryopreserve SSCs from the immature testicles of patients. The cryopreserved SSCs of mice were actually shown to repopulate barren testes of recipients to restore them as reproductive [3]. This also seemed to work in a clinical setting. Namely, SSCs can be obtained from small fragmental testis tissues of pediatric cancer patients, taken by a biopsy procedure. The SSCs could be cryopreserved for later use, if patients survive the disease and grow to reproductive age. Thawed SSCs can be reintroduced into the original testis for recolonization and full spermatogenesis. However, this scenario not only includes several technical difficulties and invasive surgical measures, but also faces a serious risk of the possible reintroduction of malignant cells, especially when the disease is leukemia. To overcome this serious drawback, the most promising way would be the culturing of SSCs in vitro to select clones by which any other contaminated cells could be eliminated. Although this strategy may be practical in the future, the culturing of human SSCs is still at an experimental stage [19–21]. To make matters worse, the cloning of SSCs, even mouse SSCs, is very difficult. Under such circumstances, our organ culture method created a new possible scenario for the cryopreservation of the reproductive potential of pre-pubertal boys. We showed, using mouse testis tissues, that small fragments of testis tissues can be simply soaked in a cryo-protectant solution and placed in liquid nitrogen for preservation. The tissues resumed spermatogenesis after thawing. This method is simpler than the cryopreservation of SSCs. Most importantly, in vitro spermatogenesis circumvents the invasive procedure of cell transplantation, let alone the possible reintroduction of malignant cells to the patient when

SSCs are cryopreserved. These advantages are priceless when it comes to actual clinical application.

Conclusion (future of clinical applications)

In order to apply the new technologies described above to clinical settings, it is necessary to develop culture systems for human SSCs and human testis tissues.

It has taken 19 years since the appearance of mouse ES cells to develop a culture system for human ES cells. On the other hand, in the case of iPS cells, the gap between mouse and human was only one year. Progress in biological sciences is speeding up rapidly, but it is always difficult to predict the future. Culturing of mouse SSCs became possible in 2003. Thus, 8 years have already passed since then, but a culture system for human SSCs has yet to be faithfully established. In vitro human spermatogenesis, just after the development of mouse in vitro spermatogenesis, on the other hand, might be a focus for research interest. However, it may not be easy to achieve. In particular, the duration of spermatogenesis is longer in humans (64 days) than in mice (35 days). In addition, the human testis, as it undergoes a pre-pubertal period of many years, may need particular hormonal induction for spermatogenesis. Although these problems regarding human spermatogenesis in vitro seem tough to overcome, we believe it is possible, and it will bring about plenty of new discoveries concerning the unseen nature of human spermatogenesis.

Acknowledgment

The author thanks Takuya Sato for Figure 4.2 and his comments on the manuscript.

References

1. Brinster, R.L., Zimmermann, J.W. Spermatogenesis following male germ-cell transplantation. *Proceedings of the National Academy of Sciences of the United States of America*. 1994; 91: 11298–11302.

2. Nagano, M., Avarbock, M.R., Leonida, E.B., Brinster, C.J., Brinster, R.L. Culture of mouse spermatogonial stem cells. *Tissue Cell*. 1998; 30: 389–397.

3. Avobock, M.R., Avarbock, M.R., Brinster, C.J., Brinster, R.L. Reconstitution of spermatogenesis from frozen spermatogonial stem cells. *Nature Medicine*. 1996; 2: 693–696.

4. Clouthier, D.E., Avarbock, M.R., Maika, S.D., Hammer, R.E., Brinster, R.L. Rat spermatogenesis in mouse testis. *Nature*. 1996; 381: 418–421.

5. Ogawa, T., Dobrinski, I., Brinster, R.L. Recipient preparation is critical for spermatogonial transplantation in the rat. *Tissue Cell*. 1999; 31: 461–472.

6. Ogawa, T., Dobrinski, I., Avorbock, M.R., Brinster, R.L. Xenogeneic spermatogenesis following transplantation of hamster germ cells to mouse testes. *Biology of Reproduction*. 1999; 60: 515–521.

7. Nagano, M., Patrizio, P., Brinster, R.L. Long-term survival of human spermatogonial stem cells in mouse testes. *Fertility and Sterility*. 2002; 78: 1225–1233.

8. Ogawa, T., Dobrinski, I., Avarbock, M.R., Brinster, R.L. Transplantation of male germ line stem cells restores fertility in infertile mice. *Nature Medicine*. 2000; 6: 29–34.

9. Kanatsu-Shinohara, M., Ogonuki, N., Inoue, K. *et al*. Long-term proliferation in culture and germline transmission of mouse male germline stem cells. *Biology of Reproduction*. 2003; 69: 612–616.

10. Meng, X., Lindahl, M., Hyvönen, M.E. *et al*. Regulation of cell fate decision of undifferentiated spermatogonia by GDNF. *Science* 2000; 287: 1489–1493.

11. Kubota, H., Avarbock, M.R., Brinster, R.L. Growth factors essential for self-renewal and expansion of mouse spermatogonial stem cells. *Proceedings of the National Academy of Sciences of the United States of America*. 2004; 101: 16489–16494.

12. Steinberger, A., Steinberger, E. Tissue culture of male mammalian gonads. *In Vitro*. 1970; 5: 17–27.

13. Steinberger, A. In vitro technique for the study of spermatogenesis. *Methods in Enzymology*. 1975; 39: 283–296.

14. Trowell, O.A. The culture of mature organs in a synthetic medium. *Experimental Cell Research*. 1959; 16: 118–147.

15. Miura, T., Yamauchi, K., Takahashi, H., Nagahama, Y. Hormonal induction of all stages of spermatogenesis in vitro in the male Japanese eel (Anguilla japonica). *Proceedings of the National Academy of Sciences of the United States of America*. 1991; 88: 5774–5778.

16. Gohbara, A., Katagiri, K., Sato, T. *et al*. In vitro murine spermatogenesis in an organ culture system. *Biology of Reproduction*. 2010; 83: 261–267.

17. Sato, T., Katagiri, K., Gohbara, A. *et al*. In vitro production of functional sperm in cultured neonatal mouse testes. *Nature*. 2011; 471: 504–507.

18. Sato, T., Katagiri, K., Yokonishi, T. *et al.* In vitro production of fertile sperm from murine spermatogonial stem cell lines. *Nature Communications.* 2011; 2: 472.

19. Sadri-Ardekani, H., Mizrak, S.C., van Daalen, S.K. *et al.* Propagation of human spermatogonial stem cells in vitro. *Journal of the American Medical Association.* 2009; 302: 2127–2134.

20. He, Z., Kokkinaki, M., Jiang, J., Dobrinski, I., Dym, M. Isolation, characterization, and culture of human spermatogonia. *Biology of Reproduction.* 2010; 82: 363–372.

21. Sadri-Ardekani, H., Akhondi, M.A., van der Veen, F., Repping, S., van Pelt, A.M. In vitro propagation of human prepubertal spermatogonial stem cells. *Journal of the American Medical Association.* 2011; 305: 2416–2418.

Adult stem-cell population in the human testis

Ellen Goossens and Herman Tournaye

Introduction

The primary function of the mammalian testis is the production of both gametes and hormones over a reproductive lifespan. This production of gametes proceeds in the seminiferous tubules and is supported by a stem-cell population, the spermatogonial stem cells (SSC). Like other tissue-specific stem cells, SSCs are defined by their ability to balance between self-renewal and differentiation. This balance maintains the stem-cell pool and guarantees the daily production of spermatozoa from puberty onwards.

Maintaining the genetic integrity of spermatogonial stem cells is important in order to preserve the quality and function of the differentiated cells, but also to guarantee correct transmission of genetic information from one generation to the next.

Spermatogonial stem cells are thus essential for both the production of gametes and the continuation of the species. However, studying SSCs is difficult because they are very few in number (0.03% of all germ cells) and specific markers have not been identified so far. Most of our knowledge results from experiments in rodent models. Very little is known about human spermatogonial stem cells.

This chapter provides an update on SSCs, on their role in male fertility, and on (future) clinical applications using these fascinating cells.

SSC progenitors populate the testes during fetal development

Early in fetal development, the extra-embryonic ectoderm expresses bone morphogenetic protein 4 and bone morphogenetic protein 8b. These two growth factors are essential for the development of primordial germ cells (PGCs) [1]. In mice, a small cluster of PGCs is first observed one week post-coitum in the embryonal epiblast. Germ cells move, at a very early stage of embryonic life, through the primitive streak into the extra-embryonic region at the base of the allantois. In the 4th week, some cells present in the yolk sac, near the base of the allantois, differentiate into PGCs, which can be identified by their expression of alkaline phosphatase, OCT4, VASA, SSEA-1, EMA1, F9, and the tyrosine kinase receptor c-kit. In the 5th week, PGCs become embedded in the wall of the hindgut and migrate through the dorsal mesentery to reach the gonadal ridges [2]. This migration is orchestrated by a chemoattractive substance and does not require any activity of the PGCs itself. Because PGCs express the c-kit receptor, they are attracted by cells that produce soluble stem-cell factor. These stem-cell-factor-producing cells are located all along the migratory path [3]. During their journey, PGCs proliferate. By the time that the PGCs reach the gonadal ridges, their number has increased to approximately 3000 cells [4]. The germ cells colonizing the developing testes differ morphologically from the migratory PGCs and are therefore called gonocytes. These gonocytes become enclosed in testicular cords formed by Sertoli-cell precursors and peritubular myoid cells. Initially, gonocytes are located in the center of the testicular cords, away from the basal membrane. In rats and mice, gonocytes proliferate for a few days and then become quiescent in the G_0/G_1 phase of the cell cycle [5]. Shortly after birth, they migrate to the basement membrane and resume proliferation, giving rise to single type A (A_s) spermatogonia or spermatogonial stem cells (SSCs) [6].

In mice, Sertoli cells only express a soluble stem-cell factor until day 7 after birth. Between the 7th day and the 11th day, the Sertoli cells switch their production from a soluble into a membrane-bound stem-cell factor. This switch is accompanied by the start of spermatogonial stem-cell differentiation [7].

SSCs balance between self-renewal and differentiation

SSC proliferation is slightly different for non-primate and primate mammals. Since most of the research focuses on rodent spermatogenesis, both proliferation schemes are presented here.

In non-primate mammals, two models exist for stem-cell renewal and spermatogonial multiplication (the A_s model and the A_0/A_1 model), but the prevailing model is the A_s model, as proposed by Huckins and Oakberg in 1971 [8,9]. Spermatogenic proliferation and differentiation is accompanied by incomplete cell division, resulting in daughter cells, which remain interconnected by intercellular bridges. The A_s or single, undifferentiated type A spermatogonia are considered to be the most primitive cell or "true" spermatogonial stem cell. When A_s spermatogonia divide into two A_s cells, they usually migrate separately. If they remain connected to each other by cytoplasmic bridges, they become paired type A (A_{pr}) spermatogonia. The production of type A_{pr} spermatogonia is the first step towards differentiation. Normally, about one half of the spermatogonial stem cells divides to form A_{pr} spermatogonia, while the other half goes through self-renewing divisions, thereby maintaining the size of the spermatogonial stem-cell population. Type A_{pr} spermatogonia divide once more to produce groups of four aligned type A (A_{al}) spermatogonia, also connected to one another. The A_{al} cells proliferate resulting in chains of 8, 16, and occasionally 32 cells. A_s, A_{pr}, and A_{al} spermatogonia have the same morphology and can only be distinguished according to their topographical arrangement on the basement membrane of the seminiferous tubules. Most of the A_{al} spermatogonia will undergo a morphological change and transform into type A_1 spermatogonia. These A_1 spermatogonia are the first generation of differentiating A and B spermatogonia.

However, a revision of this A_s model might be necessary. Recently, it was found by several research groups that the A_s population and spermatogonial chains of the same length are heterogeneous in respect to their gene expression [10–12]. Using a transplantation assay, it was possible to demonstrate that

stem-cell activity is limited to the undifferentiated spermatogonia A_s, A_{pr}, and A_{al} [13]. Nevertheless, a few years later, it was demonstrated that the differentiating spermatogonia still have a weak potential to self-renew. In damaged testes, not only A_s spermatogonia have the capacity to self-renew. A_{pr} and A_{al} spermatogonia are able to revert to the A_s state and start spermatogenesis [14].

In primates, two morphologically different classes of type A spermatogonia are observed: the dark A_d (or "reserve" stem cells) and the pale A_p spermatogonia (or "renewing" stem cells), named after their staining intensity with hematoxylin. In general, there are equal numbers of A_d and A_p spermatogonia. A_p spermatogonia cycle continuously, whereas A_d spermatogonia normally do not divide. The self-renewal of the type A_p spermatogonia is analogous to that in the A_s model, because most of the A_p spermatogonia appear in clones of two, four, and eight cells, but single A_p cells also exist [15]. Furthermore, the A_d and A_p cells can transform into each other. A_d spermatogonia are often found in clusters. Such a cluster of A_d cells could be the result of a transformation of A_p into A_d at low renewal frequency. Conversely, after cytotoxic injury, the A_d may transform into A_p, which start to proliferate and form type B spermatogonia. In monkeys, there are four generations of B spermatogonia (B_1–B_4), whereas in humans, there is only one [16]. Spermatogenesis is initiated by two divisions of pairs or quadruplets of A_p cells: a first division, after which clones of A_p separate, and a second division, which leads to clones of B_1 spermatogonia, as well as pairs or quadruplets of A_p cells. These latter cells are responsible for the maintenance of the original size of the type A population. Because the A_p, which are found in clones of two or four cells, cycle continuously, the "true" stem cells are probably the rarely dividing single A_p and A_d spermatogonia [17] (Figure 5.1).

The identity of SSCs is becoming elucidated

Spermatogonial stem cells are single triangle-shaped cells, located on the basement membrane of the seminiferous tubules in close contact with the Sertoli cells. They have an ovoid nucleus with the nucleoli close to the nuclear membrane. The dense cytoplasm contains a small Golgi apparatus, a few mitochondria, and many free ribosomes. The population of SSCs is a small subpopulation of the spermatogonia.

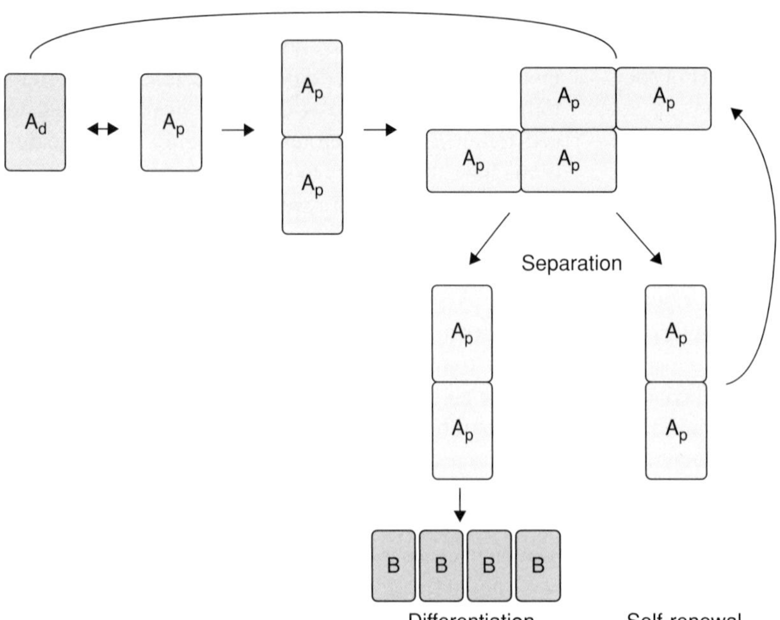

Figure 5.1 Schematic representation of the A_d/A_p model for primate spermatogonial differentiation. (See also color plate.)

A commonly used method to identify surface markers of SSCs is fluorescence-activated cell sorting in combination with SSC transplantation. This approach revealed that SSCs expressed β_1-integrin (CD29), α_6-integrin (CD49f), THY1 (CD90), CD9, GFRα1, and E-cadherin, but did not express α_v-integrin (CD51), MHC-I, C-KIT, and CD45 [18]. Although it is possible to highly enrich cell populations for SSCs using combinations of positive and negative markers (100- to 200-fold), a pure SSC suspension has not been obtained so far.

Because fluorescence-activated cell sorting is limited to the study of surface markers, other techniques have been employed to identify cytoplasmic and nuclear SSC markers. In mice, the expression of green fluorescent protein (GFP) under the promoter of OCT4 enabled the isolation and transplantation of OCT4-expressing germ cells from a heterogeneous suspension of testicular cells [13]. Cells expressing OCT4 (GFP$^+$) showed higher stem-cell activity compared with the OCT4$^-$ (GFP$^-$) cells [19]. Alternative approaches to reveal SSC-specific genes or proteins are transgenic, knock in or knock out mice. Using these models, the expression of glial-cell-line-derived neurotropic factor and its receptor, GFRα1, PLZF, SOX3, neurogenin 3, NANOS2, and STRA8 was determined in undifferentiated spermatogonia. Other genes that are expressed in spermatogonia, but not in somatic cells, are MAGE-A4, UBE1Y, USP9Y, RBMY, OTT, DDX4, TEX14, USP26, Piwil2, and Pramel1 [18]. Since transplantation experiments showed that only 11% of transplantable SSCs were neurogenin$^+$, the idea arose that the SSC population might be heterogeneous [14]. This heterogeneity among A_s spermatogonia was confirmed by a study using whole-mount immunohistochemistry. SALL4, which is important to maintain pluripotency in mouse embryonic stem cells, is specifically expressed in undifferentiated spermatogonia. While SALL4 expression mostly overlaps with PLZF, its co-expression with GFRα1 revealed heterogeneity in the SSC population. SALL4$^+$/GFRα1$^-$ and SALL4$^+$/GFRα1$^+$ populations could be identified, with GFRα1 expression being more limited (clones of 1–4 cells) than the expression of PLZF and SALL4 (also clones of 8 and 16 cells) [18].

Very recently, a new marker for rodent SSCs was proposed by Oatley *et al.* [12]. Inhibitor of DNA-binding 4 has the most restricted expression pattern observed to date. However, not all single spermatogonia express this marker, confirming the heterogeneity amongst the pool of single spermatogonia. The implications of this heterogeneity on SSC function remain to be elucidated. Although the phenotype of rodent SSCs is being unraveled, the search for markers limited to single A_s spermatogonia is still ongoing.

Table 5.1 Markers for human and rodent spermatogonia.

Marker	Human	Rodent
α_6-integrin (CD49f)	+	+
β_1-integrin (CD29)	–	+
GFRα1	+	+
STRA8	?	+
THY1	+	+
CD9	?	+
OCT4	+	–
SSEA-4	+	–
ID4	+	+
TSPY1	+	–
CD133	+	–

During the last few years a lot of progress has been made concerning the characterization of human SSCs. Human spermatogonia express many markers equivalent to those of rodent spermatogonia, e.g., α_6-integrin, GFRα1, and THY1. However, other markers are not shared. For example, human SSCs do not express β_1-integrin, but are positive for TSPY1, CD133, and SSEA-4 [20] (Table 5.1).

SSCs are housed in specialized niches

Spermatogonial stem cells can develop in three different ways: they can renew themselves, they can differentiate, or they can go into apoptosis. The mechanism determining which pathway will be followed is the subject of a great deal of investigation. The discovery of the germline stem-cell niche in *Drosophila* 12 years ago has accelerated the understanding of this regulatory system.

Niches are defined as specialized microenvironments regulating tissue homeostasis by controlling stem-cell self-renewal and differentiation. The SSC niche in the mammalian testis is located on the basal membrane of the seminiferous tubules and comprises Sertoli cells, Leydig cells, peritubular myoid cells, and extracellular matrix components. Each niche houses one stem cell, which is connected to the basement membrane through adhesion molecules (integrins). This close contact with the basement membrane allows the SSCs to respond to diffusing paracrine factors secreted by Leydig cells or myoid cells in the interstitial space. Sertoli cells have large contact areas with the germ cells through desmosome-gap junction complexes. Because these intercellular contacts are rarely seen on type A spermatogonia, Sertoli cells have to regulate spermatogonial proliferation by secreting paracrine factors. A key regulator of SSC self-renewal is glial-cell-line-derived neurotropic factor, which is secreted by Sertoli cells and acts on A_s, A_{pr}, and A_{al} spermatogonia through the RET/GFRα1 receptor complex [21] (Figure 5.2).

Sertoli cells are polarized columnar epithelial cells dividing the seminiferous tubule into a basal and an adluminal compartment. The basal compartment comprises mainly spermatogonia, while the adluminal compartment houses the more advanced germ cells. The two compartments are separated by tight junctions between Sertoli cells, the so-called blood–testis barrier. Germ cells have to cross the blood–testis barrier during germ-cell differentiation. The opening of the blood–testis barrier regulates germ-cell development by permitting the passage of preleptotene and leptotene spermatocytes. In this way, the differentiation process from leptotene spermatocytes up to mature sperm is separated from the systemic circulation. As such, Sertoli cells can supply developing germ cells with the necessary nutrients and establish an immune-privileged environment for haploid germ cells [22].

The influence of peritubular myoid cells on germ-cell regulation has long been questioned, but recent findings have led to growing interest in this still poorly-known cell type. Its role on SSC maintenance was suggested by the fact that colony-stimulating factor 1 was detected in Leydig cells and peritubular myoid cells, while its receptor is highly enriched in spermatogonia [23].

Based on the above-mentioned data, one might assume that all germ cells located at the basal membrane are SSCs. The truth is different. Only 0.3% of the spermatogonia are SSC. Stem-cell niches are not distributed randomly along the tubule, but are thought to be localized in areas near the vasculature, implying a regulatory function for specific factors transported through the blood or produced by the vascular endothelial cells [24].

Because Sertoli cells stop dividing after puberty, the number of SSC niches is invariable. So, the expansion of SSCs, which depends on the number of available niches, is limited too. In normal seminiferous epithelium, the ratio between self-renewal and differentiation should be about 1.0. More self-renewal than differentiation would reduce the seminiferous epithelium to only SSCs. Conversely, if there is more differentiation than self-renewal, the testis

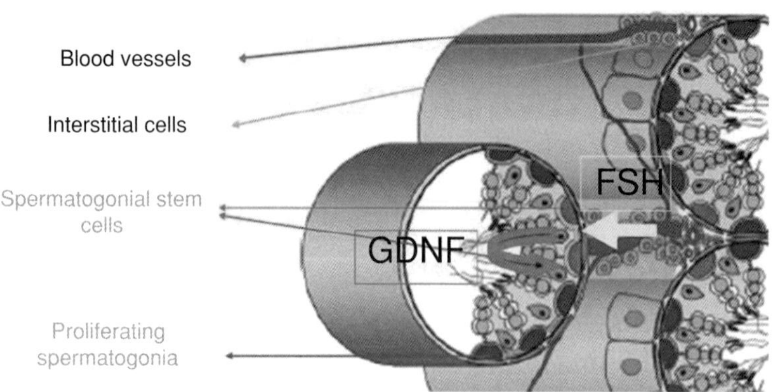

Figure 5.2 The spermatogonial stem-cell niche. Follicle-stimulating hormone is produced in the pituitary gland and is transported to the testes through the blood. FSH will bind to membrane receptors on Sertoli cells in close proximity to the interstitial tissue. Activation of the receptor will lead to the secretion of glial-cell-line-derived neurotropic factor. This factor binds to the GFRα1 receptor on SSCs and stimulates self-renewal. Sertoli cells located further away from the blood vessels will bind less FSH, resulting in a lower expression of glial-cell-line-derived neurotropic factor. SSCs in these areas are thus less stimulated to self-renew and will start differentiation. (See also color plate.)

would become depleted of SSCs. However, when the seminiferous epithelium is depleted by cytotoxic agents or irradiation, restoration of spermatogenesis must occur from stem cells. Although SSCs are less sensitive then differentiating spermatogonia, they still can be lost. In this situation, SSCs prefer self-renewal above differentiation, resulting in a much lower percentage of A_{pr} daughter cells than in the normal testis.

SSCs can survive, proliferate, and differentiate in vitro

In a first attempt to maintain SSCs in vitro, Nagano *et al.* cultured testicular cells on embryonic fibroblasts in a medium containing fetal bovine serum. This culture system allowed the survival of SSCs for 4 months [25]. The efficacy of SSC culture could be improved by enriching the cell suspension for SSCs or by using pup testicular cells [26]. The addition of glial-cell-line-derived neurotropic factor to the culture increased SSC self-renewal [21] and was a great step forward in the establishment of long-term mouse SSC culture systems [27]. Whereas fibroblast growth factor 2 was indispensable, feeder layers and serum could be omitted [28]. SSCs could survive for more than 6 months and expanded at least 1.4×10^{13}-fold from the initiation of culture to 149 days. The exclusion of feeder cells and serum is a remarkable leap forward in the establishment of any clinical application.

The culture of SSCs from other mammalian species has been reported too, but it was only very recently that human SSC culture was realized. Sadri-Ardekani *et al.* isolated and cultured testicular cells from six adult men and two pre-pubertal boys [29,30]. Frozen–thawed human SSCs could be proliferated in vitro in the presence of epidermal growth factor, glial-cell-line-derived neurotropic factor, and leukemia inhibitory factor without losing the expression of spermatogonial markers.

Several attempts have been reported on the differentiation of male germ cells in vitro, but none of these has resulted in a sufficient number of mature gametes. Culture systems using 3D matrices seem to be the most promising method for in vitro spermatogenesis, yielding morphologically normal spermatozoa from immature mouse germ cells [31]. Further research is required to reveal the applicability of this culture technique for human germ cells. In vitro tissue explants represent an alternative strategy to culture testicular cells. Functional spermatids and sperm could be produced from cryopreserved neonatal mouse testicular tissue in vitro in serum-free culture media [32].

Spermatogonial stem cells might be pluripotent

SSCs have long been considered to be unipotent with spermatogenesis as their only function, but this dogma has been challenged by new findings. Kanatsu-Shinohara *et al.* reported in vitro derivation of embryonic stem-cell-like cells from neonatal mouse testes. In their experiments, mouse embryonic stem-cell-like cells were shown to be phenotypically similar to mouse embryonic stem cells and to have the ability to differentiate in vitro into various types of somatic cells and to produce teratomas after injection into nude mice. Furthermore, these embryonic stem-cell-like cells formed germline chimeras when injected into blastocysts, proving their pluripotency [33]. Subsequently, the same was shown for adult mouse testes

[34]. Pluripotent adult germline stem cells contributed to the development of various organs after injection into blastocysts.

These results initiated a search for autologous pluripotent stem cells derived from human testis tissue for application in regenerative medicine. Several independent research groups have described the derivation of embryonic stem-cell-like cells from primary cultures of human testis [35–37]. Despite the use of different derivation methods, the cells formed colonies that morphologically resembled human embryonic stem-cell colonies. Being expanded under conditions for human embryonic stem cells, these cells expressed pluripotency-associated markers and could differentiate into multiple lineages in vitro. However, in only one of the four studies, these cells were able to form teratomas after injection into immunodeficient mice [35]. These findings resulted in a discussion about the pluripotency of these human testis-derived stem cells. Global gene expression analysis was used to compare germline stem cells, generated from adult human testis tissue, with human embryonic stem cells and human testicular fibroblasts. Surprisingly, human adult germline stem cells lacked some important characteristics of human embryonic stem cells and showed a similar gene expression profile to human testicular fibroblasts [38].

So, although pluripotent stem cells have been obtained from defined germline stem cells of mouse testis, this could not yet be accomplished using human testis cells.

Fertility restoration after SSC loss

Oncological diseases such as leukemia and Hodgkin's disease occur with an incidence of about 1 in 600 children before the age of 15 years. In recent years, remarkable progress has been made in the treatment of childhood cancers, and up to 75% of the patients can now be cured. At present, one in 1000 adults in the age group 20–30 years is a childhood cancer survivor [39]. Besides cancer, other diseases requiring gonadotoxic treatments (e.g., sickle cell disease) or genetic diseases (e.g., Klinefelter's syndrome, AZF deletions) may lead to spermatogonial stem-cell loss. It is unquestionable that prevention of sterility needs special attention in both oncology and reproductive medicine. The inability to genetically father his own children can have a high impact on the psychological well being of the patient in later adulthood. When an adult man

undergoes a gonadotoxic treatment, sperm is frozen in order to circumvent sterility after his treatment. However, no such prevention is possible before puberty since no active spermatogenesis is present. For young boys, the cryopreservation of spermatogonial stem cells followed by autologous intratesticular transplantation of these stem cells after cure is possibly the only option (Figure 5.3).

Protocols have been developed to cryopreserve SSCs

To safeguard the reproductive potential of young cancer patients, cryopreservation of testicular tissue containing SSCs is preferred above cryopreservation of SSC suspensions. Indeed, the presence of the extracellular matrix and supporting cells is critical to germ-cell survival and germ-cell function. Any cryopreservation protocol should thus aim at preserving both the stem cells and their niche cells. Undoubtedly, cryopreservation of testicular tissue is a challenging task. The complexity of the tissue architecture demands optimal conditions for each cell type. Controlled slow freezing with dimethylsulphoxide is routinely used to cryopreserve immature testicular tissue and has already led to the birth of healthy offspring in rodents [40]. Two freezing protocols have been reported for human testicular tissue [41,42]. Nevertheless, controlled slow freezing has a few drawbacks. There is the need for expensive computerized equipment and the freezing process consumes a lot of time and resources. Therefore, uncontrolled slow freezing has been explored. As with controlled freezing, uncontrolled freezing of prepubertal testicular tissue has been successfully used in different animal species, and has been fully validated in mice as a means to preserve the reproductive potential [43]. Recently, vitrification was shown to yield similar results compared to slow freezing [44]. Because both uncontrolled freezing and vitrification are inexpensive, convenient, and fast executable protocols, these methods might be considered for human testicular tissue too.

Spermatogonial stem-cell transplantation

The technique of spermatogonial stem-cell transplantation was first reported in 1994. It involves the introduction of a germ-cell suspension from a fertile donor testis into the seminiferous tubules of an infertile recipient mouse [45]. Transplanted

Before gonadotoxic treatment

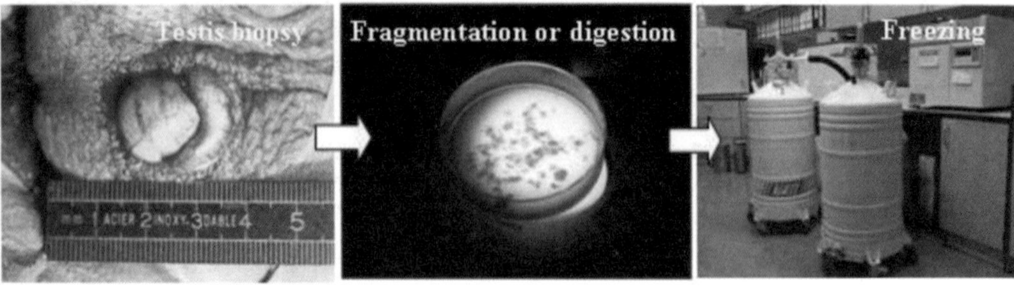

After cure

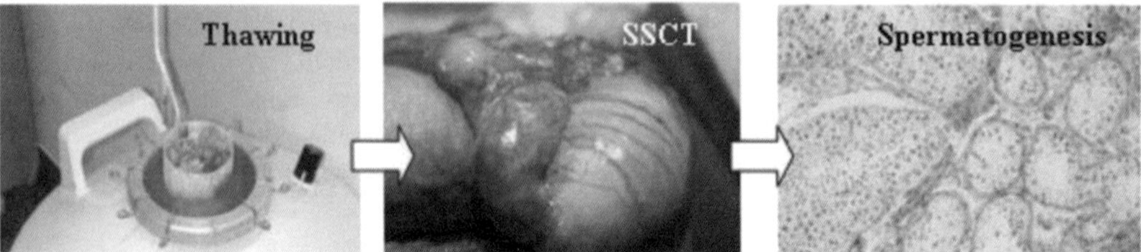

Figure 5.3 Spermatogonial stem-cell transplantation has been suggested as a method for fertility restoration after SSC loss. Before the onset of gonadotoxic treatment or before stem-cell loss occurs, testicular tissue is removed and cryopreserved. When the patient has been cured, or when the child's wish becomes apparent, the thawed tissue can be transplanted into the remaining testis. Although successful in rodents, in humans, the efficiency of spermatogonial stem-cell transplantation remains to be proven. (See also color plate.)

spermatogonial stem cells were able to relocate onto the basement membrane and colonize the tubules during the first month after transplantation. From that moment on, SSCs started to proliferate and initiate spermatogenesis. The first meiotic germ cells appear after 1 month and their number gradually increases thereafter. The recipient mice could reproduce in vivo after transplantation and produce transgenic offspring. Shortly after, this technology was performed in other mammalian species, including primates. Even the transplantation between different species with close phylogeny was proven successful (for a review, see [46]). These encouraging results, especially those from primate studies, suggest the possibility of banking and subsequently transplanting human spermatogonial stem cells to prevent sterility caused by SSC loss.

Before this application can be introduced in a clinical setting, it is important to evaluate the efficiency and safety of the procedure. In the mouse, we could show that sperm cells obtained after spermatogonial stem-cell transplantation were able to fertilize and produce normal embryos after assisted reproduction, although litter sizes were smaller compared to normal fertile control mice. A detailed analysis of the motility kinematics and concentrations of spermatozoa showed a lower sperm concentration and sperm motility after transplantation. In contrast, when donor and recipient were genetically related, the offspring showed normal genetic and epigenetic characteristics for most of the investigated modifications [47].

Testicular tissue grafting

Testicular tissue grafting has been suggested as an alternative to spermatogonial stem-cell transplantation. Testis tissue has been grafted under the back skin, in the scrotum, or in the testis. Full spermatogenesis could be obtained in grafts using immature testis tissue from different species. From the ectopic grafts, mature spermatozoa could be retrieved and used in ICSI, resulting in the birth of healthy live progeny [48]. Ectopic grafting was also performed using human testicular tissue. Adult testicular tissue showed only limited spermatogonial survival, with most of the tubules being completely regressed. Pre-pubertal and neonatal tissue, on the other hand, showed an acceptable spermatogonial survival rate and differentiation up to primary spermatocytes [49]. In an attempt to improve the results after grafting, immature testicular tissue was transplanted inside the testis. Long-term survival of spermatogonia and differentiation up to secondary spermatocytes was observed [50].

A comparison of intratesticular grafting and SSCT in a mouse model showed a better re-establishment of spermatogenesis after grafting. Cryopreservation of the grafts did not adversely affect the colonization efficiency and restoration of spermatogenesis [51]. Although intratesticular grafting seems to be more efficient, it can only be offered to patients with non-malignant diseases or non-metastasizing tumors. For patients suffering from blood or metastasizing tumors, the risk of reintroducing malignant cells would be substantial.

Contaminating malignant cells need to be removed

Many pediatric malignancies are capable of metastasizing through the blood, causing a potential risk of contamination of the collected testicular tissue. The transplantation of as few as 20 leukemic cells could cause malignant recurrence in rats [52]. In humans, the threshold number of malignant cells able to cause malignant relapse when transplanted to the testis is unknown. Therefore, it is of utter importance to detect even the slightest contamination of the testicular tissue. In case of contamination, the isolation of SSCs from malignant cells before transplantation is necessary. So far, the use of selection methods such as fluorescence-activated cell sorting and selective matrix adhesion has not been sufficiently efficient [53].

Potential applications of SSCs in cell therapy

SSCs as a source for regenerative medicine

Methods for stem-cell therapy based on embryonic stem cells or induced pluripotent stem cells have important disadvantages because of their tumorigenecity or ethical controversies. Transdifferentiation from (autologous) adult stem cells could be a more feasible and easier method. Moreover, compared to embryonic stem-cell-based research, there are less ethical constraints. SSCs share many molecular characteristics with embryonic stem cells, providing new and unique opportunities for the therapeutic use of SSCs for regenerative medicine. As the banking and transplantation of human SSCs may become a clinical routine for the preservation of male fertility in the future, there could be a clinical future for SSC-based therapies as well.

Studies in mice showed the potential of SSCs to generate tissues of all three germ layers (functional neurons, glia, cardiomyocytes, and other somatic cell types) without first converting into a less differentiated state [54]. We were able to transdifferentiate SSCs into hematopoietic cells in vivo. The donor-derived cells presented phenotypical and functional characteristics of hematopoietic cells in vitro and in vivo [55]. However, the mechanism of transdifferentiation is still unclear. Some researchers believe in cell reprogramming, others suggest that SSCs first become pluripotent before differentiating into another cell type.

SSCs at the basis of transgenerational therapy

Spermatogonial stem cells are the only stem cells in the human that can transmit parental genetic information to the offspring, making them an attractive target cell population for transgenerational gene therapy. Mouse SSCs have been successfully transfected with the use of a retroviral vector. The co-injection of retroviral particles and germ cells into recipient testes also resulted in incorporation of the reporter gene. It is now possible to transfect both adult and immature stem cells by retroviral-mediated gene delivery in vitro and in vivo by using a retrovirus vector [56,57].

Conclusive thoughts

Banking and transplantation of SSCs may become a promising method to preserve the fertility of pre-pubertal patients. According to recent discoveries, the potential of spermatogonial stem cells to become pluripotent or to transdifferentiate into other cell types is interesting and may create an additional role for spermatogonial stem cells as a source for stem-cell therapy. Nevertheless, the methods established in mice still need to be tested and adapted to human applications.

Acknowledgments

We are very grateful for the financial support received from Methusalem, the Fund for Scientific Research-Flanders (FWO-Vlaanderen, Belgium), the Flemish League against Cancer, the Research Council of the Vrije Universiteit Brussel, and the Research Council of the UZ Brussel. E.G. is a Postdoctoral Fellow of the FWO-Vlaanderen.

References

1. Ying, Y., Qi, X., Zhao, G.Q. Induction of primordial germ cells from murine epiblasts by synergistic action of BMP4 and BMP8B signalling pathways. *Proceedings of the National Academy of Sciences of the United States of America.* 2001; 98: 7858–7862.

2. Tam, P., Snow, M.H.L. Proliferation and migration of primordial germ cells during compensatory growth in the mouse embryo. *Journal of Embryology and Experimental Morphology.* 1981; 64: 133–147.

3. Fleischman, R.A. From white spots to stem cells: the role of Kit receptor in mammalian development. *Trends in Genetics.* 1993; 15: 205–206.

4. Bendel-Stenzel, M., Anderson, R., Heasman, J. *et al.* The origin and migration of primordial germ cells in the mouse. *Seminars in Cell and Developmental Biology.* 1998; 9: 393–400.

5. McLaren, A. Primordial germ cells in the mouse. *Developmental Biology.* 2003; 262: 1–15.

6. Vergouwen, R.P.F.A., Jacobs, S.G.P.M., Huiskamp, R. *et al.* Proliferative activity of interstitial cells, Sertoli cells and gonocytes during testicular development in the mouse. *Journal of Reproduction and Fertity.* 1991; 93: 233–243.

7. Manova, K., Huang, E.J., Angeles, M. *et al.* The expression pattern of the c-kit ligand in gonads of mice supports a role for the c-kit receptor in oocyte growth and in proliferation of spermatogonia. *Developmental Biology.* 1993; 157: 85–99.

8. Huckins, C. The spermatogonial stem cell population in adult rats. I. Their morphology, proliferation and maturation. *The Anatomical Record.* 1971; 169: 533–558.

9. Oakberg, E.F. Spermatogonial stem-cell renewal in the mouse. *The Anatomical Record.* 1971; 169: 515–532.

10. Suzuki, H., Sada, A., Yoshida, S. *et al.* The heterogeneity of spermatogonia is revealed by their topology and expression of marker proteins including the germ cell-specific proteins Nanos2 and Nanos3. *Developmental Biology.* 2009; 336: 222–231.

11. Zheng, K., Wu, X., Kaestner, K.H. *et al.* The pluripotency factor LIN28 marks undifferentiated spermatogonia in mouse. *BMC Developmental Biology.* 2009; 9: 38.

12. Oatley, M.J., Kaucher, A.V., Racicot, K.E. *et al.* Inhibitor of DNA binding 4 is expressed selectively by single spermatogonia in the male germline and regulates the self-renewal of spermatogonial stem cells in mice. *Biology of Reproduction.* 2011; 85: 347–356.

13. Ohbo, K., Yoshida, S., Ohmura, M. *et al.* Identification and characterization of stem cells in prepubertal spermatogenesis in mice. *Developmental Biology.* 2003; 258: 209–225.

14. Nakagawa, T., Nabeshima, Y., Yoshida, S. Functional identification of the actual and potential stem cell compartments in mouse spermatogenesis. *Developmental Cell.* 2007; 12: 195–206.

15. Clermont, Y., Hermo, L. Spermatogonial stem cells and their behavior in the seminiferous epithelium of rats and monkeys. In: Cairnie, A.B., Lala, P.K. and Osmond, D.G., eds. *Stem Cells of Renewing Cell Populations.* New York, NY: Academic Press. 1976; 273–286.

16. van Alphen, M.M.A., van de Kant, H.J.G., de Rooij, D.G. Depletion of the spermatogonia from the seminiferous epithelium of the Rhesus monkey after x-irradiation. *Radiation Research.* 1988; 113: 473–486.

17. Ehmcke, J., Simorangkir, D.R., Schlatt, S. Identification of the starting point for spermatogenesis and characterization of the testicular stem cell in adult male rhesus monkeys. *Human Reproduction.* 2005; 20: 1185–1193.

18. Phillips, B.T., Gassei, K., Orwig, K.E. Spermatogonial stem cell regulation and spermatogenesis. *Philosophical Transactions of the Royal Society of London B, Biological Science.* 2010; 365: 1663–1678.

19. Ohmura, M., Yoshida, S., Ide, Y. *et al.* Spatial analysis of germ stem cell development in Oct-4/EGFP transgenic mice. *Archives of Histology and Cytology.* 2004; 67: 285–296.

20. Dym, M., He, Z., Jiang, J. *et al.* Spermatogonial stem cells: unlimited potential. *Reproduction, Fertility and Development.* 2009; 21: 15–21.

21. Meng, X., Lindahl, M., Hyvönen, M.E. *et al.* Regulation of cell fate decision of undifferentiated spermatogonia by GDNF. *Science.* 2000; 287: 1489–1493.

22. Cheng, C.Y., Mruk, D.D. Cell junction dynamics in the testis: Sertoli-germ cell interactions and male contraceptive development. *Physiological Reviews.* 2002; 82: 825–874.

23. Oatley, J.M., Oatley, M.J., Avarbock, M.R. *et al.* Colony stimulating factor 1 is an extrinsic stimulator of mouse spermatogonial stem cell self-renewal. *Development.* 2009; 136: 1191–1199.

24. Yoshida, S., Sukeno, M., Nabeshima, Y. A vasculature-associated niche for undifferentiated spermatogonia in the mouse testis. *Science*. 2007; 317. 1722–1726.

25. Nagano, M., Avarbock, M.R., Leonida, E.B. *et al.* Culture of mouse spermatogonial stem cells. *Tissue and Cell*. 1998; 30: 389–397.

26. Nagano, M., Shinohara, T., Avarbock, M.R. *et al.* Retrovirus-mediated gene delivery into male germ line stem cells. *FEBS Letters*. 2000; 475: 7–10.

27. Kubota, H., Avarbock, M.R., Brinster, R.L. Growth factors essential for self-renewal and expansion of mouse spermatogonial stem cells. *Proceedings of the National Academy of Sciences of the United States of America*. 2004; 101: 16489–16494.

28. Kanatsu-Shinohara, M., Inoue, K., Ogonuki, N. *et al.* Serum- and feeder-free culture of mouse germline stem cells. *Biology of Reproduction*. 2011; 84: 97–105.

29. Sadri-Ardekani, H., Mizrak, S.C., van Daalen, S.K. *et al.* Propagation of human spermatogonial stem cells in vitro. *Journal of the American Medical Association*. 2009; 302: 2127–2134.

30. Sadri-Ardekani, H., Akhondi, M.A., van der Veen, F. *et al.* In vitro propagation of human prepubertal spermatogonial stem cells. *Journal of the American Medical Association*. 2011; 305: 2416–2418.

31. Stukenborg, J.B., Schlatt, S., Simoni, M. *et al.* New horizons for in vitro spermatogenesis? An update on novel three-dimensional culture systems as tools for meiotic and post-meiotic differentiation of testicular germ cells. *Molecular Human Reproduction*. 2009; 15: 521–529.

32. Sato, T., Katagiri, K., Gohbara, A. *et al.* In vitro production of functional sperm in cultured neonatal mouse testes. *Nature*. 2011; 471: 504–507.

33. Kanatsu-Shinohara, M., Inoue, K., Lee, J. *et al.* Generation of pluripotent stem cells from neonatal mouse testis. *Cell*. 2004; 119: 1001–1012.

34. Guan, K., Nayernia, K., Maier, L.S. *et al.* Pluripotency of spermatogonial stem cells from adult mouse testis. *Nature*. 2006; 440: 1199–1203.

35. Conrad, S., Renninger, M., Hennenlotter, J. *et al.* Generation of pluripotent stem cells from adult human testis. *Nature*. 2008; 456: 344–349.

36. Golestaneh, N., Kokkinaki, M., Pant, D. *et al.* Pluripotent stem cells derived from adult human testes. *Stem Cells and Development*. 2009; 18: 1115–1126.

37. Kossack, N., Meneses, J., Shefi, S. *et al.* Isolation and characterization of pluripotent human spermatogonial stem cell-derived cells. *Stem Cells*. 2009; 27: 138–149.

38. Ko, K., Araúzo-Bravo, M.J., Tapia, N. *et al.* Human adult germline stem cells in question. *Nature*. 2010; 24; 465: E1; discussion E3,

39. Hawkins, M.M., Stevens, M.C. The long-term survivors. *British Medical Bulletin*. 1996; 52: 898–923.

40. Shinohara, T., Inoue, K., Ogonuki, N. *et al.* Birth of offspring following transplantation of cryopreserved immature testicular pieces and in-vitro microinsemination. *Human Reproduction*. 2002; 17: 3039–3045.

41. Kvist, K., Thorup, J., Byskov, A.G. *et al.* Cryopreservation of intact testicular tissue from boys with cryptorchidism. *Human Reproduction*. 2006; 21: 484–491.

42. Keros, V., Hultenby, K., Borgström, B. *et al.* Methods of cryopreservation of testicular tissue with viable spermatogonia in pre-pubertal boys undergoing gonadotoxic cancer treatment. *Human Reproduction*. 2007; 22: 1384–1395.

43. Honaramooz, A., Snedaker, A., Boiani, M. *et al.* Sperm from neonatal mammalian testes grafted in mice. *Nature*. 2002; 418: 778–781.

44. Abrishami, M., Anzar, M., Yang, Y. *et al.* Cryopreservation of immature porcine testis tissue to maintain its developmental potential after xenografting into recipient mice. *Theriogenology*. 2010; 73: 86–96.

45. Brinster, R.L., Avarbock, M.R. Germline transmission of donor haplotype following spermatogonial transplantation. *Proceedings of the National Academy of Sciences of the United States of America*. 1994; 91: 11303–11307.

46. Hermann, B.P., Sukhwani, M., Hansel, M.C. *et al.* Spermatogonial stem cells in higher primates: are there differences from those in rodents? *Reproduction*. 2010; 139: 479–493.

47. Goossens, E., Tournaye, H. Fertility preservation in boys facing chemo-and radiotherapy. *Proceedings of the Belgian Royal Academies of Medicine*. 2012; 1: 1–18.

48. Schlatt, S., Honaramooz, A., Boiani, M. *et al.* Progeny from sperm obtained after ectopic grafting of neonatal mouse testes. *Biology of Reproduction*. 2003; 68: 2331–2335.

49. Sato, Y., Nozawa, S., Yoshiike, M. *et al.* Xenografting of testicular tissue from an infant human donor results in accelerated testicular maturation. *Human Reproduction*. 2010; 25: 1113–1122.

50. Van Saen, D., Goossens, E., Bourgain, C. *et al.* Meiotic activity in orthotopic xenografts derived from young adult human testicular tissue. *Human Reproduction*. 2011; 26: 282–293.

51. Van Saen, D., Goossens, E., De Block, G. *et al.* Regeneration of spermatogenesis by grafting testicular tissue or injecting testicular cells into the testes of sterile mice: a comparative study. *Fertility and Sterility.* 2009; 91(5 Suppl): 2264–2272.

52. Jahnukainen, K., Hou, M., Petersen, C. *et al.* Intratesticular transplantation of testicular cells from leukemic rats causes transmission of leukemia. *Cancer Research.* 2001; 61: 706–710.

53. Geens, M., Goossens, E., Tournaye, H. Cell selection by selective matrix adhesion is not sufficiently efficient for complete malignant cell depletion from contaminated human testicular cell suspensions. *Fertility and Sterility.* 2011; 95: 787–791.

54. Ning, L., Goossens, E., Van Saen, D. *et al.* Spermatogonial stem cells as a source for regenerative medicine. *Middle East Fertility Society Journal.* 2012; 17: 1–7.

55. Ning, L., Goossens, E., Geens, M. *et al.* Mouse spermatogonial stem cells obtain morphologic and functional characteristics of hematopoietic cells in vivo. *Human Reproduction.* 2010; 25: 3101–3109.

56. Nagano, M., Shinohara, T., Avarbock, M.R. *et al.* Retrovirus-mediated gene delivery into male germ line stem cells. *FEBS Letters.* 2000; 475: 7–10.

57. Kanatsu-Shinohara, M., Toyokuni, S., Shinohara, T. Transgenic mice produced by retroviral transduction of male germ line stem cells in vivo. *Biology of Reproduction.* 2004; 71: 1202–1207.

Meiotic recombination in human oocytes

Chapter 6

Jennifer R. Gruhn, Karl W. Broman, Patricia A. Hunt, and Terry J. Hassold

Meiosis is the specialized cell division that produces haploid gametes. Stripped to its basics, it involves one round of DNA synthesis followed by two cellular divisions. The first division (MI) is unique to meiocytes – it involves the segregation of homologous chromosomes, which reduces the number of chromosomes by one-half (i.e., in humans, from 46 to 23). The second division is analogous to a mitotic cell division and involves the segregation of sister chromatids.

The unique chromosome segregation that characterizes meiotic cell divisions depends upon complex chromosome dynamics and DNA repair mechanisms that occur during the protracted prophase stage that precedes the first cellular division. During prophase, homologous chromosome pairs find each other, align, and undergo an intimate association known as synapsis. At the same time, programmed double-strand breaks are introduced into the DNA and repaired. This repair process sets the stage for the segregation of homologous chromosomes at the first meiotic division because a subset of breaks is repaired by homologous recombination. These recombinational events become evident as physical sites of crossing-over, or chiasmata, when chromosomes condense in preparation for the first meiotic division. Importantly, the chiasmata anchor homologous chromosomes, facilitating their orientation and alignment on the first meiotic spindle, and thereby promoting proper segregation at the first meiotic division. Thus, recombination is critical for the production of genetically normal gametes.

We begin this chapter by reviewing the sexually dimorphic nature of meiosis in mammalian species, since many aspects of recombination depend on whether the gamete is proceeding through spermatogenesis or oogenesis. Next, we summarize our understanding of the recombination pathway and the proteins that are required to produce functional crossovers, outlining the basic steps that underlie this process. Finally, we focus on recombination in the human oocyte – how it is measured, how sites of recombination are chosen, and most importantly, what happens when the process goes awry.

Meiosis is a sexually dimorphic process

Although the basics of meiosis are shared by mammalian males and females, the details are remarkably different between the sexes. These include not only the time of onset, duration, and outcome of meiosis, but also the stringency of the control mechanisms and the propensity for errors that give rise to genetically abnormal gametes. In males, meiosis is a continuous process that commences at sexual maturation and generates millions of gametes per day during the entire adult lifespan. Stringent control mechanisms eliminate cells that are genetically damaged from errors occurring during either prophase or in the cell divisions; thus, under normal circumstances, human male meiosis yields relatively few aneuploid sperm. In contrast, female meiosis is a protracted process in mammalian species: oocytes complete prophase during fetal development, but the first meiotic division does not occur until just prior to ovulation in the adult ovary, and the second meiotic division occurs only if the ovulated egg is fertilized. Thus, depending on the species, female meiosis may take months, years or – as in humans – decades to complete. Further, in humans the process is remarkably error-prone, with an estimated 10–30% of all oocytes containing too many or too few chromosomes [1]. Recent data suggest that these errors are a reflection of differences in cell cycle control

Stem Cells in Reproductive Medicine 3rd edition, ed. Carlos Simón, Antonio Pellicer and Renee Reijo Pera.
Published by Cambridge University Press. © Cambridge University Press 2013.

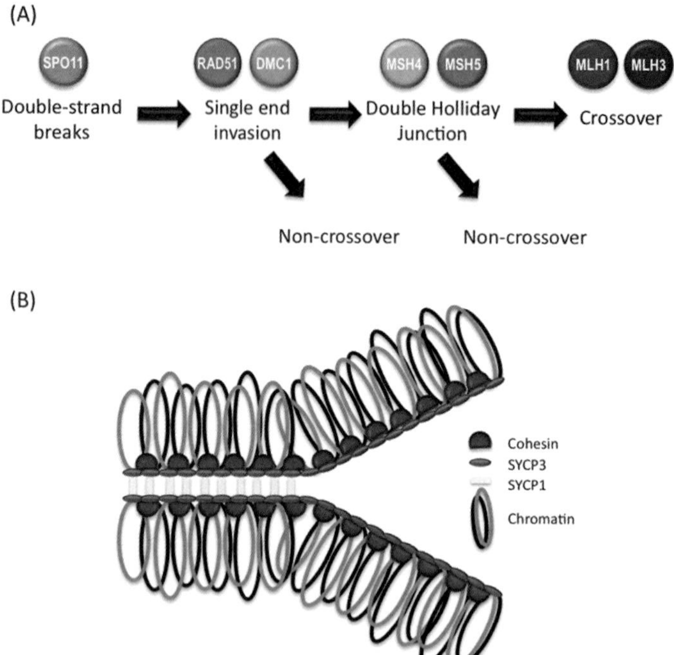

Figure 6.1 Recombination and synapsis: the defining events of meiotic prophase. (A) Overview of the main events and some of the major proteins involved in the class I meiotic recombination pathway. Meiotic recombination is initiated by the formation of programmed double-strand breaks (DSBs) by a complex of proteins, including the topoisomerase-like protein SPO11. The single-stranded DNA is then resected and single end invasion (SEI) is facilitated by the strand invasion proteins RAD51 and DMC1. This leads to formation of a D-loop and, following DNA synthesis and extension of the D-loop, an intermediate structure, a double Holliday junction (dHJ) is formed and is stabilized by the mismatch repair (MMR) proteins MSH4 and MSH5. The dHJ is resolved into a crossover by multiple proteins, including MMR proteins MLH1 and MLH3. Note that non-crossover products can also form from recombination events, either at an early step in the pathway or as an alternative mechanism of resolution of the dHJ. (B) The synaptonemal complex (SC). Meiotic recombination occurs in the context of the SC, a meiosis-specific structure that binds the homologous chromosomes to one another. Several of the protein components of the SC are now known, including SYCP3 (which contributes to the outer, axial elements of the SC) and SYCP1 (which localizes to the central region, and helps to "zipper" the homologous chromosomes together). Sister chromatid cohesion proteins (e.g., SMC1β, REC8, STAG3, and SMC3) form an initial meiotic scaffold and complex with the axial element proteins as part of the mature SC. (See also color plate.)

mechanisms that result in inefficiency in the culling of cells with errors. However, a constellation of other factors likely also contribute; e.g., events during prophase that predispose some chromosome pairs to segregation errors, the degradation of essential protein components during the period of protracted meiotic arrest, and age-associated or environmental effects that affect the complex process of oocyte growth that precedes ovulation (reviewed in [1]). In this chapter we focus on a critical and sometimes underappreciated aspect of human female meiosis, recombination and its association with aneuploidy.

The basics of recombination: how crossovers are made

Over the past two decades, studies of lower eukaryotes, especially *S. cerevisiae*, have led to a general understanding of the molecular events that result in the generation of meiotic crossovers (for reviews, see [2,3,4]). While the details vary among species, the basics are remarkably conserved and depend on interactions between at least three protein complexes – recombination machinery proteins, sister chromatid cohesions, and synaptonemal complex proteins.

The generation and processing of double-strand breaks (DSBs; Figure 6.1A) via the homologous recombination pathway is at the heart of the meiotic crossover pathway. In contrast to somatic tissues, where DNA damage is an unwanted challenge to normal cellular function, programmed DSBs are a crucial component of the meiotic process. The DSBs are generated by SPO11, a type II topoisomerase-like protein that typically yields many more DSBs than are converted into crossovers; e.g., in the human female several hundred DSBs are introduced in an oocyte, but fewer than 100 crossovers result [5]. The DSBs are then resected by nucleolytic degradation to yield long 3′ single-stranded overhangs. These are acted on by strand invasion proteins (e.g., DMC1, RAD51), allowing the single-stranded DNA to complex with the intact DNA strands from the homologous partner. The breaks can then be repaired by different mechanisms: they can be quickly repaired by the synthesis-dependent strand-annealing pathway, a process that yields only non-crossover products or, alternatively, they can be acted on by the double-strand break repair pathway. This latter pathway involves the generation of intermediate recombination structures (double Holliday junctions) that can be cut and religated in different ways, yielding either crossover or non-crossover products.

The generation and resolution of DSBs involves a number of proteins with crossover-promoting (e.g., MSH4, MSH5, MLH1, MLH3) or crossover-limiting (e.g., BLM) properties. However, optimal distribution and location of crossovers depends on protein complexes that are not part of the recombination pathway per se. The most important of these are proteins involved in the assembly of the meiotic scaffold called the synaptonemal complex (SC) that facilitates the synapsis of homologous chromosomes and plays a critical role in DSB repair (Figure 6.1B). During pre-meiotic S-phase, sister chromatid cohesin proteins are assembled on replicating DNA, providing not only the cohesion that tethers replicated sister chromatids and is a feature of replication in mitotic cells, but also providing an initial meiotic axis to which the DNA of the individual chromosomes is linked. The subsequent interaction of cohesins with the meiosis-specific components of the SC forms the outer, or axial, elements of the SC. As meiotic prophase proceeds, the axial elements of each homolog pair come into alignment with one another, and eventually are "zippered up" by the transverse filament, resulting in the intimate association (synapsis) of the homologs. In mammals, processing of DSBs occurs in the context of the SC, and any disturbances in its formation or maintenance have profound effects on crossing over. For example, female mice that are homozygous for null mutations in meiotic cohesins (e.g., *Smc1β* or *Rec8*) or genes encoding SC proteins (e.g., *Sycp3*) are characterized by reduced crossing over and by defects in chromosome segregation [6,7,8]. Thus, while recombination machinery proteins are directly responsible for

generating and processing DSBs, it is clear that the formation of functional exchanges depends on the orderly assembly of at least two other meiosis-specific protein complexes.

Measuring recombination

Because meiotic recombination occurs at prophase during fetal development in mammalian females, few investigations of human recombination have focused on this stage. Instead, most analyses of recombination have examined transmission of allelic variants through pedigrees or, more recently, comparison of haplotype blocks among individuals and populations. In this section we summarize the main attributes of the major genetic mapping techniques that have been applied to humans, three involving retrospective analyses of recombination, and two direct, cytological examinations of crossing-over-associated proteins or chiasmata in meiocytes (Table 6.1).

Retrospective analyses of recombination

Linkage analysis

Most data on human recombination come from conventional genetic linkage studies of families. The technique relies on analysis of the transmission of allelic variants, optimally involving multigeneration pedigrees, since this facilitates determinations of phase of alleles at adjacent loci. Early linkage analyses involved examination of enzyme or blood-group polymorphisms (e.g., [9,10]), and simply resulted in the identification of linkage groups (e.g., [11]). The introduction of genome-based technologies in the 1980s, however, made new classes of DNA polymorphisms available that allowed for the generation of chromosome-specific genetic maps. The first of these were relatively crude maps based on analysis of two or three allele restriction-fragment length polymorphisms [12], but subsequent identification of multiallelic minisatellites and microsatellites [13,14] led to the development of higher-resolution maps. More recently, these polymorphisms have been almost completely replaced by single nucleotide polymorphisms (SNPs), a class of variation involving single base-pair substitutions. At first glance, it might seem that SNPs are less useful than minisatellites or microsatellites, since they are two-allele polymorphic systems, while the latter are multiallelic systems.

Table 6.1 Approaches to measuring human meiotic recombination.

Method	Description	Pros	Cons
		Retrospective analysis:	
Linkage	Recombination determined by inheritance of allelic variants	– High resolution – DNA samples easily obtained	– Limited by number of progeny – Only one-half of all exchanges detectable – Two or more generations required
LD mapping	Recombination determined by variation in haplotype structure among individuals	– High resolution – DNA samples easily obtained – Only one generation required	– Cannot be used to create sex-specific maps
Centromere mapping	Recombination determined by changes from heterozygosity to homozygosity for alleles inherited from same parent	– Provides information on origin of non-disjunctional events	– Only applicable when offspring inherits more than one meiotic product from one parent (i.e., trisomy or triploidy)
		Cytological analysis:	
Immunofluorescence	Visualization of crossover-associated protein (e.g., MLH1) in pachytene stage meiocytes	– Allows direct visualization of crossover sites when first formed in prophase	– Gametic tissue difficult to obtain – Provides snapshot of recombination – Relatively low resolution
Diakinesis/MI	Visualization of chiasmata in diakinesis/MI meiocytes	– Allows direct visualization of chiasmata/crossover sites	– Gametic tissue difficult to obtain – Low resolution – Technically demanding

However, the sheer number of SNPs (i.e., in excess of 1 000 000 per genome) makes up for this deficiency and has made possible the generation of extremely high-resolution genetic maps [15], as described in the following section.

Conventional linkage analysis has a number of important strengths, including easy access to appropriate tissue samples (e.g., mouth swabs, hair samples, and peripheral blood or skin samples) and a virtually inexhaustible supply of DNA polymorphisms to examine. However, the approach also suffers from some notable limitations. For example, it is most efficient when three or more generations are available, allowing determination of the parental origin of recombination events. Furthermore, the relatively small number of children per human family limits the number of informative meioses per individual. Finally, because only two of the four chromatids in a bivalent are involved in a crossover, only one-half of all crossovers are detectable; therefore, computational methods must be employed to infer the other one-half of all crossover events.

Linkage disequilibrium (LD) mapping

Like conventional linkage studies, LD analysis provides a powerful tool for the generation of high-resolution genetic maps [16]. The two approaches, however, are markedly different. In LD mapping, the measured variable is the maintenance or change in allelic combinations at adjacent loci ("haplotypes"); i.e., the likelihood that specific combinations of alleles at nearby loci remain together more frequently than would be expected by chance alone. The extent of LD depends on multiple factors, but is largely a reflection of recombination – in general, high LD values are associated with tight linkage between loci, and lower levels or absence of LD, with the separation of allelic combinations through recombination. By studying haplotype structures of multiple individuals, the recombination landscapes of chromosome regions or whole chromosomes can be elucidated, and "hot" spots of recombination identified [16].

Importantly, LD mapping does not require analysis of multiple generations in a family. Rather it is a simple assessment of haplotype blocks among different individuals. With the recent development of large libraries of SNPs, LD studies have provided valuable genetic insight in two different types of studies. First, they have been used to examine variation in haplotype structure among different populations to study human evolution. Second, LD studies are a key component of genome-wide association studies (GWAS) to identify disease-associated genes (e.g., [17]). However, from the standpoint of understanding recombination, LD mapping has a major limitation – it simply documents the occurrence of past recombination events, but it is not able to determine the parental source of the event. Thus, while LD analysis can generate extremely high-resolution genetic maps, these reflect pooled data from oogenesis and spermatogenesis and provide no specific information on female recombination.

Centromere mapping

Centromere mapping applies one of the oldest approaches to the study of recombination – tetrad analysis – to humans. In many fungi (e.g., *Neurospora crassa*) all four products of meiosis (a "tetrad") are housed within a single sac, or ascus, making it possible to compare the genetic content among the gametes and to identify recombinant and non-recombinant meiotic products. Clearly, this situation does not apply to humans, since normally we receive only one meiotic product or gamete from each parent, with each gamete containing 23 chromosomes. However, in exceptional circumstances, a gamete may contain an extra chromosome, resulting in the production of a trisomic conception. In such situations it is possible to analyze the recombinational history of the two chromosomes inherited from the same parent. That is, by comparing DNA polymorphisms of the father, mother, and trisomic offspring, it is possible to specify the parent of origin of the extra chromosome. With this information, we can determine whether recombination occurred between the non-disjoined homologs and if so, the location of the exchange(s) [18,19,20,21,22,23]. As discussed in the final section of this chapter, this approach has been used widely over the past two decades to investigate the origin of trisomies in humans, and has provided valuable information on the relationship between altered recombination and meiotic non-disjunction in our species [24].

Cytological analysis

Recombination can be directly visualized in meiocytes using two different methods: by analyzing crossover-associated proteins in prophase cells or by analyzing chiasmata in cells preparing to undergo the first meiotic division. For studies of human female meiosis, both approaches are technically challenging. Studies of prophase cells require ovarian tissue from appropriately aged fetuses, and can only be accomplished using tissue from intentional terminations of pregnancy. Chiasmata analysis requires the fixation of adult oocytes undergoing the first meiotic division. Because this division is normally completed just prior to ovulation, these studies can only be conducted on oocytes that are meiotically matured in vitro, hence effectively restricting the analyses to oocytes obtained in the clinical setting for assisted reproduction. These limitations notwithstanding, both methods allow detection of crossovers in individual oocytes, information that is impossible to obtain using any of the retrospective analyses of recombination described above.

Analysis of crossover-associated proteins

Immunofluorescence technology provides a straightforward approach to the analysis of recombination events as they occur during pachytene of meiosis. This approach is based on the recognition that certain proteins, including the DNA mismatch repair proteins MLH1 and MLH3 [25,26] and the exonuclease Exo1 [26], localize to the sites of crossovers. MLH1 in particular has been intensively investigated, and there is now convincing evidence that it recognizes the vast majority of meiotic exchanges in pachytene stage cells of mice and humans [27,28]. By using appropriate antibodies (e.g., SYCP3) to identify the synaptonemal complex (SC), and antibodies against MLH1 to identify the exchange points on SCs, it becomes possible to examine the number and location of crossovers in the cell (Figure 6.2). Further, by combining this approach with fluorescence *in situ* hybridization (FISH) probes to specific chromosomes, detailed chromosome-specific exchange maps can be generated. The approach has a relatively modest resolution level of several megabases (Mb), much lower than the kb resolution afforded by retrospective analytic techniques, but is nevertheless much better than that associated with analyses of chiasmata in diakinesis/ MI preparations. Further, because hundreds, if not thousands, of prophase stage cells can be collected in fetal ovarian samples, it provides a sensitive approach to analyzing interindividual differences in the levels of meiotic recombination.

Analysis of chiasmata

The physical consequences of crossovers, chiasmata, can be analyzed in diakinesis/MI stage meiocytes, and this has been a useful tool in meiotic studies of human males [29]. In the human female, however, the first meiotic division resumes and is completed just prior to ovulation, and typically only a single oocyte

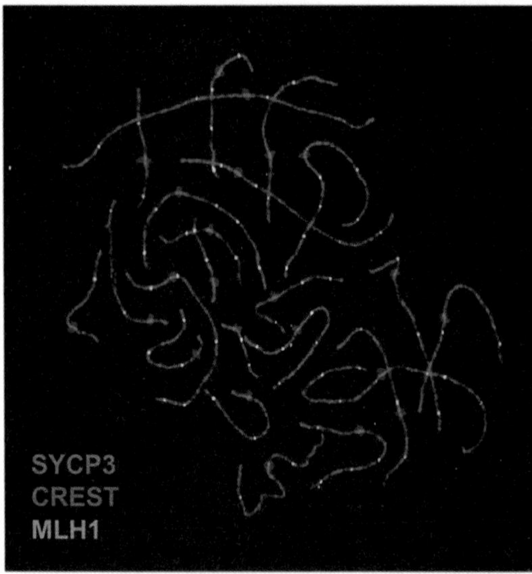

Figure 6.2 Representative image of a human pachytene stage oocyte. Antibodies against SYCP3 (in red) identify the synaptonemal complexes of the 23 pairs of homologs, antibodies against MLH1 (in green) the locations of crossovers, and CREST antisera (in blue) the centromeric regions. (See also color plate.)

reaches this stage per ovarian cycle. Consequently, few attempts have been made to acquire the appropriate tissue samples and, in the studies that have been conducted, poor quality of the preparations has precluded accurate determinations of the number of chiasmata per cell [30].

Recombination in the human female

While the different approaches to the analysis of recombination in humans and the pros and cons of each are discussed in detail above, in reality, only three have yielded useful data on human female recombination. In this section we summarize available information from two of the three, discussing data obtained from conventional linkage studies and studies of pachytene stage oocytes. In the following section we discuss the third approach, summarizing data on centromere mapping of human trisomies.

What we have learned from linkage studies

Because the first phase of the Human Genome Project involved the generation of a human genetic map [31], linkage analysis has been the primary source of data on human recombination. Due to the availability of several large family collections, to improvements in genotyping methodologies, and to the availability of

ever-increasing numbers of polymorphic loci (e.g., SNPs), information from linkage studies has increased remarkably over the past 20 years. Based on the data generated, several general features of human female recombination have emerged. For example, on average, there are 80–90 crossovers in a human oocyte. This translates to a female genome-wide genetic map of approximately 4000–4500 cM (Table 6.2), some 1.6-fold longer than that observed for the human male [15,16,32,33,34,35,36,37]. In general, each chromosome arm contains at least one exchange; the only exceptions are the short arms of acrocentric chromosomes, where exchanges are virtually absent. It is also clear that crossovers are placed non-randomly in the oocyte, with interstitial chromosomal locations predominating [35,37].

Beginning in the late 1990s, investigators extended their analyses of recombination to the analysis of interindividual variation. In an initial study, Broman and colleagues identified significant differences in genome-wide recombination levels among females from eight of the Centre d'Etude du Polymorphisme Humain (CEPH) families [35]. While the relatively small sample size limited this analysis, a subsequent study utilizing an expanded CEPH population confirmed the conclusions, finding significant interindividual variation in recombination among 34 women [37]. Similarly, Kong *et al.* identified highly significant differences in recombination rates in studies of 62 Icelandic mothers [38].

Subsequent studies have investigated the possibility of variation among racial groups as well as among women of different ages. Initially, racial differences were suggested by apparent variation in the maps generated using racially distinct populations [34,39]. This sparked interest in conducting a systematic analysis of different racial groups and, in 2005, Jorgenson and colleagues compared male and female linkage maps among Asian, Caucasian, and African American populations [33]. This study identified relatively "low," "medium," and "high" recombination rates in males and females of Asian, Caucasian, and African American populations, respectively [33], implying a genetic component in the control of the overall levels of recombination.

Other investigators have analyzed variation in recombination levels in oocytes from women of different ages, providing data to test the validity of the "production line" model of maternal age and aneuploidy. In 1968, Henderson and Edwards postulated

Table 6.2 Estimates of genome-wide levels of recombination in human females.

Method of analysis	No. meioses	Mean no. MLH1 foci	Genetic length (cM)	Reference
MLH1 foci:	3	95.0 ± 12.3	4750	[65]
	95	70.3 ± 10.5	3515	[50]
	c. 250	50.3 ± 24.7	2515	[5]
	1035	69.3 ± 14.3	3465	[28]
Genetic linkage:	–	–	4967	[66]
	–	–	4435	[35]
	–	–	4460	[38]
	–	–	4415	[67]
	–	–	4600	[39]
	–	–	4415 (African American)	[33]
	–	–	4320 (Caucasian)	
	–	–	4306 (Asian)	
	–	–	3840	[37]
	–	–	4596	[32]
	–	–	3960	[16]
	–	–	3906	[34]
	–	–	4110	[42]
	–	–	3790	[15]
	–	–	4170	[36]

that oocytes ovulated later in life have lower genome-wide recombination rates, thus contributing to higher meiotic error rates with increasing maternal age [40]. Studies comparing maternal age at the time of birth and recombination rates in offspring now have been conducted in multiple populations, but a consistent correlation between older mothers and offspring with lower recombination rates has not been found [35,36]. Thus, the production line model does not appear to explain the link between increasing maternal age and aneuploidy.

In addition to characterizing the patterns of recombination among individuals and different populations, recent studies have focused on identification of loci important in "setting" the levels of recombination events. To date, only two such loci have been identified by more than one group of investigators – a small, 900 kb inversion on chromosome 17 and the gene encoding the ring finger protein *RNF212*. The effect of the inversion (at 17q21.31) was first reported by Stefansson *et al.* in 2005 [41] and subsequently confirmed by others [42,43]. In the initial report, Stefansson *et al.* [41] noted a slight increase in fecundity and an approximate 1% increase in recombination per copy of the inversion; i.e., by comparison with non-carriers, inversion heterozygotes had a 1% increase in global recombination rates and inversion homozygotes a 2% increase. Intriguingly, the frequency of the inversion varies among populations, being relatively common in Europeans, rare in Africans, and virtually absent in East Asians. Thus, the importance of the inversion to variation in recombination may well be group-specific. Further, its impact is likely restricted to oogenesis, since there is no evidence that the presence or absence of the inversion influences male recombination rates.

In a subsequent analysis, Kong and colleagues [44] published the first report linking a specific gene to recombination rates, as genetic-mapping data from an Icelandic population correlated allelic differences at *RNF212* to variation in genome-wide recombination levels. Specifically, overall rates of recombination changed by approximately 3–4%, depending on the genotype at SNPs associated with *RNF212*. Intriguingly, the genotypic effects on recombination operated differently in males and females; i.e., SNP haplotypes associated with high levels of recombination in females were associated with low levels in males, and vice versa. The mechanism by which *RNF212* affects recombination levels is unclear. It is a putative ortholog of the *C. elegans ZHP-3* gene, known to be crucial for recombination in that species, but its function in human recombination is not yet known. Nevertheless, two subsequent studies [42,43] have confirmed the observations of Kong *et al.* [44], verifying the importance of *RNF212* in the regulation of genome-wide recombination rates in humans.

While the above genes have been linked to variation in genome-wide recombination levels, a third gene – encoding the zinc finger protein PRDM9 – has been intensively studied for its association with recombination hot spots; i.e., narrow genomic regions where recombination occurs at much higher than expected rates. PRDM9 is a histone methyltransferase that is responsible for trimethylation of histone H3K4, a so-called "permissive" chromatin mark that is associated with recombination hotspots in both mice and humans [45,46,47,48]. *PRDM9* is highly polymorphic, especially in its zinc finger arrays, and this variation has been linked to differences in hotspot utilization between the sexes and among populations of different ethnicity [15]. However, intriguingly, while there is a clear connection between *PRDM9* polymorphisms and hotspot activity, no such link has been demonstrated for overall levels of recombination. Thus, unlike *RNF212* and the chromosome 17 inversion discussed above, variation in *PRDM9* appears to affect the location, but not the overall number, of crossovers.

Watching recombination as it happens: cytological studies of pachytene oocytes

Early cytological studies of human female meiosis were hampered by difficulties in acquisition of the fetal ovarian material but, perhaps more importantly, by the lack of appropriate imaging methodologies with which to examine the material. Fortunately, with improvements in immunostaining techniques and the increasing availability of antibodies capable of detecting meiosis-acting proteins, it has now become possible to analyze the processes of pairing, synapsis, and recombination in human fetal oocytes. In pioneering studies conducted in the 1990s, Hulten and her colleagues analyzed a small series of pachytene-stage

oocytes, and demonstrated overall levels of recombination similar to those inferred by genetic linkage studies [49]. Subsequently, a number of groups have applied this approach to analyze larger series of fetal ovarian samples [5,28,50,51]. Several basic principles have emerged from these analyses.

Importantly, the general features of recombination that have been elucidated by genetic linkage analyses have been replicated by the analysis of MLH1, the cytological marker most often employed to identify exchange events in pachytene-stage cells. For example, similar to observations from linkage studies, chromosome arms typically contain at least one MLH1 focus, with a relative paucity of foci located near the telomeres or centromeres. Further, on chromosomes containing two or more MLH1 foci, the foci are widely spaced from one another; i.e., they display interference, a well-known property of meiosis that has previously been observed in linkage studies. Finally, in the study with the largest sample size, the mean number of MLH1 foci per cell was approximately 65–75, similar to, although slightly lower than, the value of 80–85 crossovers per cell predicted from linkage studies [28]. The reason for this difference is not clear, but may reflect the dynamic nature of recombination in human female meiosis. That is, based on analysis of oocytes at different stages of prophase, it appears that recombination events may resolve as crossovers at some sites before the process is completed at other sites [28]. Thus, examination of the number of MLH1 foci may just provide a snapshot of exchanges at a specific time in prophase, missing those sites where recombination has already been completed or those that have not yet reached the stage of DNA repair where MLH1 is detectable.

In addition, the cytological approach has yielded several new insights concerning human female recombination. For example, the number of meiotic events per fetal sample has made it possible to assess intra- and interindividual variation in crossover number and the results have been striking. In contrast to the situation for human males, in which the number of MLH1 foci appears to be tightly regulated [52], there is a remarkable range in the number of crossovers per oocyte [28]. For some individuals, the number of MLH1 foci per oocyte ranges from a low of approximately 50 to a high in excess of 100, and the same situation applies to interindividual variation, with mean MLH1 values ranging from 53 to 88 [28]. Thus, despite the importance of recombination to normal meiotic chromosome segregation, the overall number of exchanges per cell is extraordinarily variable in the human female. Further, the number of cells in which one or more homologs lack an MLH1 focus – i.e., an exchangeless bivalent – is also remarkably high in females. Indeed, in analyses of six representative medium and small chromosomes, Cheng and colleagues suggested that as many 10% of cells might contain at least one such exchangeless homologous pair [28]. Since such chromosomes are expected to non-disjoin 50% of the time, this suggests that at least 5% of all oocytes are pre-destined to mis-segregate because of recombination errors in meiotic prophase. This is perhaps not unexpected since, as discussed in the following section, retrospective centromere mapping studies of human trisomies have also implicated errors in recombination in the genesis of maternal meiotic non-disjunction.

Recombination and non-disjunction

Beginning about two decades ago, human geneticists initiated a series of studies to understand the relationship between recombination and human trisomies. Because the vast majority of human trisomies are attributable to errors in oogenesis, most studies have focused on maternally derived cases. The results have been striking, as all trisomic conditions that have been appropriately studied have been linked to altered recombination. However, as detailed below and as summarized in Table 6.3, the effects vary remarkably among the different chromosomes.

Initial studies of recombination and human non-disjunction focused on trisomy 21, clinically the most important of all human chromosome abnormalities. Following an initial study in 1987 [53], several groups demonstrated that absence of recombination between the homologous chromosomes 21 was an important contributor to non-disjunction (e.g., [54,55,56]). Indeed, from the most extensive data set, Sherman and colleagues estimated that over 40% of maternal MI-derived cases involve failure to cross over [55,57,58]. However, other crossover configurations were also linked to trisomy 21: some cases of maternal meiosis I origin apparently involve meioses with single, distally placed crossovers, while cases scored as arising at maternal meiosis II are frequently associated with extremely proximal crossovers [57].

Table 6.3 Recombination and maternal meiotic non-disjunction: chromosome-specific differences in the effects of altered recombination (data from [18,20,22,68]).

Trisomy	Association with number or location of exchanges
13	Estimated 25–33% of cases involve "achiasmate" (exchangeless) chromosomes
15	Estimated 20% involve achiasmate chromosomes
16	Increase in distally located exchanges; no evidence for achiasmate chromosomes
18	Estimated 30% of cases involve achiasmate chromosomes
21	Estimated 40% of cases involve achiasmate chromosomes; extremely proximal or distal exchanges associated with majority of other cases
22	Estimated 25% of cases involve achiasmate chromosomes
XXX/XXY	Estimated 30% of cases involve achiasmate chromosomes; another 10% of cases associated with pericentromeric exchanges

Thus, failure to cross over or suboptimally located exchanges appear to be important in the genesis of the vast majority of cases of trisomy 21 [57].

Studies of model organisms also provide evidence that alterations in the level or location of the sites of recombination can affect the likelihood of non-disjunction at the first meiotic division. For example, studies of mutations in genes encoding meiotic recombination proteins [59,60], of artificial chromosomes in which crossing-over is abolished or disturbed [61,62], or of spontaneous non-disjunction events [63,64] indicate that failure to cross over or crossovers located too close to the centromere or telomere increase MI non-disjunction levels.

By comparison with trisomy 21, much less information is available for other human trisomies, but alterations in recombination have been linked to the origin of these conditions as well. The most common correlate has been failure of recombination, which has been observed in cases of trisomies 13, 15, 18, and sex chromosome trisomies 22 [18,19,20,21,22,23]. However, curiously, this association does not extend to the most commonly occurring human trisomy – +16 – for which distally placed crossovers appear to be the most important contributor. Finally, while failure to recombine is important in the genesis of sex chromosome trisomies, approximately 10% of these cases have been ascribed to another unusual class of crossover in which the exchange(s) appears to occur at or near the centromere [23].

Taken together, these studies indicate that – in both humans and model organisms – alterations in recombination are an important component of meiotic non-disjunction. Thus, in humans, events that occur in the fetal ovary may predispose to non-disjunction many years later, when the oocyte is ovulated and completes the first meiotic division. This raises an obvious question: how does altered recombination correlate with the only other known risk factor for human trisomy, namely advancing maternal age? The simple answer is that we do not yet know but, from studies of trisomy 21, it is clear that the relationship is complex. For example, Sherman and colleagues [58] found no obvious age-related difference in the proportion of cases with single, distally located crossovers, suggesting that this configuration confers a similar susceptibility over all age groups. However, the proportion of cases with "crossover-less" chromosomes was increased in women 35 years and older by comparison with those 29–34 years of age, suggesting an age-related decline in the ability to properly segregate such chromosomes. Similarly, the likelihood of extremely proximal exchanges in cases of apparent MII origin was increased in the oldest age group, suggesting an interaction between recombination abnormalities and maternal-age-related risk factors.

These observations are consistent with smaller data sets from other trisomies, in which the relative importance to non-disjunction of some (e.g., [19]) but not other [18,22] susceptible crossover configurations appears to change with maternal age. These results reinforce an emerging view of the genesis of human trisomies: there are likely multiple routes to non-disjunction, some maternal age-independent and others age-dependent, some involving recombination errors and others in which recombination is irrelevant, and with the relative importance of the different mechanisms varying among individual chromosomes. Thus, it seems likely that an understanding of the underlying causes of human non-disjunction will only be accomplished by investigations of individual chromosomes.

Summary

The importance of homologous recombination to normal meiotic progression has long been recognized, but as recently as 1990 we had little understanding of how it worked in human oocytes – we knew virtually nothing about the number or chromosomal locations of exchanges, the potential effects of alterations in recombination on meiotic chromosome segregation, or the possible influence of genetic or environmental factors on recombination patterns. Much has changed since then. Advances in mapping methodology have led to the generation of high-resolution male and female genetic maps; it is now clear that errors in recombination are important contributors to most, if not all, human trisomies, and a small number of recombination-associated loci have now been identified. Clearly, much work is left, but we finally have a rough outline of the process to guide us in our future studies.

References

1. Nagaoka, S., Hassold, T., Hunt, P. Human aneuploidy: mechanisms and new insights to an age old problem. *Nature Reviews Genetics*. 2012; 13(7): 493–504.

2. Baudat, F., de Massy, B. Regulating double-stranded DNA break repair towards crossover or non-crossover during mammalian meiosis. *Chromosome Research*. 2007; 15(5): 565–577.

3. Longhese, M.P., Bonetti, D., Guerini, I., Manfrini, N., Clerici, M. DNA double-strand breaks in meiosis: checking their formation, processing and repair. *DNA Repair (Amsterdam)*. 2009; 8(9): 1127–1138.

4. Szekvolgyi, L., Nicolas, A. From meiosis to postmeiotic events: homologous recombination is obligatory but flexible. *FEBS Journal*. 2009; 277(3): 571–589.

5. Lenzi, M.L., Smith, J., Snowden, T. *et al.* Extreme heterogeneity in the molecular events leading to the establishment of chiasmata during meiosis I in human oocytes. *American Journal of Human Genetics*. 2005; 76(1): 112–127.

6. Revenkova, E., Eijpe, M., Heyting, C. *et al.* Cohesin SMC1 beta is required for meiotic chromosome dynamics, sister chromatid cohesion and DNA recombination. *Nature Cell Biology*. 2004; 6(6): 555–562.

7. Xu, H., Beasley, M.D., Warren, W.D., van der Horst, G.T., McKay, M.J. Absence of mouse REC8 cohesin promotes synapsis of sister chromatids in meiosis. *Developmental Cell*. 2005; 8(6): 949–961.

8. Yuan, L., Liu, J.G., Hoja, M.R. *et al.* Female germ cell aneuploidy and embryo death in mice lacking the meiosis-specific protein SCP3. *Science*. 2002; 296(5570): 1115–1118.

9. Race, R.R., Sanger, R. *Blood Groups in Man*, 6th edn. Chichester: Blackwell Science Ltd. 1975.

10. Harris, H. Enzyme polymorphisms in man. *Proceedings of the Royal Society of London B, Biological Science.* 1966; 164(995): 298–310.

11. Westerveld, A., Jongsma, A.P., Meera Khan, P., van Someren, H., Bootsma, D. Assignment of the AK1: Np: ABO linkage group to human chromosome 9. *Proceedings of the National Academy of Sciences of the United States of America.* 1976; 73(3): 895–899.

12. Hassold, T., Kumlin, E., Takaesu, N., Leppert, M. Use of restriction fragment length polymorphisms to study the origin of human aneuploidy. *Annals of the New York Academy of Science.* 1985; 450: 179–189.

13. Jeffreys, A.J., Wilson, V., Thein, S.L. Hypervariable 'minisatellite' regions in human DNA. *Nature.* 1985; 314(6006): 67–73.

14. Weber, J.L. Human DNA polymorphisms and methods of analysis. *Current Opinion in Biotechnology.* 1990; 1(2): 166–171.

15. Kong, A., Thorleifsson, G., Gudbjartsson, D.F. *et al.* Fine-scale recombination rate differences between sexes, populations and individuals. *Nature.* 2010; 467(7319): 1099–1103.

16. Coop, G., Wen, X., Ober, C., Pritchard, J.K., Przeworski, M. High-resolution mapping of crossovers reveals extensive variation in fine-scale recombination patterns among humans. *Science.* 2008; 319(5868): 1395–1398.

17. Rosenberg, N.A., Huang, L., Jewett, E.M. *et al.* Genome-wide association studies in diverse populations. *Nature Reviews Genetics.* 2010; 11(5): 356–366.

18. Hall, H.E., Chan, E.R., Collins, A. *et al.* The origin of trisomy 13. *American Journal of Medical Genetics A.* 2007; 143A(19): 2242–2248.

19. Robinson, W.P., Kuchinka, B.D., Bernasconi, F. *et al.* Maternal meiosis I non-disjunction of chromosome 15: dependence of the maternal age effect on level of recombination. *Human Molecular Genetics.* 1998; 7(6): 1011–1019.

20. Bugge, M., Collins, A., Hertz, J.M. *et al.* Non-disjunction of chromosome 13. *Human Molecular Genetics.* 2007; 16(16): 2004–2010.

21. Bugge, M., Collins, A., Petersen, M.B. *et al.* Non-disjunction of chromosome 18. *Human Molecular Genetics.* 1998; 7(4): 661–669.

22. Hall, H.E., Surti, U., Hoffner, L. *et al.* The origin of trisomy 22: evidence for acrocentric chromosome-specific patterns of nondisjunction. *American Journal of Medical Genetics A.* 2007; 143A(19): 2249–2255.

23. Thomas, N.S., Ennis, S., Sharp, A.J. *et al.* Maternal sex chromosome non-disjunction: evidence for X chromosome-specific risk factors. *Human Molecular Genetics.* 2001; 10(3): 243–250.

24. Hassold, T., Hunt, P. To err (meiotically) is human: the genesis of human aneuploidy. *Nature Reviews Genetics.* 2001; 2(4): 280–291.

25. Lipkin, S.M., Moens, P.B., Wang, V. *et al.* Meiotic arrest and aneuploidy in MLH3-deficient mice. *Nature Genetics.* 2002; 31(4): 385–390.

26. Kan, R., Sun, X., Kolas, N.K. *et al.* Comparative analysis of meiotic progression in female mice bearing mutations in genes of the DNA mismatch repair pathway. *Biology of Reproduction.* 2008; 78(3): 462–471.

27. Lynn, A., Koehler, K.E., Judis, L. *et al.* Covariation of synaptonemal complex length and mammalian meiotic exchange rates. *Science.* 2002; 296(5576): 2222–2225.

28. Cheng, E.Y., Hunt, P.A., Naluai-Cecchini, T.A. *et al.* Meiotic recombination in human oocytes. *PLoS Genetics.* 2009; 5(9): e1000661.

29. Laurie, D.A., Hulten, M.A. Further studies on chiasma distribution and interference in the human male. *Annals of Human Genetics.* 1985; 49(Pt 3): 203–214.

30. Hulten, M., Luciani, J.M., Kirton, V., Devictor-Vuillet, M. The use and limitations of chiasma scoring with reference to human genetic mapping. *Cytogenetics and Cell Genetics.* 1978; 22(1–6): 37–58.

31. Schuler, G.D., Boguski, M.S., Stewart, E.A. *et al.* A gene map of the human genome. *Science.* 1996; 274(5287): 540–546.

32. Matise, T.C., Chen, F., Chen, W. *et al.* A second-generation combined linkage physical map of the human genome. *Genome Research.* 2007; 17(12): 1783–1786.

33. Jorgenson, E., Tang, H., Gadde, M. *et al.* Ethnicity and human genetic linkage maps. *American Journal of Human Genetics.* 2005; 76(2): 276–290.

34. Ju, Y.S., Park, H., Lee, M.K. *et al.* A genome-wide Asian genetic map and ethnic comparison: the GENDISCAN study. *BMC Genomics.* 2008; 9: 554.

35. Broman, K.W., Murray, J.C., Sheffield, V.C., White, R.L., Weber, J.L. Comprehensive human genetic maps: individual and sex-specific variation in recombination. *American Journal of Human Genetics.* 1998; 63(3): 861–869.

36. Hussin, J., Roy-Gagnon, M.H., Gendron, R., Andelfinger, G., Awadalla, P. Age-dependent recombination rates in human pedigrees. *PLoS Genetics.* 2011; 7(9): e1002251.

37. Cheung, V.G., Burdick, J.T., Hirschmann, D., Morley, M. Polymorphic variation in human meiotic recombination. *American Journal of Human Genetics*. 2007; 80(3): 526–530.

38. Kong, A., Gudbjartsson, D.F., Sainz, J. *et al.* A high-resolution recombination map of the human genome. *Nature Genetics*. 2002; 31(3): 241–247.

39. Kong, X., Murphy, K., Raj, T. *et al.* A combined linkage-physical map of the human genome. *American Journal of Human Genetics*. 2004; 75(6): 1143–1148.

40. Henderson, S.A., Edwards, R.G. Chiasma frequency and maternal age in mammals. *Nature*. 1968; 218(5136): 22–28.

41. Stefansson, H., Helgason, A., Thorleifsson, G. *et al.* A common inversion under selection in Europeans. *Nature Genetics*. 2005; 37(2): 129–137.

42. Chowdhury, R., Bois, P.R., Feingold, E. *et al.* Genetic analysis of variation in human meiotic recombination. *PLoS Genetics*. 2009; 5(9): e1000648.

43. Fledel-Alon, A., Leffler, E.M., Guan, Y. *et al.* Variation in human recombination rates and its genetic determinants. *PLoS One* 2011; 6(6): e20321.

44. Kong, A., Thorleifsson, G., Stefansson, H. *et al.* Sequence variants in the RNF212 gene associate with genome-wide recombination rate. *Science*. 2008; 319(5868): 1398–1401.

45. Borde, V., Robine, N., Lin, W. *et al.* Histone H3 lysine 4 trimethylation marks meiotic recombination initiation sites. *EMBO Journal*. 2009; 28(2): 99–111.

46. Buard, J., Barthes, P., Grey, C., de Massy, B. Distinct histone modifications define initiation and repair of meiotic recombination in the mouse. *EMBO Journal*. 2009; 28(17): 2616–2624.

47. Hayashi, K., Yoshida, K., Matsui, Y. A histone H3 methyltransferase controls epigenetic events required for meiotic prophase. *Nature*. 2005; 438(7066): 374–378.

48. Hayashi, K., Matsui, Y. Meisetz, a novel histone tri-methyltransferase, regulates meiosis-specific epigenesis. *Cell Cycle*. 2006; 5(6): 615–620.

49. Barlow, A.L., Hulten, M.A. Combined immunocytogenetic and molecular cytogenetic analysis of meiosis I oocytes from normal human females. *Zygote*. 1998; 6(1): 27–38.

50. Tease, C., Hartshorne, G.M., Hulten, M.A. Patterns of meiotic recombination in human fetal oocytes. *American Journal of Human Genetics*. 2002; 70(6): 1469–1479.

51. Robles, P., Roig, I., Garcia, R. *et al.* Pairing and synapsis in oocytes from female fetuses with euploid and aneuploid chromosome complements. *Reproduction*. 2007; 133(5): 899–907.

52. Lynn, A., Ashley, T., Hassold, T. Variation in human meiotic recombination. *Annual Review of Genomics and Human Genetics*. 2004; 5: 317–349.

53. Warren, A.C., Chakravarti, A., Wong, C. *et al.* Evidence for reduced recombination on the nondisjoined chromosomes 21 in Down syndrome. *Science*. 1987; 237(4815): 652–654.

54. Peterson, M.B., Frantzen, M., Antonarakis, S.E. *et al.* Comparative study of microsatellite and cytogenetic markers for detecting the origin of the nondisjoined chromosome 21 in Down syndrome. *American Journal of Human Genetics*. 1992; 51(3): 516–525.

55. Lamb, N.E., Freeman, S.B., Savage-Austin, A. *et al.* Susceptible chiasmate configurations of chromosome 21 predispose to non-disjunction in both maternal meiosis I and meiosis II. *Nature Genetics*. 1996; 14(4): 400–405.

56. Ghosh, S., Bhaumik, P., Ghosh, P., Dey, S.K. Chromosome 21 non-disjunction and Down syndrome birth in an Indian cohort: analysis of incidence and aetiology from family linkage data. *Genetic Research (Cambridge)*. 2010; 92(3): 189–197.

57. Lamb, N.E., Feingold, E., Savage, A. *et al.* Characterization of susceptible chiasma configurations that increase the risk for maternal nondisjunction of chromosome 21. *Human Molecuar Genetics*. 1997; 6(9): 1391–1399.

58. Oliver, T.R., Feingold, E., Yu, K. *et al.* New insights into human nondisjunction of chromosome 21 in oocytes. *PLoS Genetics*. 2008; 4(3): e1000033.

59. Molnar, M., Parisi, S., Kakihara, Y. *et al.* Characterization of rec7, an early meiotic recombination gene in Schizosaccharomyces pombe. *Genetics*. 2001; 157(2): 519–532.

60. Roeder, G.S. Meiotic chromosomes: it takes two to tango. *Genes and Development*. 1997; 11(20): 2600–2621.

61. Sears, D.D., Hegemann, J.H., Hieter, P. Meiotic recombination and segregation of human-derived artificial chromosomes in Saccharomyces cerevisiae. *Proceedings of the National Academy of Sciences of the United States of America*. 1992; 89(12): 5296–5300.

62. Sears, D.D., Hieter, P., Simchen, G. An implanted recombination hot spot stimulates recombination and enhances sister chromatid cohesion of heterologous YACs during yeast meiosis. *Genetics*. 1994; 138(4): 1055–1065.

63. Koehler, K.E., Boulton, C.L., Collins, H.E. *et al.* Spontaneous X chromosome MI and MII nondisjunction events in Drosophila melanogaster

oocytes have different recombinational histories. *Nature Genetics.* 1996; 14(4): 406–414.

64. Rockmill, B., Voelkel-Meimau, K., Roeder, G.S. Centromere-proximal crossovers are associated with precocious separation of sister chromatids during meiosis in *Saccharomyces cerevisiae. Genetics.* 2006; 174(4): 1745–1754.

65. Barlow, A.L., Hulten, M.A. Crossing over analysis at pachytene in man. *European Journal of Human Genetics.* 1998; 6(4): 350–358.

66. Matise, T.C., Perlin, M., Chakravarti, A. Automated construction of genetic linkage maps using an expert system (MultiMap): a human genome linkage map. *Nature Genetics.* 1994; 6(4): 384–390.

67. Matise, T.C., Sachidanandam, R., Clark, A.G. *et al.* A 3.9-centimorgan-resolution human single-nucleotide polymorphism linkage map and screening set. *American Journal of Human Genetics.* 2003; 73(2): 271–284.

68. Hassold, T., Sherman, S., Hunt, P. Counting cross-overs: characterizing meiotic recombination in mammals. *Human Molecular Genetics.* 2000; 9(16): 2409–2419.

Chapter

7

Gene expression dynamics during human embryonic development

Carlos Simón and Renee A. Reijo Pera

Introduction to human embryo development and reprogramming

Human embryo development begins in transcriptional silence with an oocyt-to-embryo transition that encompasses the fusion of the egg and sperm, migration and fusion of the germ-cell pronuclei, and a series of cleavage divisions that culminate with the activation of the unique human embryonic genome, compaction of the blastomeres to form a morula, and subsequent differentiation of the first cell lineages – the trophectoderm and inner cell mass (see review by Niakan *et al.* [1]). Human embryo development is remarkable in that the oocyte provides all of the required mRNA and protein resources to carry out the complex developmental pathways of the first three days of development, in the absence of genome-wide transcription [2,3,4,5]. Consider further that the process of epigenetic modification that culminates in expression of the major wave of transcription in the human embryo occurs in transcriptional silence and involves one of the most difficult sets of chromosomes to reprogram from a differentiated to a pluripotent state – those inherited from the sperm. These chromosomes are highly condensed, highly methylated, and organized around a protamine rather than a histone scaffold. Yet, the nascent embryo formed after fertilization is capable of reprogramming these chromosomes from sperm patterns of gene expression to that associated with embryonic genome activation by day 3 in >75% of embryonic blastomeres [6].

Induced pluripotency

The observations described above are useful to contrast with induced reprogramming to generate induced pluripotent stem cells. Induced reprogramming is a powerful technology that allows the production of patient-specific stem-cell lines with properties very similar to embryonic stem cells [7,8,9]. In induced reprogramming, in contrast to embryonic reprogramming during the oocyte-to-embryo transition, transcriptional factors are generally used to epigenetically reprogram somatic cells to an embryonic stem-cell-like fate [7,8,9]. Moreover, the induction of pluripotency is relatively inefficient with efficiencies that may vary from 0.1% to approximately 5% over approximately 10–30 days depending on the age of the somatic cell donor and the method of reprogramming [7,8,9,10,11,12]. Clearly, the technology is important for understanding human development and pathology; further there is potential for novel cell-based therapies. Nonetheless, it is informative to compare the process of induced reprogramming to that occurring natively during the oocyte-to-embryo transition. As noted, the latter occurs in approximately 3 days, in transcriptional silence, with an efficiency that exceeds 75% [6].

Our lack of knowledge of human embryo development carries a heavy burden in terms of health and finance. Consider that the success rate of assisted reproductive techniques such as IVF is approximately 40% and that in some countries success is associated with multiple births in up to one-third of cases (www.cdc.gov/art/ART2009). In addition, in some cases of multiple pregnancies, fetal reduction may be recommended in order to increase the chances of live birth and/or reduce risks to the mother. Notably, multiple births may also result in premature birth, low birth weight, lung and heart problems, increased risk of cerebral palsy and chromosomal abnormalities, and developmental delay. These risks beg the

---

Stem Cells in Reproductive Medicine 3rd edition, ed. Carlos Simón, Antonio Pellicer and Renee Reijo Pera.
Published by Cambridge University Press. © Cambridge University Press 2013.

question: What are the underlying factors that contribute to adverse outcomes? The answer certainly has contributions stemming from our limited knowledge of human embryo development; in order to increase pregnancy rates, multiple embryos (two to five, in general) may be transferred. Costs of multiples include health-care costs that are estimated to be 5 to 50-fold increased relative to singleton births [13].

Significance of elucidating gene expression patterns during pre-implantation development extends to pluripotent stem-cell biology

Knowledge of human embryo development will inform our understanding of the basic science of embryology and clinical applications in assisted reproduction, and may also impact our understanding of pluripotent stem-cell biology. For example, it is clear that human pluripotent stem cells are genetically and epigenetically prone to errors; in isolation, this might imply that derivation or reprogramming techniques are prone to inducing errors [14,15,16,17,18]. However, when we consider human embryo development *per se*, it is clear that the human embryonic genome is also prone to genetic errors in chromosome segregation [18,19,20,21,22,23,24,25,26]; and furthermore, very little is known of epigenetic programs. Nonetheless, we lack sufficient information regarding fundamental aspects of the embryonic stem-cell cycle and chromosome segregation. Consequently, we lack a comparator for alternative stem-cell types, such as iPSCs, and have little evidence to support or reject the hypothesis that induced pluripotency results in lines that are genetically and epigenetically stable and capable of executing native pathways of human lineage development. Thus, it is beneficial to improve our understanding, diagnostics, and predictive capabilities regarding outcomes of pluripotent stem-cell biology and regenerative medicine.

Gene expression in the oocyte-to-embryo transition

Historically, it has been difficult to obtain reliable human embryo gene expression data due to: (1) limitations of techniques for analyzing single oocyte,

embryo, or blastomere expression, and (2) variable quality of available human embryos, which can compromise data reliability. Nonetheless, recent findings from several groups have provided a framework for our understanding of gene expression in pre-implantation human development.

A survey of human embryo development and gene expression

Human development begins with fusion of the egg and sperm, migration and fusion of the gametic pronuclei, and a rapid genome-wide demethylation that passes over the marks of imprinted loci, and reprograms development from that of the gametes to that of an embryo. By day 3 of development, eight embryonic cells have formed through a series of cleavage divisions. At this time, the embryonic genome is activated and transcription begins for the first time [2,3]. The purpose of this period of pre-implantation development is to transition from oocyte/sperm to embryo programs. Thus during this transition, messages that function in differentiation and maintenance of the germ cells must be degraded, while those required for growth and differentiation of embryonic cells must be expressed for the first time [6,27]. During this time, the unique patterns of human genome methylation and gene expression become established and provide the foundation for developmental regulation that is perpetuated throughout the differentiation of the human cell lineages; indeed, errors in this early development may have devastating consequences to the embryo, fetus, and adult. In 2004, Dobson *et al.* described gene expression in single oocytes and embryos (not single cells, however) through the first three days of development [3]. This work established that more than 1800 genes were modulated, up- or down-regulated, during the oocyte-to-embryo transition. Most remain of unknown function.

Transcription profiling of the human oocyte

Kocabas and colleagues described in detail the unique transcriptome of the human oocyte in order to shed light on the processes of oogenesis, folliculogenesis, fertilization, and embryonic development [27]. In this study, fresh oocytes were processed for gene expression analysis immediately after removal from the ovary. The authors compared the gene expression profiles to mouse oocytes, embryonic stem cells, and normal human tissues (not including the ovary). They observed that there were 5331 transcripts significantly up-regulated and 7074 transcripts significantly down-regulated in the oocyte relative to other human tissues. Furthermore, a core group of 66 transcripts was up-regulated in both mouse and human oocytes, as well as in mouse and human embryonic stem cells. Notably, the most highly overexpressed genes in the oocyte, relative to other human tissues, were those that were implicated in RNA metabolism followed by protein metabolism, DNA metabolism, and epigenetic modification. Most significantly, the vast majority of genes specifically up-regulated in the oocyte samples were of unknown function (and remain largely unknown in function to date).

Cell cycle drivers and checkpoints in the human eight-cell embryo

In 2008, Kiessling *et al.* described data obtained from whole-genome expression analysis of normal eight-cell embryos, in more detail [29]. In this study, the authors sought to focus on cell cycle controls in the eight-cell embryo relative to human fibro-blasts, induced pluripotent stem cells (iPSCs), and human embryonic stem cells (hESCs). The authors analyzed a subset of data (3803 identified by high-throughput RNA knock-down studies) and observed 35 genes that were overexpressed at least sevenfold in eight-cell embryos that were enriched for cell cycle drivers and mitotic proteins involved in chromosome adhesion, spindle function, and DNA and centro-some replication. Results suggest that there is a heavy reliance of human embryo development on cycling of key cell cycle proteins rather than cell cycle check-points. Moreover, the results suggest that the unique susceptibility of human embryos to errors in chro-mosome segregation may be linked to the unique reliance on cycling of proteins rather than checkpoint machinery.

Validation of gene expression in a large set of oocytes and embryos at six developmental stages

Subsequent studies expanded greatly our understand-ing of the transcription dynamics in the human oocyte-to-embryo transition [4]. The authors observed

that there were two major transitions in gene expres-sion: the first occurred during the metaphase II oocyte-to-four-cell-embryo stage with the expression predominantly of maternal genes; the second occurred from the eight-cell embryo stage to the blastocyst stage with the up-regulation of embryonic genes. In addition, the authors examined properties of con-servation and found that genes expressed in mice and humans during the oocyte-to-embryo transition maintained a high degree of conservation (were not undergoing rapid evolution as some studies of germ-cell development have suggested [30]). Overall, the database of gene expression analysis provides a rich resource for understanding human embryo develop-ment, in comparison to other tissue types and other species.

Analysis of single blastomeres from five- to eight-cell embryos

Galan *et al.* sought to examine gene expression in sin-gle blastomeres in order to shed light on genes and pathways that may regulate blastomere fate and con-tribute to embryonic genome activation [31]. These authors examined 49 individual blastomeres from five- to eight-cell embryos and used high-density microarray analysis to assay gene expression (with 120 probes for inner cell mass transcripts, 190 for stemness, 45 for trophectoderm, and 46 housekeep-ing genes). They observed that all single cells appeared to display a common gene expression pattern with regard to inner cell (e.g., *DDX3, FOXD3, LEFTY1, MYC, NANOG, POU5F1*), stemness (e.g., *POU5F1, DNMT3B, GABRB3, SOX2, ZFP42, TERT*), and TE markers (e.g., *GATA6, EOMES, CDX2, LHCGR*). Results at the single-cell level also further confirmed the timing of embryonic genome activation and the identity of the genes activated with several new fea-tures presented.

Correlating molecular data with imaging data and developmental potential

Recently, Wong *et al.* performed experiments in devel-opment of 242 embryos from zygote (day 1, one cell) to blastocyst stage and correlated imaging and molecular characteristics [6]. These studies allowed

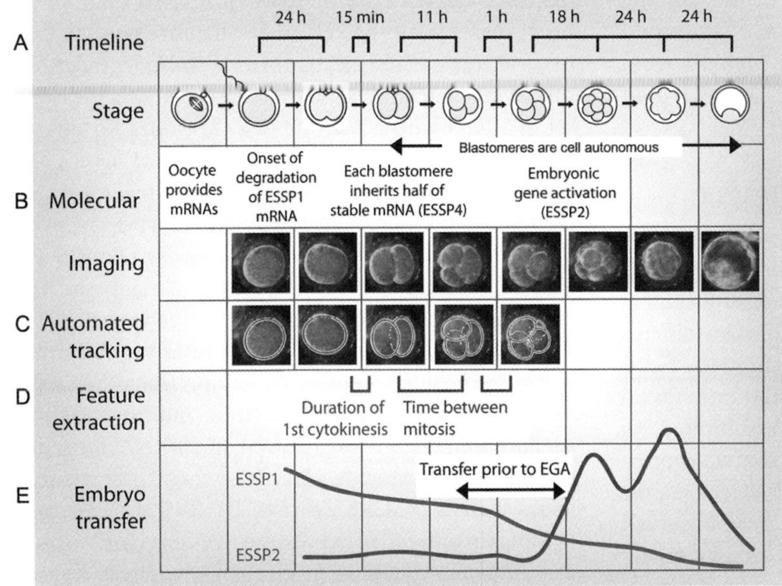

Figure 7.1 Imaging human embryo development and predicting developmental potential. (A) Timeline of human embryo development from the zygote to the blastocyst stage, highlighting critical times between stages that predict successful development. (B) Time-lapse images of human embryo development obtained. Essentially, imaging was performed on multiple systems that consisted of custom-built three-channel miniature microscope arrays that were accommodated in standard incubators, equipped with white-light Luxeon LEDs and apertures for darkfield illumination. Darkfield allowed optimal contrast of cell membranes for automated tracking and also decreased light intensity to a level significantly lower than the light typically used on an ART microscope due to the low power of the LEDs (relative to a typical 100W halogen bulb) and high sensitivity of camera sensors (estimated light exposure is equivalent to roughly 1 minute of exposure under a typical assisted-reproduction microscope). Images were captured at a 1 second exposure time every 5 minutes for up to 5 or 6 days, resulting in approximately 24 minutes of continuous light exposure. (C) Automated tracking demonstrates modeling via computer algorithms to predict success or failure. (D) Critical features that influence developmental success include the duration of first cytokinesis, the time between the first and second mitotic division, and the synchronicity of appearance of the third and fourth blastomeres. (E) Potential application in prediction of embryo developmental potential in ART. (From [6].) (See also color plate.)

construction of a model of human embryo development that correlated imaging and molecular data (Figure 7.1).

Imaging parameters prospectively diagnose embryo fate in in vitro experiments

In order to build a model of human embryo development with applications to reproductive stem-cell biology and regenerative medicine, a major goal is to identify quantitative morphological markers that predict success in embryo development. Wong *et al.* extracted and analyzed several parameters from time-lapse imaging, including blastomere size, thickness of the zona pellucida, degree of fragmentation, length of the first cell cycles, time intervals between the first few mitoses, and duration of the first cytokinesis [6]. We found a set of three parameters that collectively predicted blastocyst formation with 94.1 and 93.1%

sensitivity and specificity, respectively: (1) duration of the first cytokinesis, (2) time interval between the end of the first cleavage and the initiation of the second, and (3) synchronicity of the blastomeres in the second cleavage division to yield a four-cell embryo from a two-cell embryo. All normal embryos that successfully developed into a blastocyst exhibited similar values in all three parameters, whereas arrested embryos were highly variable. This suggested that embryos that follow strict timing in cytokinesis and mitosis during the first two cleavage divisions are much more likely to successfully develop to blastocyst stage. Considering that the embryonic genome is not activated until 1–2 days later [2], this data indicated that the fate of an embryo may be pre-determined by inherited factors rather than by genes activated in the nascent embryo. Subsequent studies in a clinical setting further validated use of these time-lapse parameters (especially the time interval between the end of the first cleavage and the initiation of the second, and the synchronicity of the blastomeres in the second cleavage division to yield a four-cell embryo from a two-cell embryo) in predicting implantation [32].

Embryo stage-specific gene expression

In parallel studies with time-lapse imaging, Wong *et al.* correlated gene expression profiling for each imaged embryo. Embryos were analyzed as either single intact embryos or were disassociated into single blastomeres followed by gene-specific RNA amplification. Gene expression analysis revealed several key findings as described [6]. First, without prior assumption of which genes might fall into similar shared expression patterns, four unique embryonic stage-specific patterns (ESSPs) of gene expression were observed (Figure 7.2A). ESSP1 was comprised of maternally inherited mRNAs that are destined for degradation; this group of genes has a high expression level at the zygote stage and subsequently declined with a half-life of just 21 hours. ESSP2 included the genes that are activated at the time of embryonic genome activation; these genes are first transcribed at approximately the eight-cell stage. ESSP3 genes are those that are activated at a later stage – at the morula-blastocyst stage – and the ESSP4 group contained stable transcripts with the half-life of ESSP4 transcripts being 193 hours, nine times longer than that of ESSP1 transcripts (Figure 7.2B). For many of the genes in these groups, the expression patterns were revealed for the first time in embryos in this study.

Individual blastomeres show cell autonomy

In addition to assaying gene expression at the whole-embryo level, Wong *et al.* also examined individual blastomeres. It is commonly assumed that blastomeres of an early human embryo are at the same developmental stage with the view that the embryo *per se* will succeed or die. However, these authors observed approximately 25% of embryos contained blastomeres of different ages (Figure 7.2C), with a subset of embryos containing maternal transcripts that were not degraded in some blastomeres, while the embryonic genome had been activated in other blastomeres. This observation suggested two properties of human embryo development: *first, degradation of maternal transcripts is unlikely to be a spontaneous process that simply occurs through time.* Instead,

maternal degradation of RNA in human embryonic blastomeres is more likely to be an active process that may rely on specific mechanisms of RNA degradation. These mechanisms selectively target a specific subset of RNAs with a half-life of *c.* 21 hours for degradation. *Second, the lack of co-existence of high levels of maternal transcripts and embryonic transcripts in the same blastomere suggested that the proper degradation of maternal transcripts may be a pre-requisite for activation of the embryonic genome.* Notably, in line with previous studies, genes that were expressed at significantly different levels in normal vs. abnormal embryos included some of those implicated in previous studies, as described above, including cytokinesis components, genes involved in miRNA biogenesis, and mRNA storage and processing. In particular, genes such as DGCR8, DICER, TARBP2, CPEB1, and Symplekin differed in expression in embryos of normal vs. abnormal dynamic morphology, whereas housekeeping genes were not different between the two groups.

The promise of novel analytic tools

Finally, we note that gene and pathway identification, and more informed analysis of genes and pathways, may be optimized through the studies of Sahoo and colleagues [33]. These studies report development of a novel set of tools (termed MiDReG for mining developmentally regulated genes) to first examine Boolean distributions of gene expression and conserved patterns and then to predict intermediate, developmental genes, and gene sets that function specifically to determine fate [33,34]. This method was recently validated with application to B-cell development [21]. The algorithm predicted 62 genes that are expressed after the KIT progenitor cell stage and remain expressed through CD19 and AICDA germinal center B cells. Both qRT-PCR and published literature of knockout mice revealed that the predicted genes have defects in B-cell differentiation and function. Novel genes are under further investigation. Data demonstrate the power of MiDReG in predicting functionally important intermediate genes in a given developmental pathway that is defined by a mutually exclusive gene expression pattern. RNAseq and epigenetic studies that model human embryo development will benefit from use of this methodology, and others under development, to validate data and capture relevant studies from other species [33,34,35].

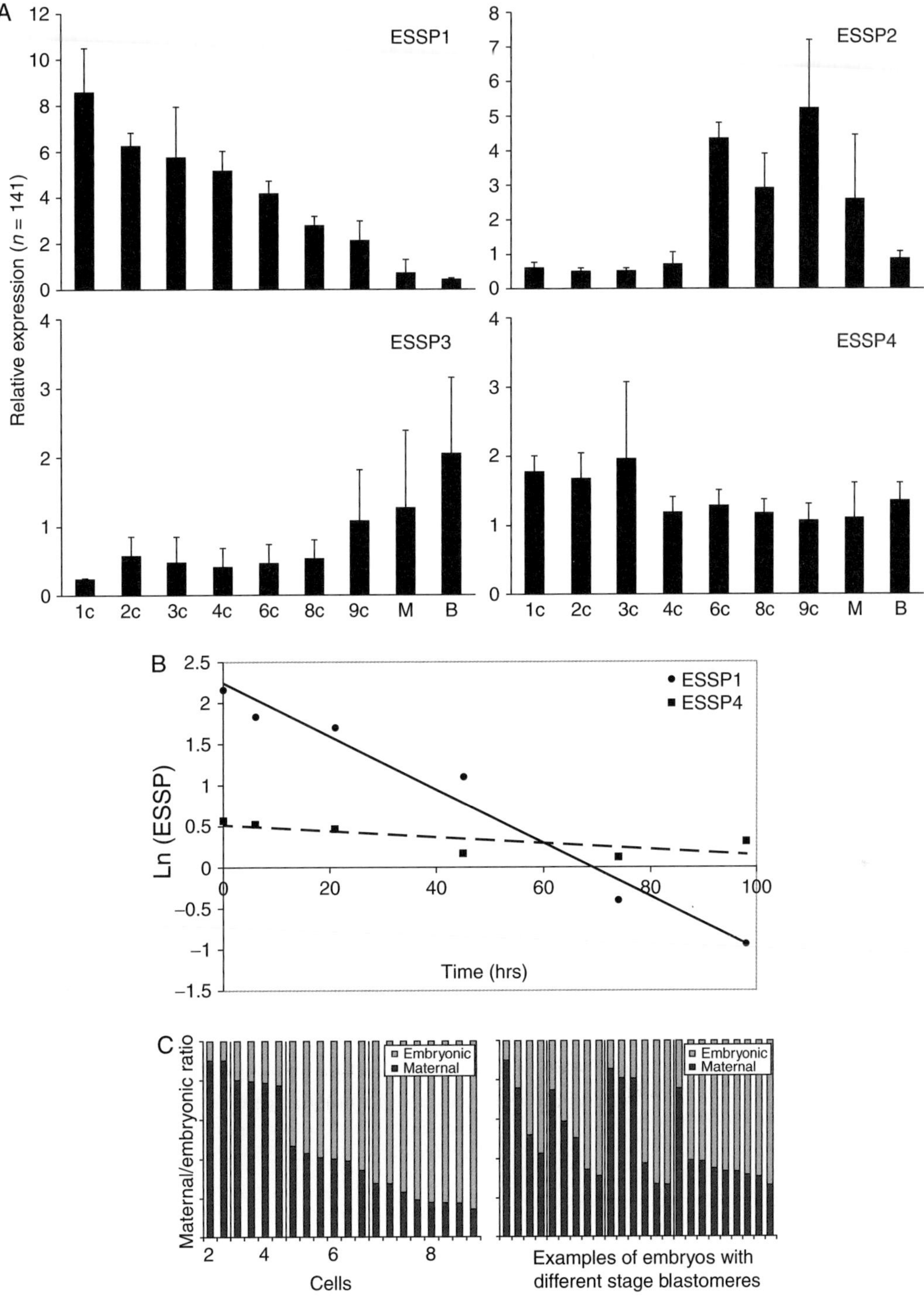

Figure 7.2 Gene expression analysis of single human embryos and blastomeres. (A) Four distinct embryo stage-specific gene expression patterns (ESSPs) exist in human pre-implantation embryos throughout development. (B) The half-lives of ESSP1 and ESSP4. (C; left) The ratio of maternal to embryonic genes in embryos changes during pre-implantation development. (C; right) Some embryos contained blastomeres of different developmental ages. (From [6].)

Summary

Recent studies of human embryo development, gene expression, and correlated imaging, are increasing our knowledge of basic stem-cell biology and both basic and clinical applications in assisted reproduction. Further use of computer-assisted diagnosis of cell fate and the use of expression analysis to generate large databases for mining of data holds great promise to further clarify fundamental aspects of human development.

References

1. Niakan, K., Han, J., Pedersen, R., Simón, C., Reijo Pera, R.A. Human pre-implantation embryo development. *Development*. 2012; 139: 829–841.

2. Braude, P., Bolton, V., Moore, S. Human gene expression first occurs between the four- and eight-cell stages of preimplantation development. *Nature*. 1988; 332(6163). 459–461.

3. Dobson, A.T., Raja, R., Abeyta, M.J. *et al*. The unique transcriptome through day 3 of human preimplantation development. *Human Molecular Genetics*. 2004; 13: 1461–1470.

4. Zhang, P., Zucchelli, M., Bruce, S. *et al*. Transcriptome profiling of human preimplantation development. *PLoS One*. 2009; 4: e7844.

5. Vassena, R., Boué, S., González-Roca, E. *et al*. Waves of early transcriptional activation and pluripotency program initiation during human preimplantation development. *Development*. 2011; 138: 3699–3709.

6. Wong, C., Loewke, K., Bossert, N. *et al*. Non-invasive imaging of human embryos before embryonic genome activation predicts development to the blastocyst stage. *Nature Biotechnology*. 2010; 28: 1115–1121.

7. Takahashi, K., Tanabe, K., Ohnuki, M. *et al*. Induction of pluripotent stem cells from adult human fibroblasts by defined factors. *Cell*. 2007; 131: 861–872.

8. Yu, J., Vodyanik, M., Smuga-Otto, K. *et al*. Induced pluripotent stem cell lines derived from human somatic cells. *Science*. 2007; 318: 1917–1920.

9. Nakagawa, M., Koyanagi, M., Tanabe, K. *et al*. Generation of induced pluripotent stem cells without Myc from mouse and human fibroblasts. *Nature Biotechnology*. 2008; 26(1): 101–106.

10. Sommer, C., Stadtfeld, M., Murphy, G. *et al*. Induced pluripotent stem cell generation using a single lentiviral stem cell cassette. *Stem Cells*. 2009; 27: 543–549.

11. Sommer, C., Sommer, A., Longmire, T. *et al*. Excision of reprogramming transgenes improves the differentiation potential of iPS cells generated with a single excisable vector. *Stem Cells*. 2010; 28: 64–74.

12. Warren, L., Manos, P., Ahfeldt, T. *et al*. Highly efficient reprogramming to pluripotency and directed differentiation of human cells with synthetic modified mRNA. *Cell Stem Cell*. 2010; 7: 618–630.

13. Chambers, G., Chapman, M., Grayson, N., Shanahan, M., Sullivan, E. Babies born after ART treatment cost more than non-ART babies: a cost analysis of inpatient birth-admission costs of singleton and multiple gestation pregnancies. *Human Reproduction*. 2007; 22: 3108–3115.

14. Gore, A., Li, Z., Fung, H. *et al*. Somatic coding mutations in human induced pluripotent stem cells. *Nature*. 2011; 471: 63–67.

15. Hussein, S., Batada, N., Vuoristo, S. *et al*. Copy number variation and selection during reprogramming to pluripotency. *Nature*. 2011; 471: 58–62.

16. Laurent, L., Ulitsky, I., Slavin, I. *et al*. Dynamic changes in the copy number of pluripotency and cell proliferation genes in human ESCs and iPSCs during reprogramming and time in culture. *Cell Stem Cell*. 2011; 8: 106–118.

17. Lister, R., Pelizzola, M., Kida, Y. *et al*. Hotspots of aberrant epigenomic reprogramming in human induced pluripotent stem cells. *Nature*. 2011; 471: 68–73.

18. Peterson, S.E., Westra. W.J., Rehen, S.K. *et al*. Normal human pluripotent stem cell lines exhibit pervasive mosaic aneuploidy. *PLoS One*. 2011; 6: e23018.

19. Kearns, W., Pen, R., Richter, K. *et al*. Aneuploidy rates of human preimplantation embryos in relation to morphology and development. *Fertility and Sterility*. 2006; 86: S474.

20. Mantzouratou, A., Mania, A., Fragouli, E. *et al*. Variable aneuploidy mechanisms in embryos from couples with poor reproductive histories undergoing preimplantation genetic screening. *Human Reproduction*. 2007; 22: 1844–1853.

21. Lathi, R., Westphal, L., Milki, A. Aneuploidy in the miscarriages of infertile women and the potential benefit of preimplanation genetic diagnosis. *Fertility and Sterility*. 2008; 89: 353–357.

22. Vanneste, E., Voet, T., Caignec, C.L. *et al*. Chromosome instability is common in human cleavage-stage embryos. *Nature Medicine*. 2009; 15: 577–583.

23. Gabriel, A., Thornhill, A., Ottolini, C. *et al*. Array comparative genomic hybridisation on first polar bodies suggests that non-disjunction is not the predominant mechanism leading to aneuploidy in humans. *Journal of Medical Genetics*. 2011; 48: 433–437.

24. Kuliev, A., Zlatopolsky, Z., Kirillova, I., Spivakova, J., Janzen, J. C. Meiosis errors in over 20,000 oocytes studied in the practice of preimplantation aneuploidy testing. *Reproductive Biomedicine Online*. 2011; 22: 2–8.

25. Selesniemi, K., Lee, H., Muhlhauser, A., Tilly, J. Prevention of maternal aging-associated oocyte aneuploidy and meiotic spindle defects in mice by dietary and genetic strategies. *Proceedings of the National Academy of Sciences of the United States of America*. 2011; 108: 12319–12324.

26. Vialard, F., Boitrelle, F., Molina-Gomes, D., Selva, J. Predisposition to aneuploidy in the oocyte. *Cytogenetic and Genome Research*. 2011; 133: 127–135.

27. Schultz, R.M. The molecular foundations of the maternal to zygotic transition in the preimplantation embryo. *Human Reproduction Update*. 2002; 8: 323–331.

28. Kocabas, A. M., Crosby, J., Ross, P. J. *et al.* The transcriptome of human oocytes. *Proceedings of the National Academy of Sciences of the United States of America*. 2006; 103: 14027–14032.

29. Kiessling, A., Bletsa, R., Desmarais, B. *et al.* Evidence that human blastomere cleavage is under unique cell cycle control. *Journal of Assisted Reproduction and Genetics*. 2009; 26: 187–195.

30. Swanson, W.J., Vacquier, V. D. The rapid evolution of reproductive proteins. *Nature Reviews Genetics*. 2002; 3: 137–144.

31. Galan, A., Montaner, D., Poo, M. *et al.* Functional genomics of 5- to 8-cell stage human embryos by blastomere single-cell cDNA analysis. *PLoS One*. 2010; 5: e13615.

32. Meseguer, M., Herrero, J., Tejera, A. *et al.* The use of morphokinetics as a predictor of embryo implantation. *Human Reproduction*. 2011; 26: 2658–2671.

33. Sahoo, D., Dill, D., Gentles, A., Tibshirani, R., Plevritis, S. Boolean implication networks derived from large scale, whole genome microarray datasets. *Genome Biology*. 2008; 9: R157.

34. Sahoo, D., Seita, J., Bhattacharya, D. *et al.* MiDReG: a method of mining developmentally regulated genes using Boolean implications. *Proceedings of the National Academy of Sciences of the United States of America*. 2010; 107: 5732–5737.

35. Seita, J., Sahoo, D., Rossi, D. *et al.* Gene expression commons: an open platform for absolute gene expression profiling. *PLoS One*. 2012; 7: e40321.

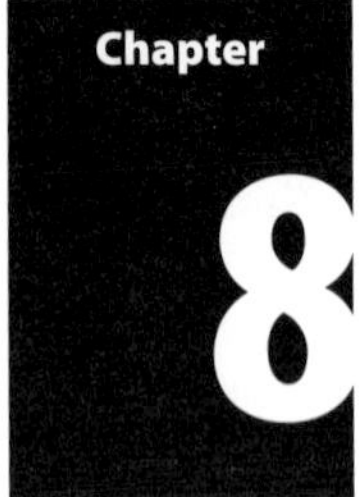

Chapter

Embryonic stem cells from blastomeres maintaining embryo viability

Irina Klimanskaya

Introduction

Since the first derivation of embryonic stem cells (ES cells) in 1981 by Evans and Kaufman [1], these cells have been studied extensively as a model of mammalian development and differentiation. Isolation of human ES (hES) cells from leftover IVF embryos in 1998 [2] has boosted the research in this field, leading to great hopes for cell therapies along with setting grounds for multiple debates in the society about the ethics of this research. ES cells are derived from the inner cell mass (ICM) of a blastocyst and remain pluripotent, maintaining normal karyotype through multiple passages in culture; they can differentiate into derivatives of all three germ layers in vitro and in vivo [3,5]. Many differentiation derivatives of therapeutic value have been produced in vitro, such as cardiomyocytes, neurons, oligodendrocytes, retinal pigment epithelium (RPE), insulin-producing cells, and other cell types [4,6–11]. Such cells and tissues, if robustly produced from ES cells, would satisfy an unmet medical need for tissue and organ repair and could be generated to decrease the risk of immune rejection, either through banking a variety of genetically diverse cell lines or via patient-specific technologies.

Two hESC derivatives have now entered human clinical trials. The first Phase I/II clinical trial was initiated by California company Geron and is aimed at testing the safety of hESC-derived oligodendrocyte progenitors in patients with a spinal cord injury. Two patients received injections of these derivatives in 2010 and reported no side effects, but the company decided not to recruit more patients for reasons associated with their business model (www.geron. com), although the injected patients will be followed up for a number of years. Another human clinical trial was started by Advanced Cell Technology, Inc., a California–Massachusetts company, in 2011, and the preliminary results reported no adverse effects associated with the cells injected in the first two patients and an improvement of vision in one of the patients [12]. These very promising advances in regenerative medicine have now brought hESC research to a new level, and answers to multiple speculations about safety and efficacy of cell therapy will hopefully be coming before long.

However, the need to use leftover IVF embryos for generation of hES cells, as well as the donation of oocytes not intended for fertilization and pregnancy, but for cloning aimed at generation of hES cells for regenerative medicine applications [10,13–15], have somewhat impeded human ES cell research. As a result of these controversies, several bills were passed by the legislators of different countries putting a number of restrictions on research in this field, one of which being the limitation on the availability of government funds, along with strict guidelines on oocyte and leftover embryo use [10,15–22].

Finding an alternative to using embryos for sourcing cells and tissues for regenerative medicine applications would add vigor to embryonic stem-cell research and satisfy its most zealous opponents [23]. Most of the human ES cell lines available today were derived from IVF blastocysts, but several approaches are being developed which could potentially allow the creation of pluripotent cells without embryo destruction. At present, there are several promising possibilities to generate pluripotent cells without harming an embryo: deriving hES from activated unfertilized oocytes which are developmentally incompetent (but can form a blastocyst) – parthenogenetic ES cells, reprogramming of somatic cells to pluripotent state – induced

Stem Cells in Reproductive Medicine 3rd edition, ed. Carlos Simón, Antonio Pellicer and Renee Reijo Pera.
Published by Cambridge University Press. © Cambridge University Press 2013.

pluripotent cells (iPS), and a single blastomere-based derivation of ES cells – using the blastomere biopsy technique that leaves the embryo alive and is widely used for pre-implantation diagnosis of genetic diseases.

ES cells via parthenogenesis

Parthenogenetically activated oocytes are a very attractive source for ES cell derivation, not only because they have been shown to be unable to produce developmentally competent mammalian blastocysts, but also because such cells would only carry maternal HLA genes, which would reduce the variability and number of lines required for immune-matching the patients. Due to genetic imprinting and deficiencies of maternal and paternal haploid gene sets, their combined action is required for normal development of an embryo, so parthenote mammalian embryos are unable to develop to birth. However, pluripotent cells were produced from primate (including human) parthenote embryos and seem to have the same phenotype, behavior, and differentiation potential as "normal" ES cells [24–33]. From an ethical viewpoint, parthenote ES cells may be less controversial because no life is destroyed, and such embryos or ES cells can be seen as advanced derivatives of an ovarian teratoma which is an in vivo analog of a parthenote. While in recent years more progress has been made in generating parthenote ES cell lines from human-activated oocytes, derivatives of such ES cell lines still need to be extensively evaluated for their safety and functionality in vivo. If the derivatives of pathenote ES cells prove to be similar to ES derivatives in their functionality and safety, a lot of our knowledge gained through research into hES will probably be transferable to the derivation of parthenote ES cell derivatives for patients.

Transdifferentiation or reprogramming

It has been an old dogma that after a cell undergoes terminal differentiation, it is committed to this particular fate; however, this has been constantly challenged since the possibility of reprogramming (aside form SCNT) the genome of an adult somatic – or "terminally" differentiated – cell was shown in the pioneering experiments of a Norwegian group [34,35], who used the bacterial toxin streptolysin-O to permeabilize the cellular membrane and load the cell with cellular extracts of another cell type. After the the cellular membrane was resealed, the reprogramming of the recipient cell was achieved by the cytoplasmic "cocktail" of the donor cells. Such experiments produced putative pluripotent cells which showed up-regulation of such pluripotency genes as Oct4, Sox2, Nanog, and Rex1, and down-regulation of somatic-cell gene expression over time. These cells could also differentiate along the neural lineage and into adipocytes, osteoblasts, and endothelial cells. Other studies explored the reprogramming ability of karyoplasts and cytoplasts, as well as whole cells in cell–cell fusion experiments, and when pluripotent donor cells were used, the pluripotency marker Oct4 was shown to be up-regulated in recipient cells [36–39]. However, all these attempts did not produce any pluripotent cell line with properties similar to ES cells as far as being immortal, karyotypically stable, and able to give rise to derivatives of all three germ layers. Nevertheless, the possibility of turning a somatic cell into a pluripotent state remained very attractive as this would allow the creation of patient-specific cell types on demand without using embryos to create ES cells.

The real revolution in the reprogramming field happened in 2006, starting a new era in cell therapy, when groundbreaking work by the Yamanaka group demonstrated that somatic cells can be reprogrammed to a pluripotent state by expression of several genes associated with pluripotency [40–42]. This study gave a huge boost to this field which resulted in the development of rather robust procedures of generating "induced pluripotent stem," or iPS, cells from both human and mouse somatic cells [43–58]. The transcription factors used in the original studies, Oct4, c-Myc, Klf4, Lin28, were delivered into the cells via retroviruses or lentiviruses, and the resulting iPS cells appeared similar to ES cells in many ways. They had ES cell morphology, expressed markers of pluripotency, differentiated into the derivatives of all three germ layers, and had normal karyotype.

However, the obvious safety questions were immediately raised because of the use of oncogenes and the need to use retro- or lentiviruses. Studies showed that the derivatives of iPS cells formed tumors in mice after transplantation, possibly due to reactivation of *c-Myc*, as well as teratomas, perhaps because of the presence of undifferentiated iPS cells among the derivatives [42,59,60]. Nevertheless, the "reprogramming quest" continued, and later studies showed the feasibility of deriving iPS cells in a safer way. It appeared that reprogramming of somatic cells, especially cells of progenitor type which could still be multipotent, to pluripotent state can be accomplished without *c-Myc*, using a combination of Oct4 (which is currently considered to be absolutely essential for pluripotency and reprogramming) and one or more other factors [61–67]. Other promising strategies include reprogramming somatic cells to pluripotent state using an siRNA- and mRNA-based approach, non-integrating episomal vectors, removal of factors used for reprogramming, or protein-based reprogramming [61–77].

However, there are other potential roadblocks to application of iPS cell derivatives for regenerative medicine, such as cell senescence [78,79], which limits reprogramming efficiency and expansion of the derivatives in culture, chromosomal aberrations, deletion of tumor-suppressive and duplication of oncogenetic genes during reprogramming and culture of iPS, and errors in GC methylation [80–82]. These and other [83] epigenetic and genetic alterations found in iPS cells raise concerns about their safe application in the future, especially considering that iPS cells are relatively new and less studied compared to ES cells, and more research is needed to better assess the safety of these man-made cells. Nevertheless, iPS cell technology, with its potential, can be compared to the derivation of ES cells in their possible impact on the regenerative medicine field, especially when solutions to all the problems and questions are found. Meanwhile, the strategies for derivation, maintenance, differentiation, and safety assessment of iPS cells keep coming from research on hES cells, and a lot of data generated from this research are likely to be transferrable to the iPS cell field. Therefore, as with parthenote ES cells, data collected through research into hES cells and their derivatives are likely to be valuable for iPS cell technology, and this brings back the issue of "ethical hES cells."

Single blastomere-derived ES cells

While iPS technology remains very promising for future clinical applications, the only safe and efficient derivatives of pluripotent cells for transplantation so far have been produced from ES cells, which, as discussed above, remains a controversial technology. In our lab we developed an approach to derive ES cells without embryo destruction using the blastomere biopsy procedure [84–87], similar to a procedure routinely used for pre-implantation diagnostics (PGD). In IVF clinics such procedures have become routine, and one or two blastomeres are removed and analyzed without depriving the embryo of its developmental potential. Such biopsied embryos remain fully viable and have produced many babies [88]. Multiple studies exploring the developmental potential of a single blastomere showed that it can contribute to all tissues and organs if aggregated with other blastomeres in a mouse embryo [89–90]. However, it was also shown that there is a possible predisposition of blastomeres to a trophoblast or ICM fate even at the two-cell stage [91–93] that depends on the spatial arrangement and order of their second cleavage division; therefore, the potential of blastomeres to form all tissues may depend on them being in the proper environment, i.e., surrounded by other blastomeres. In our earlier experiments single blastomeres from 129/Sv-*ROSA26: LacZ* mice were aggregated in micro-depressions (similar to making aggregation chimeras) with GFP-labeled mouse ES cells which seemed to support their division. After a day or two GFP-negative "buds" were observed on the sides of GFP-positive cell clumps which were separated from GFP-positive cells under a fluorescent microscope [84], either at this stage or later, after such mixed clumps were plated on mitomycin C-inactivated mouse embryonic fibroblasts (MEF) and produced a mixed outgrowth. Using mechanical passaging controlled under the fluorescent microscope, GFP-negative cells were selected and mechanically passaged until a pure population of GFP-negative ES cells was obtained. Several ES cell lines were generated which had normal karyotype, expressed Oct4, Nanog, SSEA-1, stained positive for alkaline phosphatase activity, and showed germline transmission, generating normal mouse pups in the second generation. The origin of these ES cells was confirmed by positive LacZ labeling and negative DNA PCR for GFP.

This work has been repeated [94–98] by other groups, generating ES cell lines from mouse single blastomeres and even polar bodies using different stage embryos with various efficiencies for different stage blastomeres, ranging from 5% to almost 79%.

Derivation of human hES cell lines from single blastomeres appeared more challenging. One group attempted to derive hES cells from pairs of human blastomeres, but their study [99] reported these attempts as unsuccessful. At the same time, our own experiments showed that while derivation of such lines was possible, it had very low efficiency [85]. In our experiments, the blastomeres were cultured for two days in blastocyst medium, which led to the formation of hollow spheroid structures which were then plated on feeders in ES cell culture medium in close proximity to GFP-labeled ES cells that presumably secreted some critical factors to support the progression of spheroids to ES cells. Most of such outgrowths rapidly differentiated, possibly due to a commitment already made by the cells comprising these vesicles to trophectoderm, and only two lines from single blastomeres were established. It was previously shown [100–103] that in pre-implantation mouse embryos, polarization of blastomeres is involved in specification of the polarized trophectoderm and non-polarized inner cell mass (ICM). Observed polarization of hES cells in culture can be a later event, determined by the microenvironment, and may even reflect a partial loss of ICM features, and it could be reversed by adding laminin, a component of the basement membrane, to the medium [104]. To prevent the polarization of cells in blastomere outgrowths (and subsequent commitment to trophectoderm), laminin was added to the blastomere culture medium, and no embryonic vesicles formed under these conditions. Instead, dividing blastomeres formed cell clumps that were later transferred into microdrops with feeder cells, as was previously described [86]. The efficiency of hES cell derivation was significantly improved under these conditions, reaching a rate of 20%, comparable with those reported for hES cell derivation from blastocysts [2,5]. Because in the first series of experiments [85] the embryos were not preserved, our next goal was to create hES cell lines from single blastomeres without embryo destruction, and in subsequent experiments only one blastomere from each embryo was used, and the embryos were allowed to develop to blastocyst stage, at which time they were frozen [87].

Five such cell lines established from single blastomeres (with a matching frozen blastocyst) appeared similar or identical to conventional hES cells by multiple criteria. They had typical hES cell morphology and growth rates, expressed markers of pluripotency, Oct4, Nanog, SSEA-3/4, TRA 1–60/1–81, and alkaline phosphatase, differentiated into the derivatives of all three germ layers in vivo (formed teratomas in NOD-SCID mice) and in vitro, and maintained

normal karyotype over multiple passages [87]. Among the derivatives of single-blastomere hES cell lines were cells of potential clinical value: hemangioblasts and their progeny and retinal pigment epithelium. Although the efficiency of generating hES cell lines from single blastomeres has been shown to be about the same as for the generation of ES cells, and the conditions and reagents being used for both are similar, it is more challenging for the research team because of the greater demand for a "perfect" microenvironment of the blastomere and its outgrowth at the earliest stages. hESC derivation has become a rather robust procedure for many laboratories, but a lot depends on close attention to detail, and the success often relies on each factor and each step being extensively tested in prior experiments, and the optimal combinations of media components, growth factors, extracellular matrix, or feeder cells (with attention to their preparation) must be established. In the author's experience with the derivation of many hESC lines, including those originating from a single blastomere [85–87,105], even seemingly minor modifications of the derivation procedures and components have resulted in significantly different outcomes. For instance, many hESC lines can be successfully cultured for multiple passages on differently prepared feeder cells, or feeder-free, or in different media, but at the arly stages of hESC derivation, when only a few pluripotent cells exist at a time, factors such as, for instance, concentration of bFGF, or timing of the colony dispersion, or quality of the feeder cells, can result in either deriving a cell line or losing the outgrowth to differentiation [106], especially when the outgrowth comes from a blastomere and is significantly smaller than ICM- or blastocyst-originating outgrowth.

Several studies by different groups since the derivation of the first hESC lines from a single blastomere have proved the feasibility of this technology [107–110], including derivation of an hESC line from a single blastomere of a four-cell growth-arrested embryo [108], and derivation of four hESC lines from single blastomeres on human feeders with minimal exposure to animal products and derivation efficiencies ranging from 12.5% to 50%, which is comparable to and even exceeds derivation efficiency from blastocysts [107]. Multiparameter comparison of blastomere-derived and blastocyst-derived hESC under the same conditions showed that blastomere-derived hES cells had a virtually identical transcription profile as hESC, independent of the stage of the embryos, with only 1% increase in unique genes associated with the cell cycle and 2.9% increase in genes involved in regulation of transcription in single blastomere lines [110]. The authors also found no differences in expression of pluripotency markers, morphology, karyotype, and differentiation into three germ layers in vivo and in vitro. Our laboratory's experience with blastocyst- and blastomere-derived hESC lines shows that these lines are very similar in their ability to make differentiated derivatives, such as RPE or hemangioblast, although the yields vary slightly from cell line to cell line. RPE from several single blastomere-originated hESC have been generated robustly, including RPE from hESC line MA09, which has now been produced under cGMP (which includes extensive testing for animal and human pathogens and a strictly controlled manufacturing process), and these RPE cells were shown to be functional and safe in animal models [111], demonstrating photoreceptor rescue similar to that previously shown using RPE derived from hESC [113], integrating into the host's RPE layer, expressing RPE maker bestrophin, and being almost indiscernible form the host's own RPE [12]. If more derivatives of single blastomere hESC lines are to be generated, it would be very interesting to learn about their similarity to the same types of cell derived from hESC.

At this moment, there are only two derivatives of two hESC cell lines that have been used in clinical trials in human patients after getting FDA clearance (which means that they demonstrated safety and efficacy in pre-clinical animal models): oligodendrocyte progenitors derived from H9 (WA09) hESC and RPE derived from the progeny of a single blastomere – hES cell line MA09 [85].

In conclusion, the most promising technologies to bring cell therapy to the patients without destroying human embryos are induced pluripotent cells, parthenogenetic pluripotent cells, and generation of hESC from a single blastomere. The first two have great potential because the derivatives could be immune-matched with the patient, but they are still very far from human studies, as there are too many unknowns and more data are needed on safety and functionality of their derivatives. Meanwhile, derivation of hES cells from a single blastomere is the only technology to date capable of the generation of pluripotent hES cells and subsequent derivatives of clinical value without embryo destruction.

References

1. Evans, M.J., Kaufman, M.H. Establishment in culture of pluripotential cells from mouse embryos. *Nature*. 1981; 292: 154.

2. Thomson, J.A., Itskovitz-Eldor, J., Shapiro, S.S. *et al.* Embryonic stem cell lines derived from human blastocysts. *Science*. 1998; 282: 1145.

3. Carpenter, M.K., Rosler, E., Rao, M.S. Characterization and differentiation of human embryonic stem cells. *Cloning and Stem Cells*. 2003; 5(1): 79–88.

4. Lanza, R., Gearhart, J., Hogan, B. *et al.* eds. *Handbook of Stem Cells. Vol. 1: Embryonic Stem Cells*. San Diego, CA: Elsevier/Academic Press. 2004.

5. Hoffman, L.M., Carpenter, M.K. Characterization and culture of human embryonic stem cells. *Nature Biotechnology*. 2005; 23(6): 699–708.

6. Smith, A.G. Embryo-derived stem cells: of mice and men. *Annual Review of Cell and Developmental Biology*. 2001; 17: 435–462.

7. Passier, R., Denning, C., Mummery, C. Cardiomyocytes from human embryonic stem cells. *Handbook of Experimental Pharmacology*. 2006; (174): 101–122.

8. Ben-Hur, T. Human embryonic stem cells for neuronal repair. *Israeli Medical Association Journal*. 2006; 8(2): 122–126.

9. Klimanskaya, I., Hipp, J., Rezai, K.A. *et al.* Derivation and comparative assessment of retinal pigment epithelium from human embryonic stem cells using transcriptomics. *Cloning and Stem Cells*. 2004; 6(3): 217–245.

10. Klimanskaya, I., Rosenthal, N., Lanza R. Derive and conquer: sourcing and differentiating stem cells for therapeutic applications. *Nature Reviews Drug Discovery*. 2008; 7(2): 131–142.

11. Kroon, E., Martinson, L.A., Kadoya, K. *et al.* Pancreatic endoderm derived from human embryonic stem cells generates glucose-responsive insulin-secreting cells in vivo. *Nature Biotechnology*. 2008; 26(4): 443–452.

12. Schwartz, S.D., Hubschman, J.P., Heilwell, G. *et al.* Embryonic stem cell trials for macular degeneration: a preliminary report. *Lancet*. 2012; 379(9817): 713–720.

13. Hug, K. Sources of human embryos for stem cell research: ethical problems and their possible solutions. *Medicina (Kaunas)*. 2005; 41(12): 1002–1010.

14. Hug, K. Therapeutic perspectives of human embryonic stem cell research versus the moral status of a human embryo–does one have to be compromised for the other? *Medicina (Kaunas)*. 2006; 42(2): 107–114.

15. Evans, M. Ethical sourcing of human embryonic stem cells–rational solutions? *Nature Reviews Molecular Cell Biology.* 2005; 6(8): 663–667.

16. Lanza, R.P., Cibelli, J.B., West, M.D. *et al.* The ethical reasons for stem cell research. *Science.* 2001; 292(5520): 1299.

17. McLaren, A. A scientist's view of the ethics of human embryonic stem cell research. *Cell Stem Cell.* 2007; 1(1): 23–26.

18. Winston, R.M. Does government regulation inhibit embryonic stem cell research and can it be effective? *Cell Stem Cell.* 2007; 1(1): 27–34.

19. Denker, H.W. Human embryonic stem cells: the real challenge for research as well as for bioethics is still ahead of us. *Cells Tissues Organs.* 2008; 187(4): 250–256.

20. Intemann, K.K., de Melo-Martín, I. Regulating scientific research: should scientists be left alone? *FASEB Journal.* 2008; 22(3): 654–658.

21. The President's Council on Bioethics.White Paper: Alternative Sources of Human Pluripotent Stem Cells. Washington, DC: National Academic Press. 2005.

22. Hyun, I. The bioethics of stem cell research and therapy. *Journal of Clinical Investigation.* 2010; 120(1): 71–75.

23. Tweedell, K.S. New paths to pluripotent stem cells. *Current Stem Cell Research and Therapy.* 2008; 3(3): 151–162.

24. Cibelli, J.B., Grant, K.A., Chapman, K.B. *et al.* Parthenogenetic stem cells in nonhuman primates. *Science.* 2002; 295(5556): 819.

25. De Sousa, P.A., Wilmut, I. Human parthenogenetic embryo stem cells: appreciating what you have when you have it. *Cell Stem Cell.* 2007; 1(3): 243–244.

26. Dighe, V., Clepper, L., Pedersen, D. *et al.* Heterozygous embryonic stem cell lines derived from nonhuman primate parthenotes. *Stem Cells.* 2008; 26(3): 756–766.

27. Mai, Q., Yu, Y., Li, T. *et al.* Derivation of human embryonic stem cell lines from parthenogenetic blastocysts. *Cell Research.* 2007; 17(12): 1008–1019.

28. Lin, G., OuYang, Q., Zhou, X. *et al.* A highly homozygous and parthenogenetic human embryonic stem cell line derived from a one-pronuclear oocyte following in vitro fertilization procedure. *Cell Research.* 2007; 17(12): 999–1007.

29. Revazova, E.S., Turovets, N.A., Kochetkova, O.D. *et al.* HLA homozygous stem cell lines derived from human parthenogenetic blastocysts. *Cloning and Stem Cells.* 2008; 10(1): 11–24.

30. Brevini, T.A., Gandolfi, F. Parthenotes as a source of embryonic stem cells. *Cell Proliferation.* 2008; 41 Suppl 1: 20–30.

31. Sung, L.Y., Chang, C.C., Amano, T. *et al.* Efficient derivation of embryonic stem cells from nuclear transfer and parthenogenetic embryos derived from cryopreserved oocytes. *Cell Reprogramming.* 2010; 12(2): 203–211.

32. Turovets, N., D'Amour, K.A., Agapov, V. *et al.* Human parthenogenetic stem cells produce enriched populations of definitive endoderm cells after trichostatin A pretreatment. *Differentiation.* 2011; 81(5): 292–298.

33. Isaev, D.A., Garitaonandia, I., Abramihina, T.V. *et al.* In vitro differentiation of human parthenogenetic stem cells into neural lineages. *Regenerative Medicine.* 2012; 7(1): 37–45.

34. Taranger, C.K., Noer, A., Sorensen, A.L. *et al.* Induction of dedifferentiation, genomewide transcriptional programming, and epigenetic reprogramming by extracts of carcinoma and embryonic stem cells. *Molecular Biology of the Cell.* 2005; 16(12): 5719–5735.

35. Hakelien, A.M., Gaustad, K.G., Taranger, C.K. *et al.* Long-term in vitro, cell-type-specific genome-wide reprogramming of gene expression. *Experimental Cell Research.* 2005; 309(1): 32–47.

36. Do, J.T., Scholer, H.R. Nuclei of embryonic stem cells reprogram somatic cells. *Stem Cells.* 2004; 22(6): 941–949.

37. Tada, M., Tada, T., Lefebvre, L., Barton, S.C., Surani, M.A. Embryonic germ cells induce epigenetic reprogramming of somatic nucleus in hybrid cells. *EMBO Journal.* 1997; 16(21): 6510–6520.

38. Tada, M., Takahama, Y., Abe, K. *et al.* Nuclear reprogramming of somatic cells by in vitro hybridization with ES cells. *Current Biology.* 2001; 11(19): 1553–1558.

39. Strelchenko, N., Kukharenko, V., Shkumatov, A. *et al.* Reprogramming of human somatic cells by embryonic stem cell cytoplast. *Reproductive Biomedicine Online.* 2006; 12(1): 107–111.

40. Takahashi, K., Yamanaka, S. Induction of pluripotent stem cells from mouse embryonic and adult fibroblast cultures by defined factors. *Cell.* 2006; 126(4): 663–676.

41. Takahashi, K., Tanabe, K., Ohnuki, M. *et al.* Induction of pluripotent stem cells from adult human fibroblasts by defined factors. *Cell.* 2007; 131(5): 861–872.

42. Okita, K., Ichisaka, T., Yamanaka, S. Generation of germline-competent induced pluripotent stem cells. *Nature.* 2007; 448(7151): 313–317.

43. Lewitzky, M., Yamanaka, S. Reprogramming somatic cells towards pluripotency by defined factors. *Current Opinion in Biotechnology.* 2007; 18(5): 467–473.

44. Hanna, J., Wernig, M., Markoulaki, S. *et al.* Treatment of sickle cell anemia mouse model with iPS cells generated from autologous skin. *Science*. 2007; 318(5858): 1920–1923.

45. Yu, J., Vodyanik, M.A., Smuga-Otto, K. *et al.* Induced pluripotent stem cell lines derived from human somatic cells. *Science*. 2007; 318: 1917–1920.

46. Meissner, A., Wernig, M., Jaenisch, R. Direct reprogramming of genetically unmodified fibroblasts into pluripotent stem cells. *Nature Biotechnology*. 2007; 25(10): 1177–1181.

47. Jaenisch, R., Young, R. Stem cells, the molecular circuitry of pluripotency and nuclear reprogramming. *Cell*. 2008; 132(4): 567–582.

48. Stadtfeld, M., Brennand, K., Hochedlinger, K. Reprogramming of pancreatic beta cells into induced pluripotent stem cells. *Current Biology*. 2008; 18(12): 890–894.

49. Hanna, J., Markoulaki, S., Schorderet, P. *et al.* Direct reprogramming of terminally differentiated mature B lymphocytes to pluripotency. *Cell*. 2008; 133(2): 250–264.

50. Park, I.H., Zhao, R., West, J.A. *et al.* Reprogramming of human somatic cells to pluripotency with defined factors. *Nature*. 2008; 451: 141–146.

51. Park, I.H., Zhao, R., West, J.A. *et al.* Reprogramming of human somatic cells to pluripotency with defined factors. *Nature*. 2008; 451(7175): 141–146.

52. Lowry, W.E., Richter, L., Yachechko, R. *et al.* Generation of human induced pluripotent stem cells from dermal fibroblasts. *Proceedings of the National Academy of Sciences of the United States of America*. 2008; 105(8): 2883–2888.

53. Brambrink, T., Foreman, R., Welstead, G.G. *et al.* Sequential expression of pluripotency markers during direct reprogramming of mouse somatic cells. *Cell Stem Cell*. 2008; 2(2): 151–159.

54. Stadtfeld, M., Maherali, N., Breault, D.T., Hochedlinger, K. Defining molecular cornerstones during fibroblast to iPS cell reprogramming in mouse. *Cell Stem Cell*. 2008; 2(3): 230–240.

55. Wernig, M., Zhao, J.P., Pruszak, J. *et al.* Neurons derived from reprogrammed fibroblasts functionally integrate into the fetal brain and improve symptoms of rats with Parkinson's disease. *Proceedings of the National Academy of Sciences of the United States of America*. 2008; 105(15): 5856–5861.

56. Schenke-Layland, K., Rhodes, K.E., Angelis, E. *et al.* Reprogrammed mouse fibroblasts differentiate into cells of the cardiovascular and hematopoietic lineages. *Stem Cells*. 2008; 26(6): 1537–1546.

57. Yu, J., Vodyanik, M.A., Smuga-Otto, K. *et al.* Induced pluripotent stem cell lines derived from human somatic cells. *Science*. 2007; 318(5858): 1917–1920.

58. Shi, Y., Do, J.T., Desponts, C. *et al.* A combined chemical and genetic approach for the generation of induced pluripotent stem cells. *Cell Stem Cell*. 2008; 2(6): 525–528.

59. Duinsbergen, D., Salvatori, D., Eriksson, M., Mikkers, H. Tumors originating from induced pluripotent stem cells and methods for their prevention. *Annals of the New York Academy of Science*. 2009; 1176: 197–204.

60. Miura, K., Okada, Y., Aoi, T. *et al.* Variation in the safety of induced pluripotent stem cell lines. *Nature Biotechnology*. 2009; 27(8): 743–745.

61. Nakagawa, M., Koyanagi, M., Tanabe, K. *et al.* Generation of induced pluripotent stem cells without Myc from mouse and human fibroblasts. *Nature Biotechnology*. 2008; 26(1): 101–106.

62. William Lau, K.H., Baylink, D.J., Zhang, X.B. Efficient reprogramming of human cord blood CD34(+) cells into induced pluripotent stem cells with OCT4 and SOX2 alone. *Molecular Therapy*. 2012; 20(2): 408–416.

63. Liu, T., Zou, G., Gao, Y. *et al.* High efficiency of reprogramming CD34+ cells derived from human amniotic fluid intoinduced pluripotent stem cells with Oct4. *Stem Cells and Development*. 2012; 21(12): 2322–2332.

64. Zhao, H.X., Li, Y., Jin, H.F. *et al.* Rapid and efficient reprogramming of human amnion-derived cells into pluripotency by three factors OCT4/SOX2/NANOG. *Differentiation*. 2010; 80(2–3): 123–129.

65. Tsai, S.Y., Clavel, C., Kim, S. *et al.* Oct4 and klf4 reprogram dermal papilla cells into induced pluripotent stem cells. *Stem Cells*. 2010; 28(2): 221–228.

66. Wei, Z., Yang, Y., Zhang, P. *et al.* Klf4 interacts directly with Oct4 and Sox2 to promote reprogramming. *Stem Cells*. 2009; 27(12): 2969–2978.

67. Kim, J.B., Greber, B., Araúzo-Bravo, M.J. *et al.* Direct reprogramming of human neural stem cells by OCT4. *Nature*. 2009; 461(7264): 649–653.

68. Yu, J., Hu, K., Smuga-Otto, K. *et al.* Human induced pluripotent stem cells free of vector and transgene sequences. *Science*. 2009; 324(5928): 797–801.

69. Woltjen, K., Michael, I.P., Mohseni, P. *et al.* Piggyback transposition reprograms fibroblasts to induced pluripotent stem cells. *Nature*. 2009; 458(7239): 766–770.

70. Rhee, Y.H., Ko, J.Y., Chang, M.Y. *et al.* Protein-based human iPS cells efficiently generate functional dopamine neurons and can treat a rat model of

Parkinson disease. *Journal of Clinical Investigation.* 2011; 121(6): 2326–2335.

71. Kaji, K., Norrby, K., Paca, A. *et al.* Virus-free induction of pluripotency and subsequent excision of reprogramming factors. *Nature.* 2009; 458(7239): 771–775.

72. Hiratsuka, M., Uno, N., Ueda, K. *et al.* Integration-free iPS cells engineered using human artificial chromosome vectors. *PLoS One.* 2011; 6(10): e25961.

73. Okita, K., Matsumura, Y., Sato, Y. *et al.* A more efficient method to generate integration-free human iPS cells. *Nature Methods.* 2011; 8(5): 409–412.

74. Yu, J., Chau, K.F., Vodyanik, M.A., Jiang, J., Jiang, Y. Efficient feeder-free episomal reprogramming with small molecules. *PLoS One.* 2011; 6(3): e17557.

75. Hu, K., Yu, J., Suknuntha, K. *et al.* Efficient generation of transgene-free induced pluripotent stem cells from normal and neoplastic bone marrow and cord blood mononuclear cells. *Blood.* 2011; 117(14): e109–119.

76. Yu, J., Hu, K., Smuga-Otto, K. *et al.* Human induced pluripotent stem cells free of vector and transgene sequences. *Science.* 2009; 324(5928): 797–801.

77. Banito, A., Rashid, S.T., Acosta, J.C. *et al.* Senescence impairs successful reprogramming to pluripotent stem cells. *Genes and Development.* 2009; 23(18): 2134–2139.

78. Feng, Q., Lu, S.J., Klimanskaya, I. *et al.* Hemangioblastic derivatives from human induced pluripotent stem cells exhibit limited expansion and early senescence. *Stem Cells.* 2010; 28(4): 704–712.

79. Mayshar, Y., Ben-David, U., Lavon, N. *et al.* Identification and classification of chromosomal aberrations in human induced pluripotent stem cells. *Cell Stem Cell.* 2010; 7(4): 521–531.

80. Lister, R., Pelizzola, M., Kida, Y.S. *et al.* Hotspots of aberrant epigenomic reprogramming in human induced pluripotent stem cells. *Nature.* 2011; 471(7336): 68–73.

81. Laurent, L.C., Ulitsky, I., Slavin, I. *et al.* Dynamic changes in the copy number of pluripotency and cell proliferation genes in human ESCs and iPSCs during reprogramming and time in culture. *Cell Stem Cell.* 2011; 8(1): 106–118.

82. Gore, A., Li, Z., Fung, H.L. *et al.* Somatic coding mutations in human induced pluripotent stem cells. *Nature.* 2011; 471(7336): 63–67.

83. Chung, Y., Klimanskaya, I., Becker, S. *et al.* Embryonic and extraembryonic stem cell lines derived from single mouse blastomeres. *Nature.* 2006; 439(7073): 216–219.

84. Klimanskaya, I., Chung, Y., Becker, S., Lu, S.J., Lanza, R. Human embryonic stem cell lines derived from single blastomeres. *Nature.* 2006; 444(7118): 481–485.

Erratum in: *Nature.* 2006; 444(7118): 512. *Nature.* 2007; 446(7133): 342.

85. Klimanskaya, I., Chung, Y., Becker, S., Lu, S.J., Lanza, R. Derivation of human embryonic stem cells from single blastomeres. *Nature Protocols.* 2007; 2(8): 1963–1972.

86. Chung, Y., Klimanskaya, I., Becker, S. *et al.* Human embryonic stem cell lines generated without embryo destruction. *Cell Stem Cell.* 2008; 2(2): 113–117.

87. Handyside, A.H., Kontogianni, E.H., Hardy, K. *et al.* Pregnancies from biopsied human preimplantation embryos sexed by Y-specific DNA amplification. *Nature.* 1990; 344: 768–770.

88. Kelly, S.J. Studies of the developmental potential of 4- and 8-cell stage mouse blastomeres. *Journal of Experimental Zoology.* 1977; 200(3): 365–376.

89. Pedersen, R.A. Potency, lineage and allocation in preimplantation mouse embryos. In Rossant, J. and Pedersen, R.A., eds. *Experimental Approaches to Mammalian Embryonic Development.* New York, NY: Cambridge University Press. 1986; 3–33.

90. Piotrowska, K., Wianny, F., Pedersen, R.A. *et al.* Blastomeres arising from the first cleavage division have distinguishable fates in normal mouse development. *Development.* 2001; 128(19): 3739–3748.

91. Piotrowska-Nitsche, K., Zernicka-Goetz, M. Spatial arrangement of individual 4-cell stage blastomeres and the order in which they are generated correlate with blastocyst pattern in the mouse embryo. *Mechanisms of Development.* 2005; 122(4): 487–500.

92. Piotrowska-Nitsche, K., Perea-Gomez, A., Haraguchi, S. *et al.* Four-cell stage mouse blastomeres have different developmental properties. *Development.* 2005; 132(3): 479–490.

93. Lorthongpanich, C., Yang, S.H., Piotrowska-Nitsche, K., Parnpai, R., Chan, A.W. Development of single mouse blastomeres into blastocysts, outgrowths and the establishment of embryonic stem cells. *Reproduction.* 2008; 135(6): 805–813.

94. Teramura, T., Takehara, T., Kishi, N. *et al.* A mouse and embryonic stem cell derived from a single embryo. *Cloning and Stem Cells.* 2007; 9(4): 485–494.

95. González, S., Ibáñez, E., Santaló, J. Establishment of mouse embryonic stem cells from isolated blastomeres and whole embryos using three derivation methods. *Assisted Reproduction and Genetics.* 2010; 27(12): 671–682.

96. Lorthongpanich, C., Yang, S.H., Piotrowska-Nitsche, K., Parnpai, R., Chan, A.W. Development of single mouse blastomeres into blastocysts, outgrowths and the establishment of embryonic stem cells. *Reproduction.* 2008; 135(6): 805–813.

97. Wakayama, S., Hikichi, T., Suetsugu, R. *et al.* Efficient establishment of mouse embryonic stem cell lines from single blastomeres and polar bodies. *Stem Cells.* 2007; 25(4): 986–993.

98. Fong, C.Y., Richards, M., Bongso, A. Unsuccessful derivation of human embryonic stem cell lines from pairs of human blastomeres. *Reproductive Biomedicine Online.* 2006; 13(2): 295–300.

99. Johnson, M.H., McConnell, J.M. Lineage allocation and cell polarity during mouse embryogenesis. *Seminars in Cell and Developmental Biology.* 2004; 15(5): 583–597.

100. Fleming, T.P., Papenbrock, T., Fesenko, I., Hausen, P, Sheth, B. Assembly of tight junctions during early vertebrate development. *Seminars in Cell and Developmental Biology.* 2000; 11: 291–299.

101. Rossant, J. Lineage development and polar asymmetries in the peri-implantation mouse blastocyst. *Seminars in Cell and Developmental Biology.* 2004; 15: 573–581.

102. Johnson, M.H., Ziomek, C.A. The foundation of two distinct cell lineages within the mouse morula. *Cell.* 1981; 24: 71–80.

103. Krtolica, A., Genbacev, O., Escobedo, C. *et al.* Disruption of apical-basal polarity of human embryonic stem cells enhances hematoendothelial differentiation. *Stem Cells.* 2007; 25(9): 2215–2223.

104. Cowan, C.A., Klimanskaya, I., McMahon, J. *et al.* Derivation of embryonic stem-cell lines from human blastocysts. *New England Journal of Medicine.* 2004; 350(13): 1353–1356.

105. Klimanskaya, I., McMahon, J. Approaches for derivation and maintenance of human embryonic stem cells. Detailed procedures and alternatives. In: Lanza, R., Hogan, B., Pedersen, R. *et al.* eds. *Essentials of Stem Cell Biology.* London: Elsevier. 2006; 287–304.

106. Ilic, D., Giritharan, G., Zdravkovic, T. *et al.* Derivation of human embryonic stem cell lines from biopsied blastomeres on human feeders with minimal exposure to xenomaterials. *Stem Cells and Development.* 2009; 18(9): 1343–1350.

107. Feki, A., Bosman, A., Dubuisson, J.B. *et al.* Derivation of the first Swiss human embryonic stem cell line from a single blastomere of an arrested four-cell stage embryo. *Swiss Medical Weekly.* 2008; 138(37–38): 540–550.

108. Geens, M., Mateizel, I., Sermon, K. *et al.* Human embryonic stem cell lines derived from single blastomeres of two 4-cell stage embryos. *Human Reproduction.* 2009; 24(11): 2709–2717.

109. Giritharan, G., Ilic, D., Gormley, M., Krtolica, A. Human embryonic stem cells derived from embryos at different stages of development share similar transcription profiles. *PLoS One.* 2011; 6(10): e26570.

110. Lu, B., Malcuit, C., Wang, S. *et al.* Long-term safety and function of RPE from human embryonic stem cells in preclinical models of macular degeneration. *Stem Cells.* 2009; 27(9): 2126–2135.

111. Lund, R.D., Wang, S., Klimanskaya, I. *et al.* Human embryonic stem cell-derived cells rescue visual function in dystrophic RCS rats. *Cloning and Stem Cells.* 2006; 8(3): 189–199.

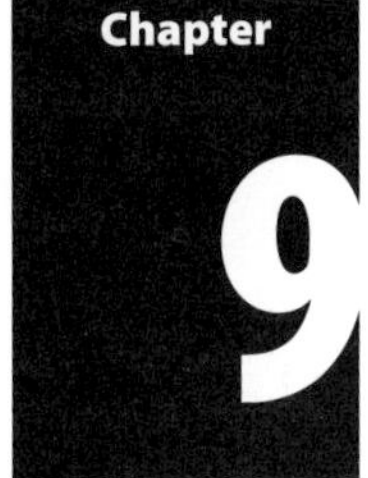

Chapter 9

Gamete generation from stem cells to avoid gamete donation and customized hESCs from blastomeres as the cellular insurance for the newborn: Will it ever be ethically acceptable?

Heidi Mertes and Guido Pennings

Introduction

A crucial facet of human embryonic stem cell (hESC) research is to gain insight into cell differentiation and how this differentiation can be directed to produce specific types of somatic cells for applications in regenerative medicine. Besides differentiation into somatic cells, hESCs can also be coaxed into becoming both male and female germ cells in the laboratory [1,2,3]. As an important proof of principle, researchers were able to produce live offspring from sperm cells derived from mouse ESCs, but the offspring were abnormal and died prematurely [4]. Germ-cell derivation from human ESCs appears to be more challenging than from mouse ESCs, which may be due to the fact that hESCs bare more resemblance to mouse epiblast-derived stem cells than to "naive" mESCs [5]. On another front, primordial germ cells have been derived from mouse induced pluripotent stem cells (iPSCs) and recently successful complete meiosis from human iPSCs was reported [6,7]. Besides gamete generation from ESCs and iPSCs, a hypothesis that is gaining ground is that germline stem cells may still be present in the adult ovary, bone marrow, and peripheral blood, which may be capable of oocyte formation [8,9,10]. Although clinical applications are not around the corner yet, these advances do inspire hope of reaching a way to produce human sperm and egg cells in the laboratory, thus avoiding the need for gamete donation.

Another topical issue is the possibility of deriving an hESC line from a single blastomere that would be biopsied from a morula [11]. If the morula is implanted and leads to a live birth, this newborn would have a genetically identical stem-cell line available that might be used for future therapeutic purposes.

In this chapter, we will discuss the ethical questions and concerns that arise in these scenarios.

Gamete generation to avoid gamete donation

Although gamete donation has been an established procedure for several years, it remains a "second best option." Drawbacks are the absence of a genetic link between parent and child, the difficulty of recruiting donors, concerns over the psychological wellbeing of donor-conceived children who are unable to trace their genetic heritage, and possible disputes about the parental role of the donor. All of these problems would be avoided if it were possible to derive gametes from the would-be parents' own tissue or from an ESC line that has the same genetic make-up. Alternatively, at least the donor shortage and, if managed well, also disputes between donors and recipients would be addressed if gametes could be "produced on demand" by deriving them from existing stem-cell lines.

Gamete generation from adult stem cells/iPS cells

The most exciting prospect for reproductive medicine is undoubtedly the generation of gametes from the

Stem Cells in Reproductive Medicine 3rd edition, ed. Carlos Simón, Antonio Pellicer and Renee Reijo Pera.
Published by Cambridge University Press. © Cambridge University Press 2013.

infertile patient's own tissue. More specifically, there have been reports about human iPSCs completing meiosis [7] and about the presence of germline stem cells in bone marrow, peripheral blood, and in the ovary for both mice and humans [8,9,10,11]. Although the latter findings have received their fair share of skepticism due to the fact that they have not yet been reproduced and are not compatible with the decades-old theory that the ovarian reserve is finite and cannot be replenished during adulthood, the existence of adult germline stem cells needs to be considered as a possibility.

The major advantage of gamete generation from adult stem cells or iPSCs over gamete generation from hESCs is that the person who needs the gametes can be his or her own tissue donor at the time when the problem of infertility presents itself (unless donor gametes are sought to avoid transmitting a genetic disease) and – even more importantly – will be 50% genetically related to his/her offspring. The only ethical concerns that pop up in this scenario are related to safety aspects. As a core rule of medicine is to cause no harm, it would be completely unacceptable to use stem-cell-derived gametes for reproductive purposes in humans at this stage. Although profound sympathy can exist for people wanting to become parents, the right to procreate is not absolute, and the welfare of the resulting children should always remain the first concern in medically assisted reproduction. Certain steps will be necessary to ensure that the transition from research to the clinic can be made in a safe manner [12]. First, further animal studies are needed, not only to assess the health of the direct offspring generated by derived gametes, but also to study possible effects in later generations. However, animal models are not always transferable to humans. Even if abnormalities in animal offspring can be avoided, one should still perform pre-clinical research on human embryos. As the goal of this research would be to evaluate the health of embryos resulting from derived gametes, the use of spare embryos is not an option and embryos will have to be created specifically for research purposes. This procedure is prohibited in many countries but it is nevertheless an indispensable step to ensure safe medical applications. The next step would be clinical trials, although these should only start when animal studies and pre-clinical embryo research have successfully eliminated most safety concerns. Such trials would require continuous evaluation with immediate feedback to ensure fast intervention if any alarming findings present themselves. Finally, if the use of stem-cell-derived gametes reaches the clinic, follow-up studies should be conducted to continually evaluate the safety of the procedure.

While following these steps, and especially before starting clinical trials, a thorough reflection is needed on the value of the genetic link. Most likely, gametes cultured in vitro will be less safe and much more expensive than naturally produced gametes. From what point are the risks and costs of this technology too high compared to the use of donor gametes? In other words, when does the right and wish to have genetically related children become unacceptable? People who are unable to produce gametes naturally may regard their condition as a fundamental injustice which should be rectified by medicine. However, their wish to have a genetically related child does not create a duty for researchers and doctors to pursue this ideal at all costs, especially not if such pursuit would endanger the welfare of the future child.

Gamete generation from embryonic stem cells

When gamete generation from hESCs is concerned, there are two possible scenarios.

First, if the goal of gamete generation (instead of relying on gamete donation) is to offer patients who cannot produce gametes the possibility to have genetically related children, then gametes will have to be created from hESC lines that are derived from a cloned embryo of the patient. This means that besides the difficult task to establish a procedure for the safe derivation of gametes from hESCs (as mentioned, live offspring from ESC-derived mouse sperm cells had irregular growth patterns and showed abnormalities that led to premature death), a safe and efficient way to create a cloned embryo from an existing person will also need to be established. Even if it is possible, it will take many years to achieve such a feat and we can again wonder if the gain – having a genetic link with a child – weighs up against the invested effort and the risks for the health of the resulting offspring.

Second, if the objective is merely to have an easily accessible source of gametes, rather than to establish a genetic link, the creation of gametes from existing hESC lines might be considered.

Each of the two scenarios presented above will have to deal with the same safety concerns as gamete generation from adult/iPS cells, but they each also present extra ethical concerns.

Moral status of the human embryo

The moral status of the human embryo is the main point of contention in the ethical debate surrounding hESC research. Broadly speaking, three positions can be discerned. One can attribute a very high moral status to an embryo. This implies that it cannot be destroyed for research purposes, irrespective of the possible benefits that may be obtained through this research. On the other side of the spectrum, one believes that a human embryo has no moral status or a very limited one, meaning that its destruction for research is no reason for moral concern. A third, intermediate position holds that a human embryo has a certain moral status, but that this status is not absolute. If a research project has a reasonable chance of leading to positive outcomes, the harm that is done by the destruction of embryos can be outweighed by the benefits and can be ethically justified.

As long as artificial gametes are only used in research, no fundamentally new elements are added to this discussion. If they are used for infertility treatments, however, the ultimate purpose of the embryo destruction becomes reproduction instead of research, which further complicates the issue. Embryos are routinely sacrificed for reproductive purposes during infertility treatments since not all created embryos are replaced. The only ethically relevant difference with reproduction through hESC-derived gametes is then that embryo destruction is a mere unintended "side-effect" of current ART, while it would be an essential component of the production procedure for hESC-derived gametes. People basing their moral judgement on the intention to destroy embryos (from the onset) will consider this distinction crucial; others, basing their moral judgement on the consequences of a procedure, will consider it irrelevant. In the discarded–created discussion regarding ESC research, some representatives of the intermediate position on the moral status of the human embryo have argued that every embryo created should at least have the possibility of becoming a human being, as this situation resembles that of embryos "in nature." This criterion is fulfilled in present ART methods, but not in embryos created for hESC research or for the production of hESC-derived gametes. In conclusion, the moral status of the human embryo may be an important issue in the discussion surrounding reproduction by means of hESC-derived gametes, even for those who do not oppose current ART.

Embryonic parents

If the cloning technique and gamete generation from hESCs are combined, a philosophical problem arises concerning the determination of parenthood. Is the provider of the somatic cell nucleus that is used to create the embryo from which the embryonic stem cells are taken to derive gametes, the genetic parent of the child? This person's DNA will match the resulting child's DNA to the same degree as a "natural" genetic parent, except for the fact that when a cultured oocyte is used, the mother's mitochondrial DNA will not correspond to the child's. The donors of the somatic cells will find their traits in the children and will pass a paternity or maternity test with flying colors. If this is the criterion for genetic parenthood, they are the genetic parents. However, given the way in which the genetic link is brought about, this particular relationship between parent and child bears more resemblance to the relationship between a person and the children of his/her identical twin (who is a natural clone). Also in this case a paternity test would be positive, although we would not consider this to be a parent–child relationship. It is equally unlikely that if a clone were to reproduce, that the "original version" of the clone would be considered as the genetic parent of the child. Given these analogies, it is not as obvious as it may seem that the donor of the original genetic material is the genetic parent of a child resulting from hESC-derived gametes [13].

One could argue that the gametes "belong" to the embryo of which they were derived and that the embryo comes closer to being the resulting child's genetic parent than the person who wants to have genetic children in the first place. If prospective parents feel the same way, than the use of ESC-derived gametes as a reproductive strategy misses its goal. If would-be parents make their peace with this drawback of ESC-derived gametes as a reproductive strategy, a concern still persists about the effect on children arising from derived gametes. They might encounter psychological problems if they consider the embryo that precedes them in their family tree as their actual parent. It is debatable whether psychological problems are more likely to develop when donor gametes are used or when ESC-derived gametes are used. In the former case, knowing that one parent is not genetically related to the child, while some other person is, might produce a rift between the (social) parent and the child. In places where donor anonymity is imposed, it might lead to a frustrating search for one's genetic origin. However, when donor gametes are used, the absent genetic parent is at least a 'full-grown' human being, while this is not the case for ESC-derived gametes. In the latter procedure, however, there is no missing family lineage; the child will know as much or as little as any other child about where some of his or her traits came from.

In the scenario where ESC-derived oocytes are used for reproduction by unrelated would-be parents, the resulting child might have the feeling of coming from "nowhere," as there is no person that might be regarded as the genetic mother/father. In many countries, there is an increasing acknowledgment of the right to know one's genetic origin. The abandonment of donor anonymity clearly illustrates this point. One may wonder whether there would be room in this climate for ESC-derived "donor" gametes. Presuming that these gametes would be derived from a spare (or otherwise naturally fertilized) embryo, the "donor" would technically never have existed. Although the identities of the child's genetic grandparents could be released, the parent's identity would be non-existent and could thus neither be kept anonymous, nor be released. A hypothetical situation that resembles this scenario is reproduction by means of oocytes or ovarian tissue from aborted fetuses. The use of fetal reproductive tissue for infertility treatments is shunned, even by countries with liberal regulations, such as the UK [14], due to concerns about safety, increased abortion rates, the psychological welfare of the resulting children and oftentimes – unfortunately – the "yuck factor" [15,16]. The use of gametes derived from embryonic stem cells could meet the same degree of opposition.

Concerns for the psychological wellbeing of the resulting child should, however, not be exaggerated. Similar concerns were voiced at the advent of IVF and conception using donor gametes, but studies have thus far failed to confirm their legitimacy [17,18,19].

Informed consent

In the scenario in which gametes would be derived from existing stem-cell lines and then used for reproductive purposes, the issue of informed consent needs careful consideration. IVF patients may agree to donate their surplus embryos to stem-cell scientists for research or – in the future – for therapeutic applications, but if gametes derived from these embryos are used for reproduction, an explicit informed consent from the donors should be sought. The necessity of this requirement might be questioned: after all, it would not be as if the embryo itself is implanted. While it is defendable that an embryo belongs to its genetic progenitors, it may be more difficult to explain why the gametes that were produced from the stem-cell line that was produced from the embryo that was created from one's tissue still belong to the original donor. The donors would not become genetic parents of the resulting offspring, "merely" genetic grandparents, and in day-to-day life, people become genetic grandparents without giving their informed consent all the time. However, as opposed to what happens in natural reproduction, in this case the resulting genetic grandchild(ren) would grow up in a different family and be unknown to the original donors, which may cause a lot of distress. Moreover, we might say that in natural reproduction, the reproductive liberty of a person wanting to become a parent takes precedence over the reproductive liberty of that person's own parents who might not want to become grandparents. In the case at hand, there are no two parties whose reproductive liberties need to be weighed against each other, and so we respect the reproductive liberty of the embryo donors.

"Non-medical" applications

Popular articles reporting on the development of ESC-derived gametes often mention "ethical issues" that will need to be resolved before they could actually be used in the clinic, but strangely enough they do not refer to any of the issues we discussed so far. Headlines such as "The prospect of all-female conception" and "Getting ready for same-sex reproduction" indicate fascination with the possibility of gay or lesbian couples having children that are genetically related to both partners [20,21]. Other possible applications that have received attention are the production of oocytes for women who have entered menopause, the creation of children with just one genetic parent, and the creation of genetically enhanced children. One argument that is used to denounce all of these applications is that doctors should limit themselves to curing diseases, rather than reinventing nature. Reproduction through

ESC-derived gametes should then only be available for those who are faced with "authentic infertility." Menopause could be described as a medical condition if it started prematurely, but this is not the case when homosexual couples cannot have children or when a person cannot impregnate him/herself. Hence it is true that helping lesbian women to have a child together does not "cure" any disease. However, as pointed out by Smajdor, in the ART setting, healthy women are undergoing medical treatments on a daily basis because their partners are infertile, rather than being told to look for a different partner [22]. This illustrates how difficult it is to draw a clear line between medical and non-medical interventions. Moreover, the idea that medicine can only be used to "repair" and not to innovate implies a leap from how things normally are to how they should be. This belief that it is unethical for people to purposely deviate from the standard has no rational foundation. There is no reason to believe that nature has any moral authority and thus we cannot conclude that medical interventions that "change the course of nature" are necessarily immoral.

However, there are some valid concerns over some of the non-medical applications. Combining an oocyte and a sperm cell from the same person into one embryo would constitute the most extreme form of inbreeding with the related safety concerns. As doctors are required to keep the best interests of the resulting child in mind, there are good reasons not to perform this kind of social and medical experiment.

For post-menopausal women, an individual evaluation of each woman's particular situation is desirable to evaluate the risks for mother and child, a procedure that does not deviate from evaluations preceding a treatment with donor oocytes [23]. Elements to be considered are health risks and whether the parents will be able to take care of the resulting child (given their age). An extra factor that will be important when ESC-derived gametes are used by menopausal women is if the age of the original somatic cell has any impact on the quality of the resulting oocyte, for example in terms of telomere length, as the cells of cloned animals appear to be "older" than their actual age [24].

Reproduction of homosexual or lesbian couples through ESC-derived gametes requires the derivation of sperm from "female" stem cells or oocytes from "male" stem cells. While experiments in mice indicate that there is a possibility to achieve the latter scenario [25], the former is subject to a number of technical difficulties that will be difficult to overcome. Scientists are divided on the theoretical question of whether or not it is possible to obtain viable sperm from female cells [26]. Even if technical roadblocks could be overcome, safety concerns are greater in this case than when oocytes are derived from female stem cells and sperm from male stem cells. These concerns are mainly caused by fears about faulty imprinting.

Besides safety issues linked to the specific technology of artificial gamete derivation, more general concerns have been voiced regarding the rearing of a child by two people of the same gender. Notably, fears about the psychological welfare of the resulting children due to a lack of either a mother-figure or a father-figure are common, and are also present in the debate about adoption by homosexual couples. Studies in this area, however, have repeatedly shown that these fears are ungrounded and that children of same-sex couples show a healthy emotional and psychological development [27].

A final possible application that raises ethical questions is the creation of genetically enhanced children. Pre-supposing that stem cells can be manipulated, this would facilitate germline gene modifications, which faces its own ethical problems and resulting opposition [28,29]. However, genetic manipulation is in no way intrinsic to the procedure of gamete derivation from ESCs, nor is reproduction through ESC-derived gametes a necessary condition for germline modifications. It has been shown that the human embryo can be genetically modified directly [30]. Thus, whether or not genetic enhancement of children is ethically troubling is a separate discussion that has no inherent link to the prospect of reproduction through derived gametes.

Conclusion

We can now draw a conclusion regarding the first question of this chapter, "Will it ever be ethically acceptable to generate gametes from stem cells to avoid gamete donation?" Although we would not go as far as to say that gamete generation from stem cells will never be ethically acceptable, we have indicated that several red flags can be raised that need to be cleared before gamete generation can find its way to the clinic. While the complexity of the proposed procedure is primarily a technical hurdle, it is also an ethical problem in terms of health risks for the resulting children and in terms of a just allocation of healthcare resources. As a society, we will need to make an assessment of how far we are willing to go to offer genetic parenthood to infertile patients. With regard to the relevant differences between gamete generation from adult or iPS cells, as compared to gamete generation from hESCs, the former incites less ethical concerns than the latter. If gamete generation from stem cells is further pursued – which it probably will be – the future will tell which of the three routes is the most promising one.

Customized hESCs from blastomeres as the cellular insurance for the newborn

As demonstrated by Chung *et al.* in mice and by Klimanskaya *et al.* and Geens *et al.* in humans, ESC lines cannot only be generated from an isolated inner cell mass or by plating an entire morula, they can also be generated from isolated blastomeres from embryos at the four-cell stage or the eight-cell stage [31,32,33]. Blastomere biopsies have been performed for many years as a means to enable pre-implantation genetic diagnosis (PGD). The loss of one blastomere from a four- or eight-cell does not have an impact on the implantation rate of the embryo and the limited data that have been gathered suggest that the procedure is safe for the resulting children [34,35], although one study found a higher perinatal death rate among PGD/PGS children in multiple pregnancies [36]. It seems plausible then that embryonic stem-cell lines could be generated from blastomeres, while the biopsied embryos are implanted. Chung *et al.* see a double advantage to this approach: "The ability to generate human ES cells from PGD blastomeres could circumvent the ethical concerns voiced by many, and allow the banking of autologous ES cell lines for children born from transferred embryos" [31].

Avoiding embryo destruction

The ethical concerns that Chung *et al.* refer to are related to the fact that in "standard" ESC derivation from an embryo at the blastocyst stage, the embryo does not survive the procedure. This is particularly problematic for people who believe that an embryo is ensouled at the time of conception. At first glance, this problem is circumvented when the biopsied embryo survives. However, at the four-cell stage and possibly also at the eight-cell stage, each of the blastomeres that make up the morula are totipotent. This means that the biopsied blastomere has the status of an embryo, and its destruction can be considered equally

problematic as the destruction of the "original" embryo. In the lingo of ESC research opponents we might say that while the original embryo goes on to become a child, its twin sibling is sacrificed in order to make the stem-cell line. This first presumed (ethical) advantage of deriving stem-cell lines from biopsied blastomeres can therefore be dismissed as unconvincing.

The advantage of having an autologous stem-cell line in storage

The second postulated advantage of the proposed procedure is that a child born after the blastomere biopsy will have a stem-cell line available for autologous transplantation, should it ever suffer from an illness that can be cured by such a transplant. This again, seems a plausible assumption, as HLA-matching grafts are often difficult to find and allografts require a lifelong intake of immunosuppressant drugs. However, in practice, the advantage may turn out to be much less impressive, at least for the time being. As was extensively argued in the context of private umbilical-cord-blood banking, the best grafts are often those with a close, but not a perfect HLA match. In autologous transplants for hematologic malignancies there is a risk of reintroducing the disease [37], and there is no graft vs. leukaemia effect [38]. Moreover, Ballen *et al.* estimated that there is only a 0.005% to 0.04% chance that an individual might benefit from a transplant of his/her own umbilical-cord-blood stem cells [39]. One might say that these estimates will be better for hESCs, which can potentially be used on many more fronts than hematopoietic stem cells as they can differentiate into all three cell-type lineages and – as discussed above – into germ cells. They may, however, also be worse: while the use of cord-blood stem cells is an established procedure, there are currently no evidence-based clinical applications using hESCs. Thus, establishing matching hESC lines, hoping that they will benefit newborns is premature at best and useless at worst.

That being said, as with private umbilical-cordblood banking, if the possible benefit to siblings is also taken into account, the cost–benefit analysis will somewhat improve, as siblings will often be a good HLA match, while not carrying the same malignancy [40].

Another application that was suggested by Geens *et al.* is to establish a matching ESC line for so-called savior siblings [33]. In this scenario, the stem cells from the umbilical cord could either be complemented with these hESCs, or the hESCs could be used to treat the sick sibling before the savior sibling is even born.

If in time it turns out that the main beneficiaries are – as is the case for umbilical-cord-blood banking – the siblings of the newborn, rather than the newborn himself/herself, this should be clearly conveyed to the prospective parents. However, although the possible advantages for the siblings improve the balance between the possible benefits and the resources needed to obtain these benefits, the balance would still be negative.

Efficiency

As experience in PGD shows, the biopsy of one blastomere of a four- or eight-cell embryo slows down the formation of the blastocyst and has an effect on the hatching process, but does not have an impact on implantation rates or live birth rates, and overall leads to healthy offspring [41,42]. The biopsy of two blastomeres, however, does have an impact on successful blastocyst formation and on the live birth rate [43]. In theory, only one blastomere is necessary to make an hESC line and thus one might say there is no problem. In practice however, the efficiency of establishing an hESC line is low, with reported rates ranging from 2% to 20% per blastomere [32,33,44]. This means that a trade-off will need to be made between the chance of successfully establishing an hESC line on the one hand, and the chance of a successful pregnancy on the other hand. On many occasions the final outcome will be either an hESC line without a newborn, or a newborn without an hESC line. A possible approach would be to create several embryos, take a blastomere biopsy of each, freeze all the embryos and implant only those for which an hESC was successfully established. The amount of resources that would be necessary for such a scenario would be out of proportion, given the slim chance that the hESC line would actually be of any benefit to the newborn.

The alternatives

At present, stem-cell treatments have only proven useful in the treatment of hematologic conditions. For these conditions, however, the alternatives of allogeneic bone-marrow transfer or treatment with cord-blood stem cells are better and cheaper. Also if hESC lines prove to be useful for other applications, the alternative of establishing an hESC line bank

from surplus embryos or embryos created for this purpose (with specific HLA configurations) will undoubtedly be a more cost-effective option than establishing personalized stem-cell lines for individual newborns. An ideal stem-cell bank for allogeneic transplantation would cover a high percentage of patients with a limited number of stem-cell lines. The best donor embryos would be those with haplotypes that are homozygous for each HLA locus [45]. A counter argument to this approach is that even in the best-case scenario, such stem-cell banks could only provide a full match for about a third of the population and a beneficial match for about two-thirds [46]. The problem of graft rejection by the immune system therefore remains important. A promising avenue in this regard is that of inducing donor-specific tolerance. Tolerance may be induced by first grafting hematopoietic stem cells from the same source as the therapeutic graft to establish mixed chimerism, which is already being studied and applied in the context of organ transplantation [47]. This possibility may become particularly appealing for stem-cell therapies if one were to succeed in coaxing hESCs from the same stem-cell line into becoming both hematopoietic stem cells and the needed cells. This way HLA types would not have to match perfectly and the disadvantages of an allogeneic transplant are significantly reduced.

The reason why research into more cost-effective options such as public hESC banks are also morally superior to the private banking of hESC lines for individual newborns is that such options promote distributive justice instead of enlarging the gap between the healthcare options of the haves and the have-nots. Moreover, the option of the tailor-made hESC line will only be available for those who pass through the fertility clinic, as the procedure cannot be performed on embryos in vivo.

Conclusion

Both new high-tech developments discussed in this chapter are focused on old problems, i.e., genetic parenthood and health. Both developments rely on great optimism in technical solutions. However, the high technicality itself holds numerous uncertainties and risks. The question is whether we should continue in this way. In a sense it is the researchers' duty to explore new avenues and to pursue possibilities that make us mesmerised about future applications. However, besides wondering if we *can* achieve certain applications, we should also wonder whether we *should*. If we want solutions that are affordable and applicable to many people, we will most likely have to look for simpler ways. Especially in the field of stem-cell research, where the hopes of patients are very high, scientists should be cautious not to promise or insinuate innovations that will never be available to the mainstream population.

References

1. Hübner, K., Fuhrmann, G., Christenson, L.K. *et al.* Derivation of oocytes from mouse embryonic stem cells. *Science.* 2003; 300: 1251–1256.

2. Toyooka, Y., Tsunekawa, N., Akasu, R. *et al.* Embryonic stem cells can form germ cells in vitro. *Proceedings of the National Academy of Sciences of the United States of America.* 2003; 100: 11457–11462.

3. Geijsen, N., Horoschak, M., Kim, K. *et al.* Derivation of embryonic germ cells and male gametes from embryonic stem cells. *Nature.* 2004; 427: 148–154.

4. Nayernia, K., Nolte, J., Michelmann, H.W. *et al.* In vitro-differentiated embryonic stem cells give rise to male gametes that can generate offspring mice. *Developmental Cell.* 2006; 11: 125–132.

5. Pelosi, E., Forabosco, A., Schlessinger, D. Germ cell formation from embryonic stem cells and the use of somatic cell nuclei in oocytes. *Annals of the New York Academy of Science.* 2011; 1221: 18–26.

6. Imamura, M., Aoi, T., Tokumasu, A. Induction of primordial germ cells from mouse induced pluripotent stem cells derived from adult hepatocytes. *Molecular Reproduction and Development.* 2010; 77: 802–811.

7. Eguizabal, C., Montserrat, N., Vassena, R. *et al.* Complete meioses from human induced pluripotent stem cells. *Stem Cells.* 2011; 29: 1186–1195.

8. Johnson, J., Canning, J., Kaneko, T., Pru, J.K., Tilly, J.L. Germline stem cells and follicular renewal in the postnatal mammalian ovary. *Nature.* 2004; 428: 145–150.

9. Johnson, J., Bagley, J., Skaznik-Wikiel, M. *et al.* Oocyte generation in adult mammalian ovaries by putative germ cells derived from bone marrow and peripheral blood. *Cell.* 2005; 122: 303–315.

10. Drusenheimer, N., Wulf, G., Nolte, J. *et al.* Putative human male germ cells from bone marrow stem cells. *Society for Reproduction and Fertility Supplement.* 2007; 63: 69–76.

11. White, Y.A.R., Woods, D.C., Takai, Y. *et al.* Oocyte formation by mitotically active germ cells purified from ovaries of reproductive-age women. *Nature Medicine.* 2012; 18; 413–421.

12. ESHRE Task Force on Ethics and Law, including Pennings, G., de Wert, G., Shenfield, F. *et al.* ESHRE Task Force on Ethics and Law 13: The welfare of the child in medically assisted reproduction. *Human Reproduction.* 2007; 22: 2585–2588.

13. Mertes, H., Pennings, G. Embryonic stem cell-derived gametes and genetic parenthood: a problematic relationship. *Cambridge Quarterly of Healthcare Ethics.* 2008; 17: 7–14.

14. Human Fertilisation and Embryology Authority. Report on the consultation on donated ovarian tissue in embryo research and assisted conception. 1994. http://www.hfea.gov.uk/en/711.html.

15. Mavroforou, A., Michalodimitrakis, E. Moral arguments on the use of ovarian tissue from aborted foetuses in infertility treatment. *Human Reproduction and Genetic Ethics.* 2005; 11: 6–11.

16. Polkinghorne, J.C. Law and ethics of transplanting fetal tissue. In Edwards, R.G., ed. *Fetal Tissue Transplantation in Medicine.* Cambridge: Cambridge University Press, 1992; 323–330.

17. Brewaeys, A. Donor insemination, the impact on family and child development. *Journal of Psychosomatic Obstetrics and Gynaecology.* 1996; 17: 1–13.

18. Golombok, S., MacCallum, F., Goodman, E. The "test-tube" generation: parent–child relationships and the psychological well-being of in vitro fertilization children at adolescence. *Child Development.* 2001; 72: 599–608.

19. Golombok, S., Jadva, V., Lycett, E. *et al.* Families created by gamete donation: follow-up at age 2. *Human Reproduction.* 2004; 20: 286–293.

20. Connor, S. The prospect of all-female conception. *The Independent,* 13 April 2007. http://www.independent.co.uk/news/science/the-prospect-of-allfemale-conception-444464.html.

21. Anonymous. Getting ready for same-sex reproduction. *New Scientist.* 2008: 2641. http://www.newscientist.com/channel/sex/mg19726413.000-editorial-getting-ready-for-samesex-reproduction.html.

22. Smajdor, A. Artificial gametes: the end of infertility? *Bionews.* 2008; 446, 26 February.

23. Pennings, G. Age and assisted reproduction. *Medicine and Law.* 1995; 14: 531–541.

24. Shiels, P.G., Kind, A.J., Campbell, K.H.S. *et al.* Analysis of telomere lengths in cloned sheep. *Nature.* 1999; 399: 316–317.

25. Kerkis, A., Fonseca, S., Serafim, R.C. *et al.* In vitro differentiation of male mouse embryonic stem cells into both presumptive sperm cells and oocytes. *Cloning and Stem Cells.* 2007; 9: 535–548.

26. Aldhous, P. Are male eggs and female sperm on the horizon? *New Scientist*. 2000: 2641. http://www.newscientist.com/channel/sex/mg19726414.000-are-male-eggs-and-female-sperm-on-the-horizon.html.

27. Golombok, S. Adoption by lesbian couples. Is it in the best interests of the child? *British Medical Journal*. 2002; 324: 1407–1408.

28. Testa, G., Harris, J. Ethics and synthetic gametes. *Bioethics*. 2005; 19: 146–165.

29. Newson, A.J., Smajdor, A.C. Artificial gametes: new paths to parenthood? *Journal of Medical Ethics*. 2005; 31: 184–186.

30. Zaninovic, N., Hao, J., Pareja, J. *et al*. Genetic modification of preimplantation embryos and embryonic stem cells (ESC) by recombinant vectors: efficient and stable method for creating transgenic embryos and ESC. *Fertility and Sterility*. 2007; 88: S310.

31. Chung, Y., Klimanskaya, I., Becker, S. *et al*. Embryonic and extraembryonic stem cell lines derived from single mouse blastomeres. *Nature*. 2006; 439: 216–219.

32. Klimanskaya, I., Chung, Y., Becker, S., Lu, S.-J., Lanza, R. Human embryonic stem cell lines derived from single blastomeres. *Nature*. 2006; 444: 481–485.

33. Geens, M., Mateizel, I., Sermon, K. *et al*. Human embryonic stem cell lines derived from single blastomeres of two 4-cell stage embryos. *Human Reproduction*. 2009; 24: 2709–2717.

34. Desmyttere, S., Bonduelle, M., Nekkebroeck, J. *et al*. Growth and health outcome of 102 2-year-old children conceived after preimplantation genetic diagnosis of screening. *Early Human Development*. 2009; 85: 755–759.

35. Desmyttere, S., De Rycke, M., Staessens, C. *et al*. Neonatal follow-up of 995 consecutively born children after embryo biopsy for PGD. *Human Reproduction*. 2012; 27: 288–293.

36. Liebaers, I., Desmyttere, S., Verpoest, W. *et al*. Report on a consecutive series of 581 children born after blastomere biopsy for preimplantation genetic diagnosis. *Human Reproduction*. 2010; 25: 275–282.

37. Greaves, M. Pre-natal origins of childhood leukemia. *Reviews in Clinical and Experimental Hematology*. 2003; 7: 233–245.

38. Urbano-Ispizua, A. Risk assessment in haematopoietic stem cell transplantation: stem cell source. *Best Practice Research in Clinical Haematology*. 2007; 20: 265–280.

39. Ballen, K.K., Barker, J.N., Stewart, S.K., Greene, M.F., Lane, T.A. Collection and preservation of cord blood for personal use. *Biology of Blood and Marrow Transplantation*. 2008; 14: 356–363.

40. Hollands, P., McCauley, C. Private cord blood banking: current use and clinical future. *Stem Cell Reviews and Reports*. 2009; 5: 195–203.

41. Kirkegaard, K., Hindkjaer, J.J., Ingerslev, H.J. Human embryonic development after blastomere removal: a time-lapse analysis. *Human Reproduction*. 2012; 27: 97–105.

42. Goossens, V., De Rycke, M., De Vos, A. *et al*. Diagnostic efficiency, embryonic development and clinical outcome after the biopsy of one or two blastomeres for preimplantation genetic diagnosis. *Human Reproduction*. 2008; 23: 481–492.

43. De Vos, A., Staessens, C., De Rycke, M. *et al*. Impact of cleavage-stage embryo biopsy in view of PGD on human blastocyst implantation: a prospective cohort of single embryo transfers. *Human Reproduction*. 2009; 24(12): 2988–2996.

44. Chung, Y., Klimanskaya, I., Becker, S. *et al*. Human embryonic stem cell lines generated without embryo destruction. *Cell Stem Cell*. 2008; 2: 113–117.

45. Bradley, J.A., Bolton, E.M., Pedersen, R.A. Stem cell medicine encounters the immune system. *Nature Reviews Immunology*. 2002; 2: 859–872.

46. Taylor, C.J., Bolton, E.M., Pocock, S. *et al*. Banking on human embryonic stem cells: estimating the number of donor cell lines needed for HLA matching. *Lancet*. 2005; 366: 2019–2025.

47. Pilat, N., Wekerle, T. Transplantation tolerance through mixed chimerism. *Nature Reviews Nephrology*. 2010; 6: 594–605.

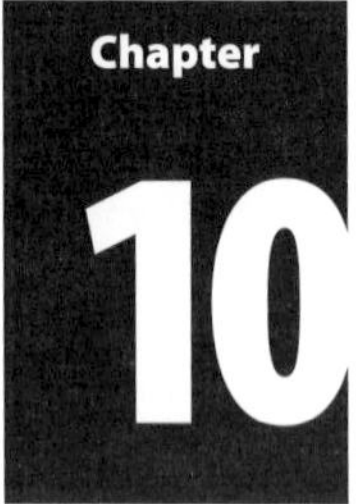

Amniotic fluid and placental membranes: Uunexpected sources of highly multipotent cells

Sean V. Murphy and Anthony Atala

Introduction

In recent years, gestational tissue such as the placenta, placental membranes, umbilical cord, and amniotic fluid have been recognized as an untapped resource for the field of regenerative medicine. These tissues have been shown to be a rich source of multipotent and pluripotent stem cells with potent immunosuppressive properties that make these cells an exciting new tool for the treatment of disease [1–5]. Gestational tissue offers a considerable advantage as a stem-cell source over "traditional sources" such as bone marrow or embryo-derived cells. Such tissue is often discarded following birth so does not require an invasive biopsy or the destruction of a human embryo. This means that there are no ethical and legal considerations associated with their collection and use.

Early investigation into gestational tissue-derived stem cells identified multipotent hematopoietic stem cells (HSCs) and mesenchymal stem cells (MSCs), stem cells from umbilical-cord blood [6]. HSCs have been shown to have important clinical applications for the treatment of blood-related disorders such as sickle cell disease, thalassemia, and leukemia. MSCs are currently being used in clinical trials for the treatment of various diseases such as graft vs. host disease and intervertebral disc disease. Recently, researchers have isolated and characterized highly multipotent cells from the amniotic fluid and placental membranes [1,2]. The highly multipotent and anti-inflammatory properties of these amniotic fluid-derived stem cells (AFSCs) suggest potential clinical applications of these cells to treat diseases including bone defects, lung disease, neurological disorders, kidney disease, and heart disease [7–11]. This chapter will focus on AFSCs isolated from the amniotic fluid and placental membranes, discussing their properties and potential clinical applications.

Development of gestational stem cells

Shortly after fertilization the zygote undergoes a series of cell divisions to form a solid ball of cells known as the morula [12]. The morula develops into a fluid-filled sphere (the blastocoel), which then compacts, forming an inner cell mass, which subsequently forms the embryo, and the outer cell mass (the trophoblast), which develops into placental tissue. At embryonic day 4–5 the inner cell mass becomes differentiated into two tissues: the hypoblast (primary endoderm), which will form most extra-embryonic structures, and the epiblast (primary ectoderm), from which the embryo will develop. The hypoblast and epiblast form a bi-layered disk, dividing the blastocyst into two chambers: a yolk sac and a fluid-filled amniotic cavity. Prior to gastrulation, epiblast cells migrate along the walls of the amniotic cavity and form the amnion epithelium [13].

The amniotic sac is a thin but tough transparent pair of membranes that contains the embryo during development. The inner membrane, the amnion, contains the amniotic fluid and the fetus. The outer membrane, the chorion, contains the amnion and is part of the placenta. During embryonic development the amnion fills with a fluid composed mainly of water [14]. Originally, it is isotonic, containing proteins, carbohydrates, lipids and phospholipids, urea, and electrolytes. Later, urine excreted by the fetus increases its volume and changes the concentrations of these components [15]. The fetus can breathe and swallow the amniotic fluid, which contributes to growth and development of the lungs and gastrointestinal tract. Amniotic fluid also passes via the fetal blood into the maternal blood. The amniotic fluid and placental membranes ensure symmetrical structural development and growth, cushions and protects the embryo, helps maintain consistent pressure and temperature,

---

Stem Cells in Reproductive Medicine 3rd edition, ed. Carlos Simón, Antonio Pellicer and Renee Reijo Pera.
Published by Cambridge University Press. © Cambridge University Press 2013.

and permits freedom of fetal movement, which is important for proper musculoskeletal development and blood flow [16].

Due to the origin of the amniotic fluid and placental membranes, these tissues are a rich source of cells that maintain highly multipotent differentiation potential. The amnion epithelium develops prior to the process of gastrulation, so does not undergo the process of lineage specialization observed in the developing embryo. The amniotic fluid comprises a heterogeneous cell population, which is reported to contain cells of all three germ layers [17,18]. These cells originate from the fetal amnion epithelium, skin, and alimentary, respiratory, and urogenital tracts. The cell population found within the amniotic fluid changes with time and reflects the changes in the developing fetus [19]. Scientists at the Wake Forest Institute for Regenerative Medicine (WFIRM) discovered a small number of stem cells in amniotic fluid specimens which represent an intermediate stage between embryonic stem (ES) cells and adult stem cells, giving rise to many of the specialized cell types found in the human body [1]. In addition to being easily obtainable, AFSCs can be grown in large quantities because they typically double every 36 to 48 hours. They also do not produce tumors, which can occur with certain other types of stem cells. AFSCs appear to have ideal properties as a cell source for the field of regenerative medicine.

Isolation and characterization of amniotic fluid stem cells

An advantage of AFSCs for regenerative therapy is their ready availability. There are more than 4 million live births each year in the United States. Amniotic fluid cells can be obtained from a small amount of fluid during amniocentesis at the second trimester. This procedure is already performed in many pregnancies in which the fetus has a congenital abnormality or when used to determine characteristics such as sex [20]. As many pregnant women already undergo amniocentesis to screen for fetal abnormalities, cells can be isolated from this test fluid and saved for future use. There is also the potential to collect amniotic fluid at term from routine cesarean sections. Another advantage of extracting cells from amniotic fluid or placenta is that it allows for autologous reimplantation, effectively bypassing the problems associated with a technique called donor–recipient HLA matching and

minimizing the chances of cell rejection [21]. Even so, a bank with 100 000 specimens theoretically could supply 99% of the US population with perfect genetic matches for transplantation.

Kaviani and co-workers reported that just 2 ml of amniotic fluid contains up to 20 000 cells, 80% of which are viable [22]. A highly multipotent subpopulation of AFSCs present in the amniotic fluid can be isolated through positive selection for cells expressing the membrane receptor c-kit (CD117) [1]. C-kit is a protein tyrosine-kinase receptor that specifically binds to the ligand stem-cell factor (SCF), and it is this complex that has critical functions in gametogenesis, melanogenesis, and hematopoiesis [23]. In addition, c-kit is expressed in a variety of stem cells, including ES cells [24], primordial germ cells, and many somatic stem cells [25]. Approximately 1% of cells present in amniotic fluid have been shown to be c-kit-positive in analysis by fluorescence-activated cell sorting (FACS). Progenitor cells maintain a round shape for 1 week postisolation when cultured in non-treated culture dishes. In this state, they demonstrate low proliferative capability. After the first week the cells begin to adhere to the plate and change their morphology, becoming elongated and proliferating rapidly, reaching 80% confluence and a need for passage every 48 to 72 h. Feeder layers are not required for maintenance or expansion. The progenitor cells show a high self-renewal capacity with over 250 population doublings. This far exceeds Hayflick's limit, which is defined as 50 doublings for most cultured somatic cells.

AFSCs maintain a normal karyotype at late passages and display normal G1 and G2 cell cycle checkpoints (Figure 10.1A and B). They also conserve a long telomere length in late passages due to continued telomerase activity (Figure 10.1C). AFSCs express human embryonic stage-specific marker SSEA-4, and the stem-cell marker Oct 4 (Figure 10.1D). Further surface-marker analysis demonstrated the presence of the mesenchymal and/or neuronal markers CD29, CD44, CD73, CD90, and CD105 (Figure 10.1E). AFSCs are also characterized by the absence of a variety of surface molecules, such as the hematopoietic lineage marker CD45, hematopoietic stem-cell markers CD34 and CD133, and markers associated with ES cells such as SSEA-3 and Tra 1–81. This expression profile is of interest as it demonstrates expression of some key markers of the ES cell phenotype, but not the full complement of markers expressed by ES cells. This indicates that AFSCs are not as primitive as ES cells, yet

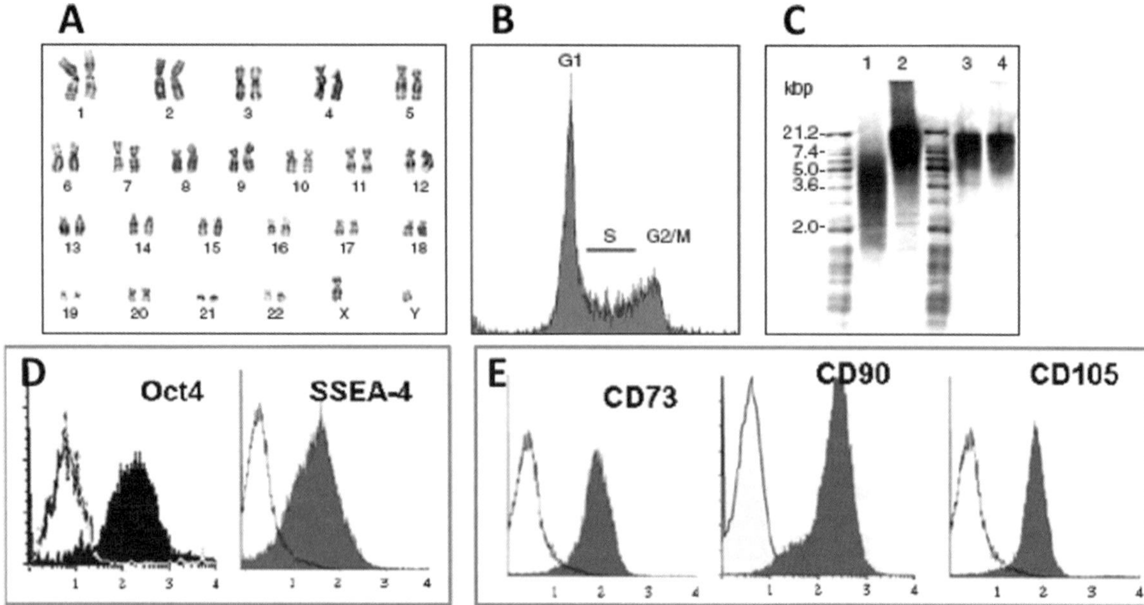

Figure 10.1 Consistent phenotype of AFSCs following long-term culture. (A) Clonal human AFSCs maintain a normal karyotype after 250 population doublings.(B) AFSCs passaged in culture show normal cell cycle control. (C) Telomere length is conserved in AFSCs between early passage (lane 3) and late passage (lane 4). Lane 1; short length telomere standards. Lane 2; high length telomere standards. (D) AFSCs express markers characteristic of embryonic stem cells, Oct4 and SSEA-4. (E) AFSCs express markers characteristic of mesenchymal stem cells, CD73, CD90, CD105. Modified from De Coppi, P., Bartsch, G., Sr., Siddiqui, M.M *et al.* Isolation of amniotic stem cell lines with potential for therapy. *Nature Biotechnology.* 2007; 25: 100–106.

they maintain greater potential than most adult stem cells.

Like ES cells, AFSCs form embryoid bodies in vitro, which stain positive for markers of all three germ layers. However, unlike ES cells, when implanted into immunodeficient mice in vivo, AFSCs do not form teratomas, an essential safety characteristic for a potential cell therapy. AFSCs have a high clonal capacity, demonstrated using a technique involving retrovirally tagged cells. In this assay, a tagged single cell gave rise to a population that differentiated along six distinct lineages from all three germ layers: adipogenic, osteogenic, myogenic, endothelial, neurogenic, and hepatic.

Multipotency of amniotic fluid stem cells

The highly multipotent differentiation potential of AFSCs opens the possibility of this cell type being utilized to treat a wide range of diseases through the generation of replacement cells in the laboratory. The specialized cell types derived from AFSCs in vitro are discussed below.

Osteocytes

An osteogenic phenotype can be induced from AFSCs utilizing culture media supplemented with dexamethasone, beta-glycerophosphate, and ascorbic acid 2-phosphate. AFSCs maintained in this medium demonstrate a phenotypic change within 4 days, including a loss of spindle-shape phenotype and development of an osteoblast-like appearance with finger-like excavations into the cytoplasm [1]. After 16 days aggregates of AFSCs form, showing typical lamellar bone-like structures, demonstrating calcium precipitation and production of alkaline phosphatase (AP), a major feature of osteoblasts. These AFSC aggregates also express specific genes implicated in mammalian bone development (AP, core-binding factor A1 (CBFA1), and osteocalcin) in a pattern consistent with the physiological analog (Figure 10.2A–C). Further studies have highlighted the importance of three-dimensional (3D) culture surfaces and visible light radiation on the osteogenic differentiation of AFSCs. Culturing of AFSCs in a 3D fibrin scaffold and osteogenic media, Maraldi *et al.* demonstrated a significant improvement in osteogenic differentiation and mineralized ECM

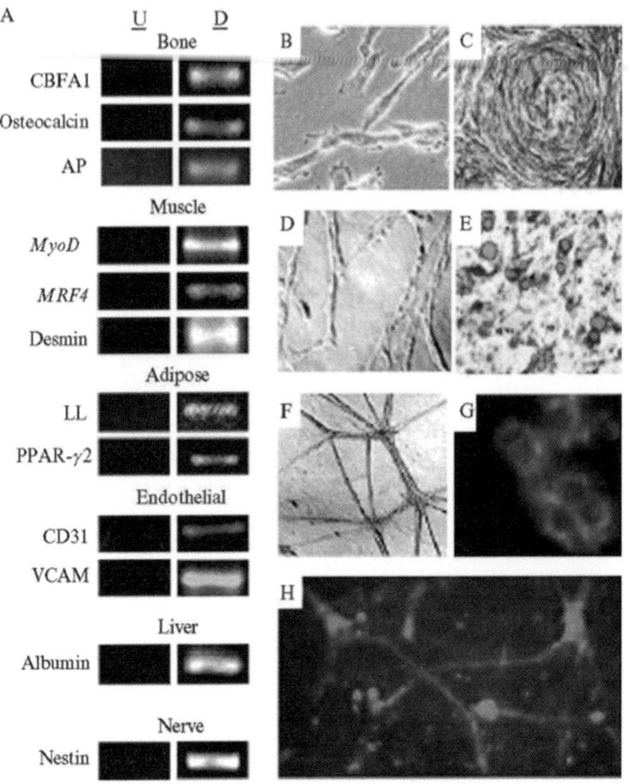

Figure 10.2 Multistage differentiation of AFSCs in vitro. (A) RT-PCR analysis of differentiation. U: Undifferentiated cells, D: Cells maintained under conditions for differentiation to: osteocytes (8 days), adipocytes (16 days), endothelial cells (8 days), hepatocytes (45 days), neurons (2 days). (B) Phase-contrast microscopy of undifferentiated AFSCs. (C) AFSC-derived osteocytes: histochemical staining for alkaline phosphatase. (D) AFSC-derived myocytes: multinucleated myotube-like cells. (E) AFSC-derived adipocytes: intracellular oil aggregation. (F) AFSC-derived endothelial cells: capillary-like structures. (G) AFSC-derived hepatocytes: immunofluorescent staining for albumin. (H) AFSC-derived neurons: immunofluorescent staining for nestin. (See also color plate.) From Delo D.M., De Coppi P., Bartsch G., Jr, Atala A. Amniotic fluid and palcental stem cells. *Methods Enzymol.* 2006; 419: 426–438.

production by AFSCs compared to two-dimensional culture conditions [26]. Culture of AFSCs on nanofibrous scaffolds with morphology similar to that of natural collagen fibers, significantly enhanced AP activity, calcium content, and osteogenic gene expression [27]. These studies also highlighted the importance of bone morphogenetic protein 7 (BMP 7) in the osteogenic induction of AFSCs. Although early in development, recent studies also suggest that exposure to visible light irradiation (470 and 525 nm) may also facilitate the osteogenic differentiation of AFSCs [28].

Myocytes

AFSCs can be induced to form a myogenic phenotype by maintenance on a thin coat of Matrigel in medium supplemented with horse serum and chick embryo extract [29]. To initiate differentiation, the presence of 5-azacytidine in the medium for 24 h is necessary. Phenotypically, AFSCs under these conditions organize themselves into bundles that fuse to form multinucleated cells (Figure 10.2D). These cells express myogenic factor 6 (Myf6), MyoD, and desmin, which are essential for muscle development. The development profile of AFSCs induction towards a myogenic phenotype closely follows a characteristic pattern of gene expression reflecting that seen with embryonic muscle development [30]. Specifically, Myf6 and MyoD gene expression is observed on day 8 and suppressed on day 16, while desmin expression is detected at day 8 and increases after 16 days.

When cultured in myogenic induction medium AFSCs up-regulate the expression of cardiac-specific genes cardiac troponin I and cardiac troponin T, redistribute connexin43, and down-regulate the stem-cell marker SRY box 2 (sox2) [31]. When co-cultured with neonatal rat cardiomyocytes (NRCs), AFSCs formed both mechanical and electrical connections with the NRCs, suggesting that AFSC-derived cardiomyocyte phenotype have the potential to be used as a cardiac cell therapy.

Adipocytes

AFSCs can be induced to form a adipogenic phenotype in culture media containing dexamethasone, 3-isobutyl-1-methylxanthine, insulin, and indomethacin. AFSCs cultured with adipogenic supplements change their morphology from elongated to round within 8 days. This coincides with the accumulation of intracellular droplets (Figure 10.2E). After 16 days in culture, over 95% of the cells contain cytoplasmic lipid-rich vacuoles. Culture with adipogenic supplements also induces the expression of peroxisome proliferation-activated receptor γ-2 (PPAR-γ2), a transcription factor that regulates adipogenesis, and of lipoprotein lipase (LPL). Expression of these genes is detected in progenitor cells under adipogenic conditions, but not in undifferentiated cells. Chen *et al.* confirmed this observation, inducing AFSCs into adipose-like cells containing lipid droplets and expressing adipose specific markers of PPARγ and C/EBPα [32].

Endothelial cells

AFSCs can be induced to form an endothelial phenotype through culture in a medium containing VEGF, hFGF-b, epidermal growth factor, insulin-like growth factor-1, heparin, ascorbic acid, and maintained on gelatin- or Matrigel-coated dishes. Phenotypic changes are observed within 1 week of initiation of the protocol [1]. Differentiated cells stain positively for human-specific endothelial cell surface marker (P1H12), factor VIII (FVIII), and kinase insert domain receptor (KDR), which are specific markers for endothelial cells. These cells also express CD31, von Willebrand factor (vWF), and vascular cell adhesion molecule (VCAM), which are important for cell adhesion and formation of junctions in epithelial cells. Additionally, mRNA and protein levels of CD31 and vWF significantly increased in response to physiological levels (12 dyne/cm^2) of shear force, suggesting that AFSCs acquire endothelial cell characteristics when stimulated by growth factors and shear force. AFSC-derived endothelial cells are able to grow in culture and form capillary-like structures in vitro [33] (Figure 10.2F). After 1 week of endothelial induction AFSCs form small capillary-like structures. After 2 weeks of differentiation, however, clear cord structures are observed, and the length of these structures is increased following exposure to physiological levels of shear force. These studies demonstrate that AFSCs display potential as a cell therapy to treat vascular diseases.

Hepatocytes

For hepatic differentiation, AFSCs can be seeded on Matrigel- or collagen-coated dishes and cultured in media supplemented with hepatocyte growth factor, insulin, oncostatin M, dexamethasone, fibroblast growth factor 4, and monothioglycerol for 45 days [34]. After 7 days of culture, cells exhibit a morphological change, shifting from an elongated to a cobblestone-like appearance. AFSCs maintained under these conditions for 45 days stain positively for albumin (Figure 10.2G) and express the transcription factor hepatocyte nuclear factor 4 (HNF4), the c-Met receptor, the multidrug resistance (MDR) membrane transporter, albumin, and alpha-fetoprotein [1]. In addition, AFS cells differentiated towards a hepatocyte phenotype secrete urea, a characteristic liver-specific function that requires co-ordinated expression of multiple enzymes and specific mitochondrial amino-acid transporters [35]. Zheng *et al.* confirmed the potential of AFSCs to be induced into a hepatic lineage, demonstrating the expression of liver-specific genes and protein for α-fetoprotein (AFP), albumin, cytokeratin-18 (CK18), hepatocyte nuclear factor (HNF1α), CCAAT-enhancer binding protein (C/EBPα), and cytochrome P450 (CYP$_1$A$_1$). Further, AFSC-derived hepatocytes produce and secrete urea and have significantly increased glycogen storage capacity, suggesting that AFSCs may prove to be a valuable and promising source of human hepatocytes for the treatment of liver diseases [36].

Chondrocytes

A chondrogenic phenotype can be induced in AFSCs in vitro by maintaining cells in a three-dimensional alginate hydrogel in medium supplemented with transforming growth factor-beta 1 (TGF-β1), bone morphogenetic protein 2 (BMP2), and insulin-like growth factor-1 (IGF1) [37]. Synthesis of sulfated glycosaminoglycan (sGAG) is an indicator of the formation of a cartilaginous matrix. AFSCs maintained under these conditions synthesize sGAG and produce type II collagen 3 weeks after induction. Further studies have identified that encapsulation of AFSCs in a fibrin hydrogel supplemented with TGF-β3 is superior in inducing a chondrogenic phenotype [38]. Maintenance under these conditions resulted in synthesis of sGAG and type II collagen, as well as cartilage-specific proteins aggrecan, COL II, and SOX9. These results suggest that TGF-β3-loaded fibrin hydrogels are suitable inducers of differentiation of AFSCs into the chondrogenic phenotype.

Neuronal Cells

Mareschi *et al.* have had success in inducing AFSCs into a neuronal phenotype [39]. Cells maintained in neural progenitor maintenance medium (NPMM) supplemented with recombinant hFGF-B, recombinant hEGF, and NSF-1 form cellular aggregates similar to neurospheres after 24 hours in NPMM. After 3 days these floating neurosphere-like clusters analyzed stain-positive for nestin. Following 3 weeks of maintenance under these conditions neurospheres are positive for nestin, GFAP, NSE, and MAP-2. Approximately 75% of total cells express both MAP-2 and GFAP. This is supported by electrophysiological data showing that AFSCs express significant densities of functioning voltage-gated Na channels.

Clinical application of amniotic fluid stem cells

The underlying aim of regenerative medicine is to utilize the available tools to aid in the regeneration of new organs and tissues. The highly multipotent differentiation potential of AFSCs is well established, and much research is now focused on utilizing this potential to generate novel therapies for a range of injuries and diseases. The ability to use AFSCs to generate large numbers of osteocytes, myocytes, adipocytes, endothelial cells, hepatocytes, chondrocytes, and neurons provides a valuable tool for the development of novel cell therapies. This section will discuss the clinical applications of AFSCs that are currently being investigated in pre-clinical animal models of disease.

Bone regeneration

Cell-based therapy for bone regeneration is an emerging technology. AFSCs have the potential to be utilized to treat craniofacial bone defects, spinal or major bone injury. Pre-clinical studies have established that 3D scaffolds containing AFSCs can generate highly mineralized bone tissue 8 weeks after transplantation into mice [1] (Figure 10.3). Micro CT scanning analysis of constructs at 18 weeks post-implantation confirmed the presence of hard tissue within the AFSC-seeded constructs. The density of the tissue-engineered bone found at the sites of implantation was found to be somewhat greater than that of mouse femoral bone. Scaffolds can be designed to produce bone to generate specific craniofacial shapes, or

at densities to facilitate the replacement of major bones damaged by car accidents or battle injuries. Although early in development, these studies demonstrate that AFSCs are a valuable tool for future therapies for bone regeneration.

Myocardial infarction

Myocardial infarction (MI) causes tissue death, and the ability to replace that lost myocardial tissue is an important goal in the field of regenerative medicine. The therapeutic potential of AFSCs for acute myocardial infarction has been demonstrated by Bollini *et al.* in a study in which Wistar rats underwent 30 min of ischemia by ligation of the left anterior descending coronary artery, followed by administration of AFSCs [40]. In this model AFSCs were shown to be cardio-protective, improving myocardial cell survival and decreasing the infarct size. Interestingly, the authors found that similar results were obtained utilizing AFSC-conditioned medium, and identified that AFSCs secrete putative paracrine factors, such as the actin monomer-binding protein thymosin β4 (Tβ4). Other studies have identified superparamagnetic micron-sized iron oxide particle (MPIO)-labeled AFSCs in the mouse heart by high-resolution magnetic resonance imaging (MRI) up to 28 days following injection [10]. This is supported by studies performed by Lee *et al.* who used a methyl-cellulose hydrogel system – enriched with extra-cellular matrices (ECM) – to cultivate AFSCs to form spherically symmetric cell bodies [41]. These AFSC bodies were xenogenically transplanted in the peri-infarct area of an immune-suppressed rat, via direct intramyocardial injection. The authors demonstrated that the retention of cell engraftment was approximately 20%, a significant improvement over disassociated cells. Most importantly, the functional benefits of cell transplantation included the attenuation of the progression of heart failure, improved the global function, and increased the regional wall motion (Figure 10.4). The authors also suggest that the injected AFSC bodies could undergo differentiation into angiogenic or cardiomyogenic lineages in vivo, and contribute to functional benefits by direct regeneration.

Renal disease

Regenerative therapy has the potential to cure certain hereditary forms of kidney disease and acute kidney

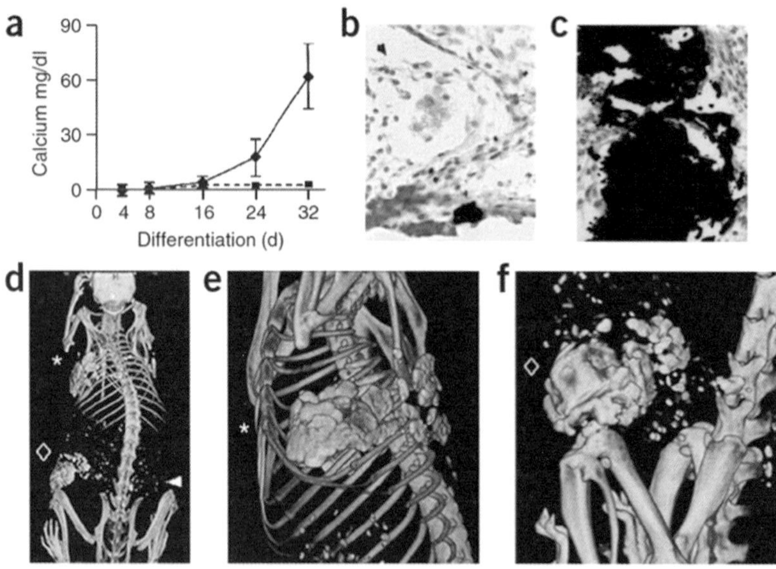

Figure 10.3 Tissue-engineered bone from AFSCs. (a) Measurement of calcium levels in AFSCs maintained in osteogenic differentiation medium (solid line) and undifferentiated AFSCs (broken line) in vitro. (b) Von Kossa staining of unseeded alginate/collagen scaffold recovered 8 weeks after implantation. (c) Von Kossa staining of AFSC seeded alginate/collagen scaffold recovered 8 weeks after implantation; black staining indicates strong mineralization. (d–f) Micro CT scan of mouse 18 weeks after implantation of printed constructs. Arrow: region of implantation of control scaffold without AFSCs. Asterisk and Diamond: scaffolds seeded with AFSCs. (See also color plate.) From De Coppi, P., Bartsch G., Jr., Siddiqui, M.M. *et al.* Isolation of amniotic stem cell lines with potential for therapy. *Nature Medicine.* 2007; 25: 100–106.

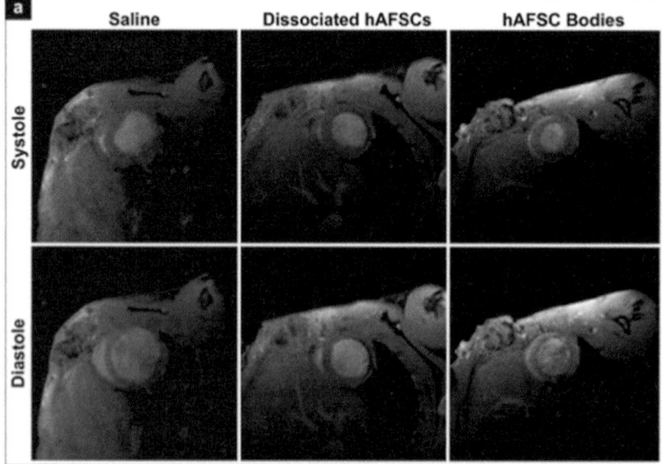

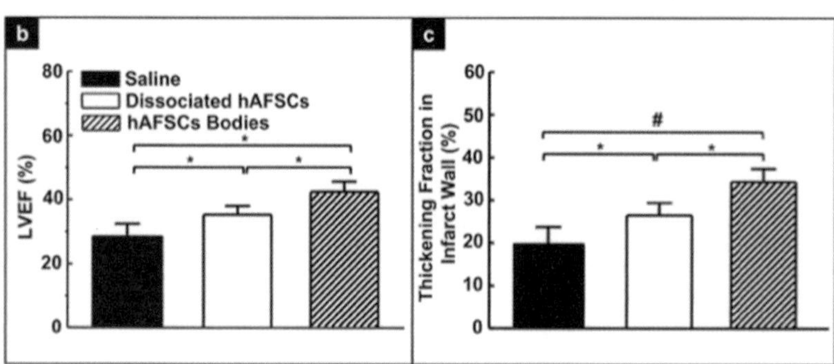

Figure 10.4 MRI functional showing how AFSCs attenuate the progression of heart failure, improve the global function, and increase the regional wall motion. (a) Increased left ventricular (LV) chamber dimensions of saline-injected hearts in both end-diastolic and end-systolic phases, whereas transplantation of dissociated AFSCs or AFSC bodies into the infarcted recipients attenuated the changes in LV geometry. (b) Greater left ventricular ejection fraction (LVEF) in rats injected with AFSC bodies compared to rats injected with dissociated AFSCs or saline. (c) In the AFSC-body group, the infarcted-wall thickening fraction was significantly greater than those hearts treated with dissociated AFSCs or saline, suggesting a superior regional contractile function in the infarct region. From Lee, W.Y., Wei, H.J., Lin, W.W. *et al.* Enhancement of cell retention and functional benefits in myocardial infarction using human amniotic-fluid stem-cell bodies enriched with endogenous ECM. *Biomaterials.* 2011; 32: 5558–5567.

injury, and could eliminate the need for dialysis and/or kidney transplants in some patients with end-stage kidney disease. Perin *et al.* have shown that AFSCs can contribute to renal development both in vitro and in vivo [11,42]. These studies demonstrated that when injected into the primordia of the developing kidney, AFSCs divide and spread throughout the organ and contribute to the embryonic tubular and glomerular structures. These cells express kidney-specific markers such as Zona occludens-1, claudin, and glial-derived neurotrophic factor (GDNF). In a mouse model of acute tubular necrosis (ATN), AFSCs integrate into the damaged tubules, and provide a protective effect, ameliorating ATN in the acute injury phase. AFSC-treated animals showed decreased creatinine and BUN blood levels and a decrease in the number of damaged tubules. This beneficial effect with AFSCs was also correlated with significant increases in proliferative activity of tubular epithelial cells, decreased cast formation, and decreased apoptosis of tubular epithelial cells. Integrated cells expressed PAX2, NPHS1 dolicholus biflorus, and peanut agglutinin, indicating AFSCs are able to commit toward renal differentiation in vivo. Interestingly, the authors demonstrate that the timing of AFSC administration is critical to the protective effect, stating that if injury is already established the damage is not attenuated. This suggests that the mechanism of action may be through protecting damaged epithelial tubular cells, preventing apoptosis. These studies also show evidence of potent immunomodulatory effects of AFSCs that appear to influence the local immune response to prevent or promote the resolution of tissue damage.

Neural regeneration

A major goal of regenerative medicine is to ameliorate irreversible destruction of brain tissue by utilizing stem cells to control the process of neurogenesis. The engraftment and survival of AFSCs within the rodent brain has been demonstrated in the "twitcher" mouse model of neurological disease [1]. These mice are deficient in the lysosomal enzyme galactocerebrosidase and undergo extensive neurodegeneration and neurological deterioration, initiating with dysfunction of oligodendrocytes. AFSCs implanted directly into the lateral ventricles of the developing brain of a newborn mouse survive and integrate into the fetal mouse brain, with over 70% of administered cells surviving 2 months following implantation. AFSCs

were present in a variety of brain regions, including periventricular areas, the hippocampus, and the olfactory bulb (Figure 10.5). Further studies have demonstrated the potential of a combination of AFSCs and granulocyte-colony stimulating factor (G-CSF) to improve peripheral nerve injury by inherited neurotrophic factor secretion [43]. In this study, peripheral nerve injury was produced in Sprauge–Dawley rats by crushing the left sciatic nerve using a vessel clamp. AFSCs were embedded in fibrin glue and delivered to the injured site concurrently with intraperitoneal injections of G-CSF over 7 days. Increased nerve myelination and improved motor function was observed in treated animals. The authors proposed AFSCs promoted neural regeneration though the suppression of apoptotic death and the attenuation of inflammatory response. Rehni *et al.* highlighted the potency of AFSCs in a mouse model of ischemic stroke [44]. In this model, middle cerebral artery occlusion and reperfusion produces ischemia and reperfusion-induced cerebral injury, and induces behavioral deficits in mice. Behavioral changes included markedly impaired memory, motor coordination, sensorimotor ability, and somatosensory functions. Intracerebroventricular administration of AFSCs had a significant neuroprotective effect, reversing the focal cerebral ischemia–reperfusion-induced behavioral deficits observed in untreated mice. These studies suggest that AFSCs may have important clinical applications for the treatment of degenerative or behavioral brain disorders, paving the way for potential treatments for disease such as stroke, Parkinson's disease, Alzheimer's disease, and spinal injuries.

Lung regeneration

Clinical applications for cell therapy for lung regeneration involve the repair of defects in the airway wall, which can result from tumors, trauma, or diseases that are associated with epithelial damage. AFSCs show the potential to be utilized in the treatment of diseases such as cystic fibrosis, acute respiratory distress syndrome, chronic obstructive lung disease, pulmonary fibrosis, pulmonary edema, and pulmonary hypertension. Carrero *et al.* demonstrated that AFSCs integrate into the epithelium of embryonic mouse lung and express the early human differentiation marker thyroid transcription factor 1 (TTF1) [45]. In the adult lung, AFSCs integrated into pulmonary

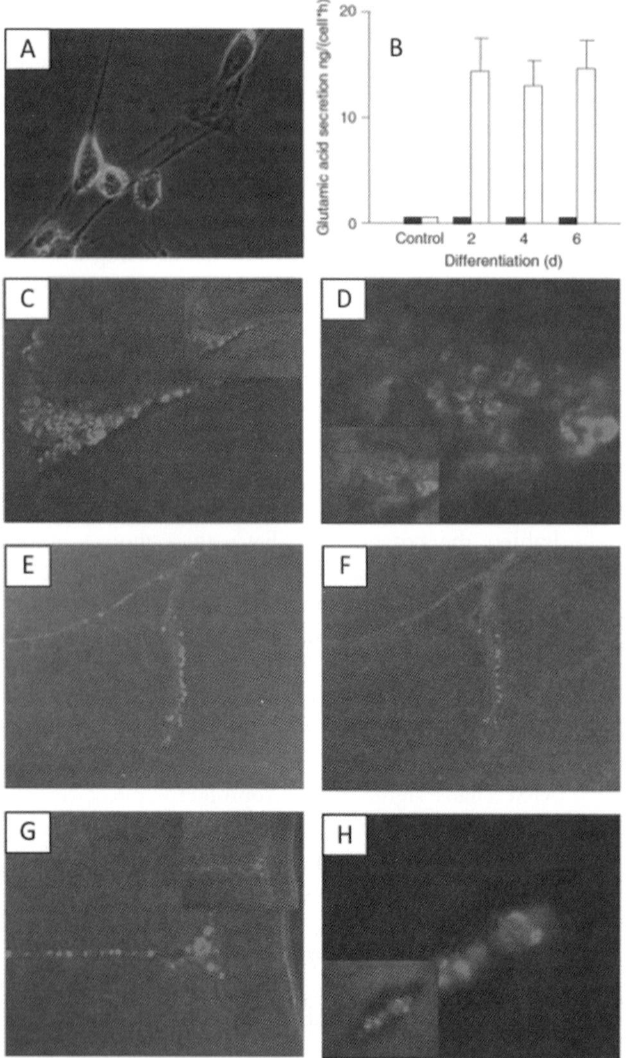

Figure 10.5 Neuronal differentiation and engraftment of AFSCs. (A) Phase-contrast micrograph showing cells after second stage of neurogenic differentiation under conditions biasing for production of dopaminergic neurons. (B) Secretion of neurotransmitter glutamic acid in response to potassium ions in cells after neurogenic differentiation in the presence of NGF (open bars) and after maintenance of undifferentiated cells in standard growth medium (closed bars). (C–H) Engraftment of neurogenetically differentiated human AFSCs 1 month after injection into the brain of newborn twitcher mice. Red staining (human mitochondrial protein) shows human cells. Blue staining (DAPI) shows cell nuclei. (C) Lateral ventricle. (D) Higher magnification view of lateral ventricle. (E) Periventricular area and hippocampus. (F) Same field as E, with DAPI staining superimposed. (G) Third ventricle. (H) Olfactory bulb. (See also color plate.) Modified from De Coppi, P., Bartsch, G., Jr., Siddiqui, M.M. *et al.* Isolation of amniotic stem cell lines with potential for therapy. *Nature Biotechnology.* 2007; 25: 100–106.

epithelium following oxygen- or naphthalene-induced injury and expressed markers associated with lung epithelium such as TTF 1 and surfactant protein C (SP-C) (Figure 10.6). Interestingly, following naphthalene injury, which specifically destroys Clara cells that express cytochrome P450, AFSCs accumulated in the upper airway, increased numbers compared with after oxygen treatment. This behavior suggests a certain level of plasticity of AFSCs in responding to different types of lung damage. Further work by this group investigated the role of AFSCs in pulmonary wound healing [46]. These studies identified mechanisms whereby damage to the pulmonary epithelium promotes the migration of AFSCs to the wound site, where they are induced to secrete macrophage migration inhibitory factor (MIF), and plasminogen activator inhibitor-1 (PAI-1), which promote epithelial wound repair. These studies also detected the integration of AFSCs into the pulmonary epithelium and their production of SP-C. These important studies highlight the potential of AFSCs for clinical and bioengineering applications for patients with lung disease.

Blood and immune system regeneration

Ditadi *et al.* have demonstrated that AFSCs display multilineage hematopoietic differentiation potential

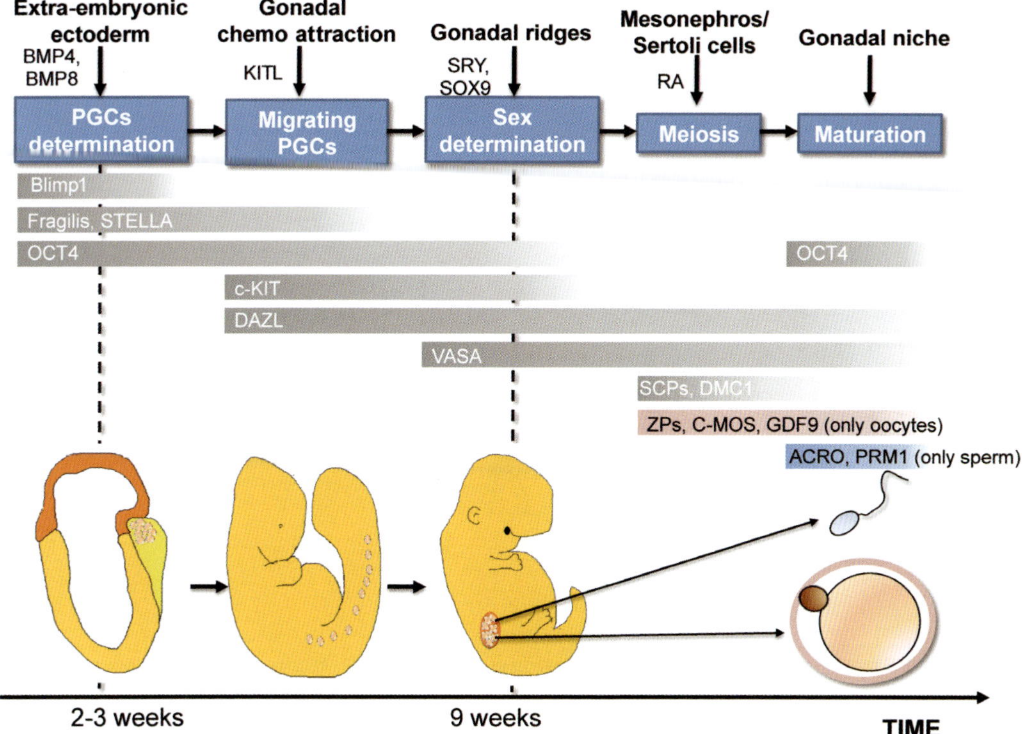

Figure 2.1 Schematic representation of the main developmental stages of human germline differentiation in vivo. Stages of germline differentiation are indicated within boxes. Tissue and/or cellular inducers with their signaling molecules are indicated above each differentiation stage and the specific molecular markers are indicated below.

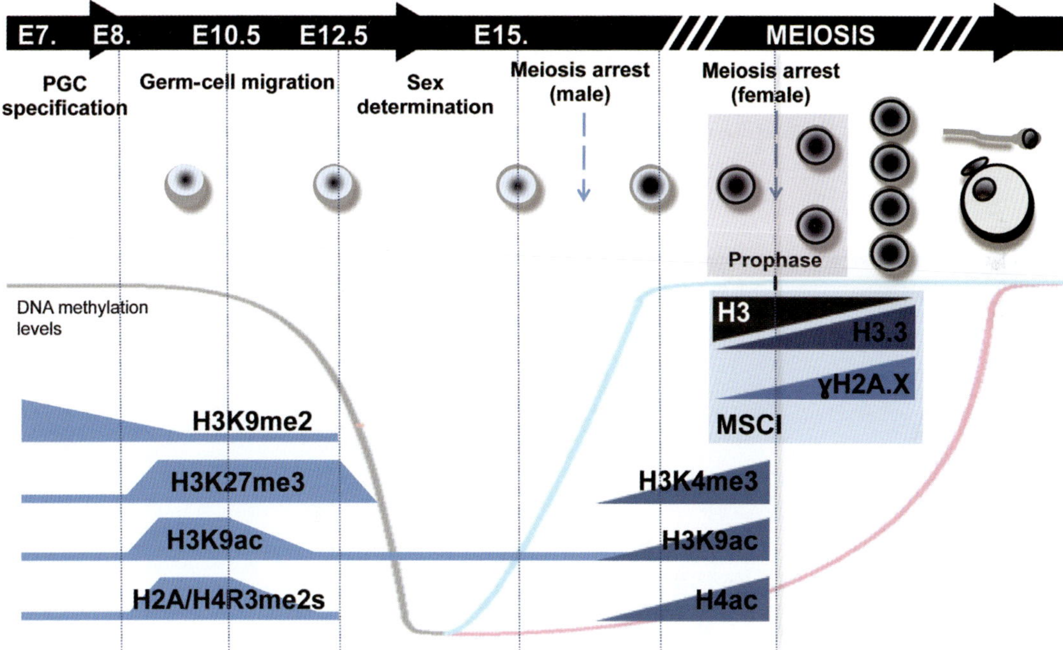

Figure 2.2 Major epigenetic changes during germ-cell differentiation in mice. DNA methylation changes decrease when germ cells start to migrate and there is a complete erasure of DNA methylation patterns once PGCs have entered the gonadal crests. In males (blue line) the DNA methylation pattern recovers before entering meiosis, while in females (pink) they are recovered during meiosis. Levels in histone modification change during germ-cell reprogramming from somatic cells (see text). Prophase I is the main checkpoint. During meiosis, there is a substitution of H3 by its variant H3.3, and the phosphorylation of H2AX is needed for correct meiotic progression, mainly in MSCI formation (see text).

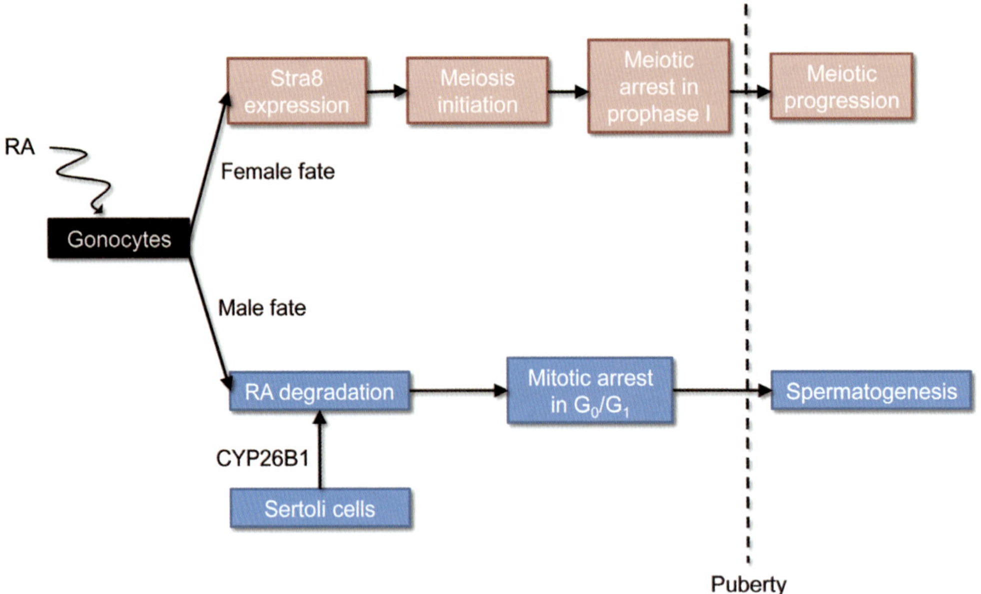

Figure 2.3 Model explanation of the divergent time point of meiotic initiation in males and females in response to the RA signaling from the adjacent mesonephros.

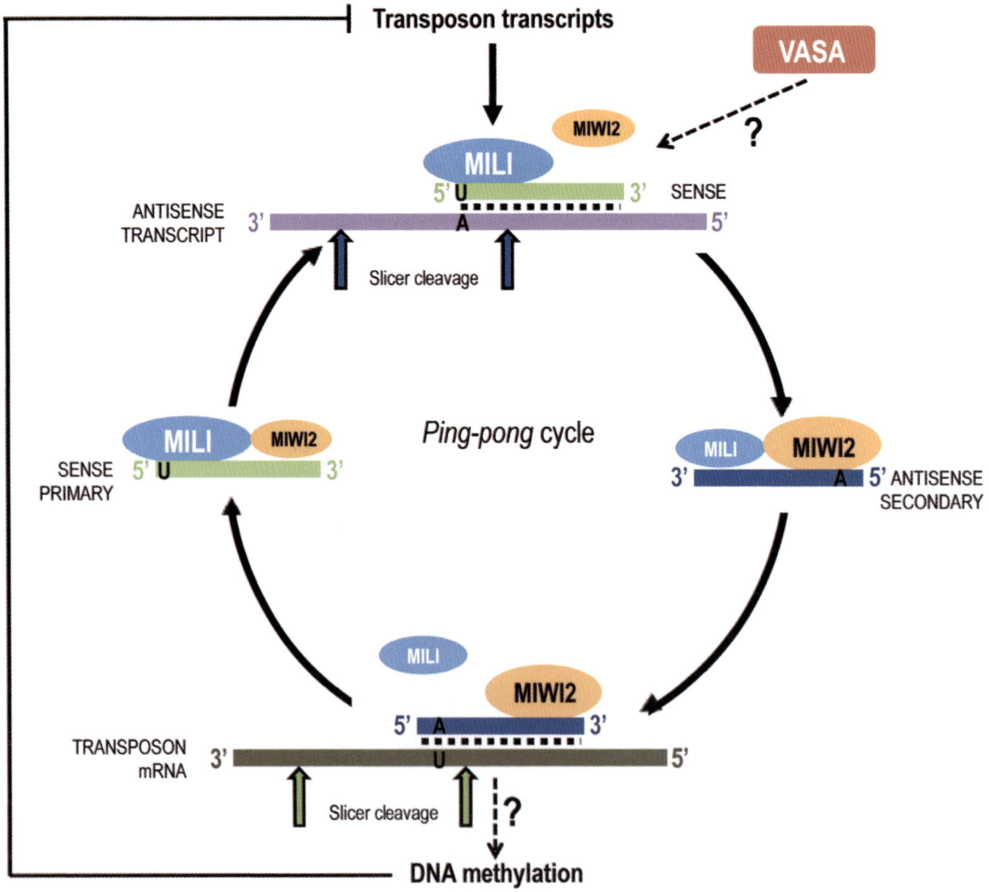

Figure 2.5 First class piRNA processing in mammals. Primary processing of mRNAs of active transposable elements are the source of sense piRNA that associate to MILI and enter a ping-pong cycle where MIWI2 binds secondary antisense piRNA. Antisense piRNA are the responsible of DNA methylation at transposable elements, even though this mechanism remains unclear. VASA may participate in promoting this cycle (see text), although the mechanism is not clear.

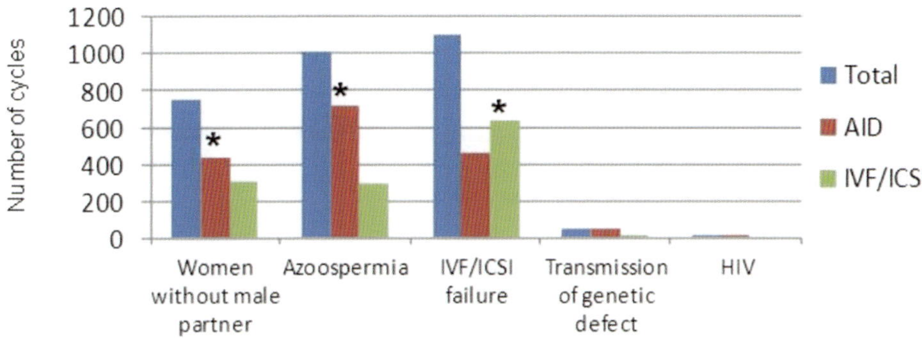

Figure 3.1 Number of cycles with donor sperm depending on the ART procedure (AID vs. IVF/ICSI) and clinical indications for donor sperm. The distribution of the proportions were compared by chi-square analysis. * denotes a statistically significant difference between proportions presented in AID vs. IVF $p < 0.0001$.

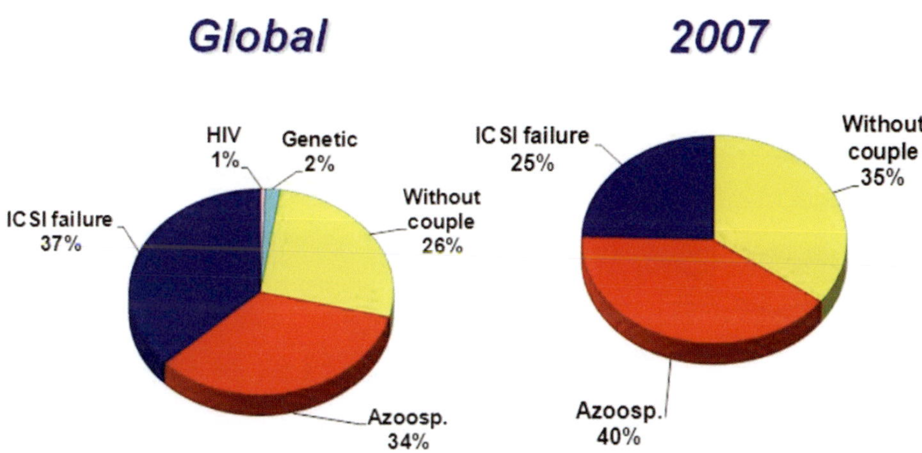

Figure 3.2 Distribution of the clinical indications for sperm donation. In the left graph the global proportion of each indication is represented (from 1999 to 2007). In the right graph the proportions observed in the last year are represented. The distribution of the proportions was compared by chi-square analysis. A statistically significant difference in the proportions presented in the two distributions was observed. $p < 0.0001$.

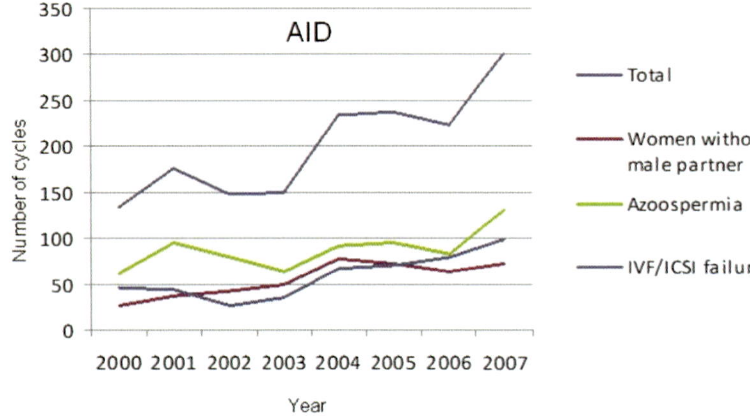

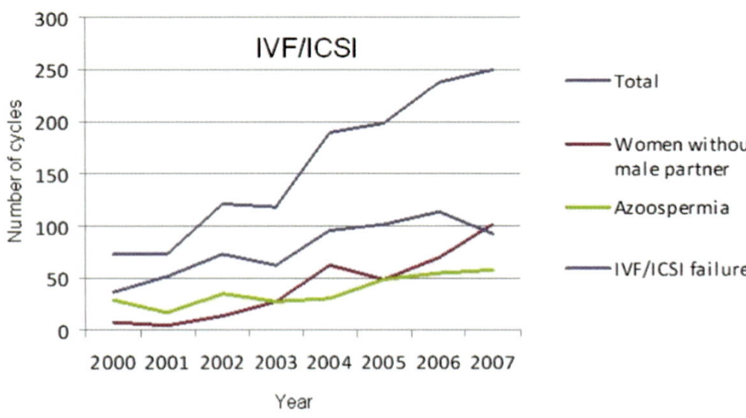

Figure 3.3 Number of cycles with donor sperm depending on the clinical indication in the ART procedure. These values are presented in a linear fashion for the years from 2000 to 2007. The upper panel represents the AID cycles and the lower panel the IVF/ICSI cycles.

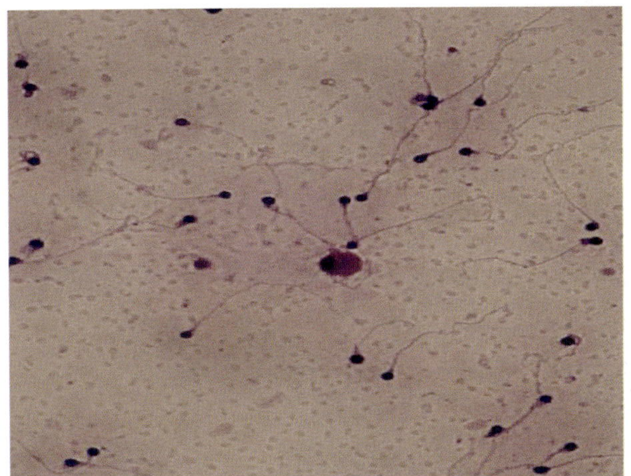

Figure 3.4 Hematoxylin-eosin staining of ejaculated spermatozoa from a patient suffering globozoospermia. Magnification 400×.

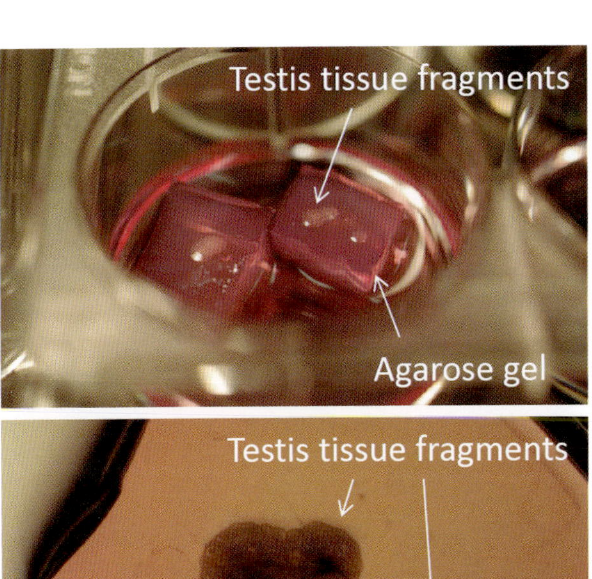

Figure 4.1 Testis tissue culture on agarose gel.

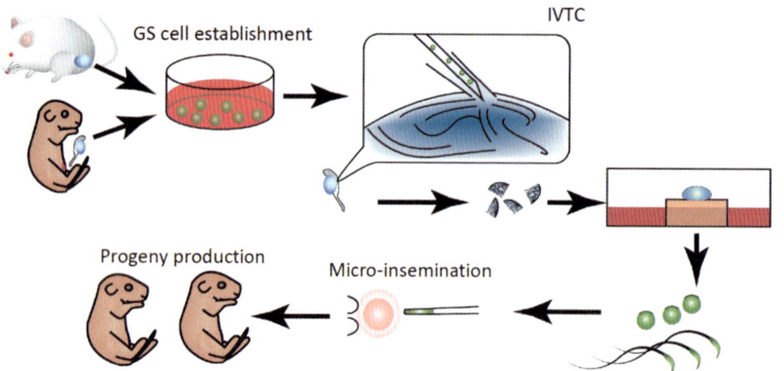

Figure 4.2 Experimental scheme of in-vitro transplantation and culture method.

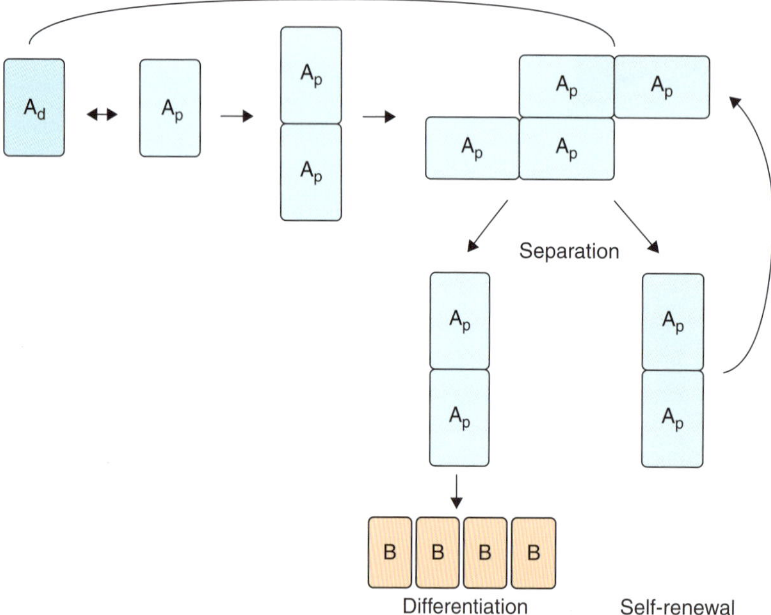

Figure 5.1 Schematic representation of the A_d/A_p model for primate spermatogonial differentiation.

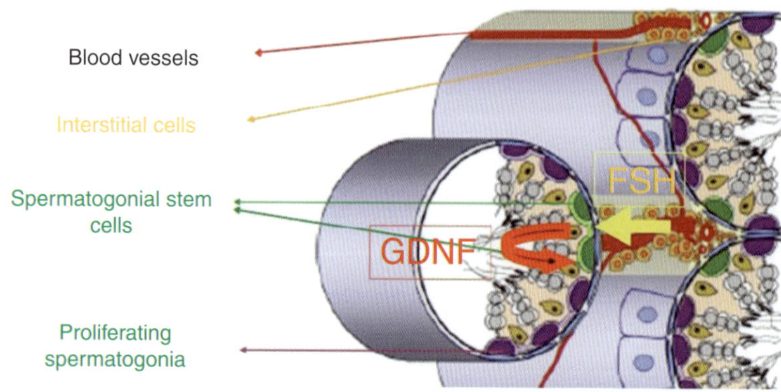

Figure 5.2 The spermatogonial stem-cell niche. Follicle-stimulating hormone is produced in the pituitary gland and is transported to the testes through the blood. FSH will bind to membrane receptors on Sertoli cells in close proximity to the interstitial tissue. Activation of the receptor will lead to the secretion of glial-cell-line-derived neurotropic factor. This factor binds to the GFRα1 receptor on SSCs and stimulates self-renewal. Sertoli cells located further away from the blood vessels will bind less FSH, resulting in a lower expression of glial-cell-line-derived neurotropic factor. SSCs in these areas are thus less stimulated to self-renew and will start differentiation.

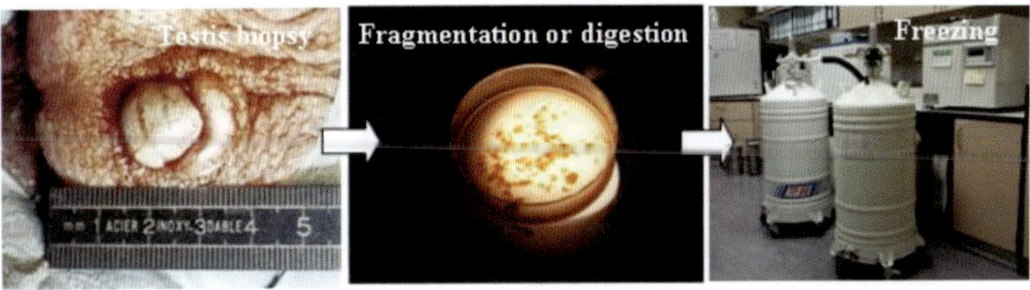

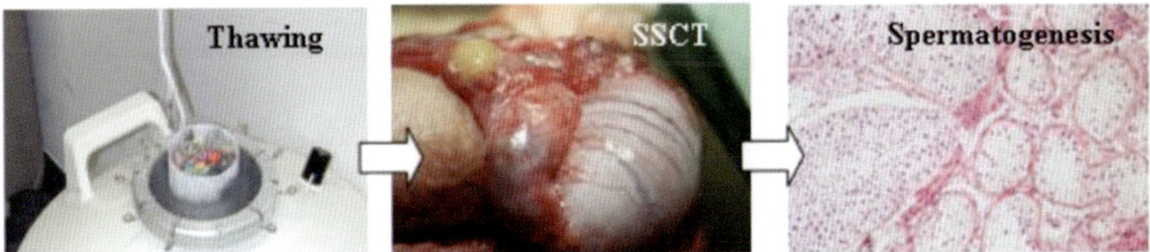

Figure 5.3 Spermatogonial stem-cell transplantation has been suggested as a method for fertility restoration after SSC loss. Before the onset of gonadotoxic treatment or before stem-cell loss occurs, testicular tissue is removed and cryopreserved. When the patient has been cured, or when the child's wish becomes apparent, the thawed tissue can be transplanted into the remaining testis. Although successful in rodents, in humans, the efficiency of spermatogonial stem-cell transplantation remains to be proven.

(A)

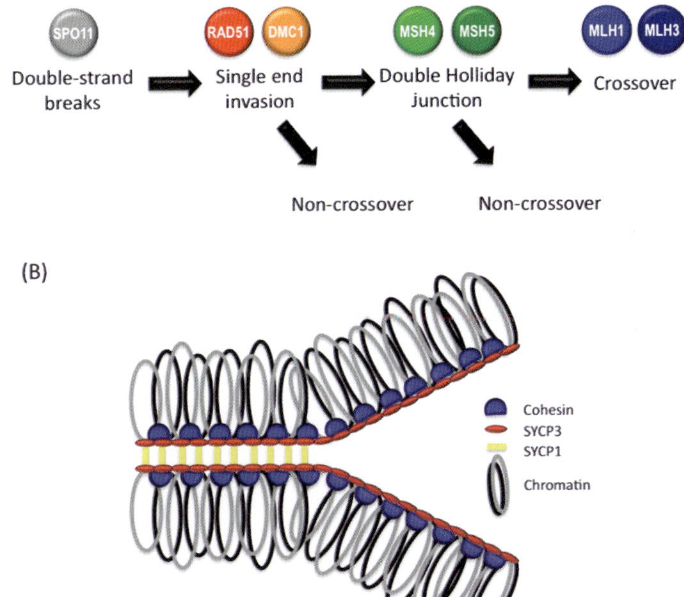

Figure 6.1 Recombination and synapsis: the defining events of meiotic prophase. (A) Overview of the main events and some of the major proteins involved in the class I meiotic recombination pathway. Meiotic recombination is initiated by the formation of programmed double-strand breaks (DSBs) by a complex of proteins, including the topoisomerase-like protein SPO11. The single-stranded DNA is then resected and single end invasion (SEI) is facilitated by the strand invasion proteins RAD51 and DMC1. This leads to formation of a D-loop and, following DNA synthesis and extension of the D-loop, an intermediate structure, a double Holliday junction (dHJ) is formed and is stabilized by the mismatch repair (MMR) proteins MSH4 and MSH5. The dHJ is resolved into a crossover by multiple proteins, including MMR proteins MLH1 and MLH3. Note that non-crossover products can also form from recombination events, either at an early step in the pathway or as an alternative mechanism of resolution of the dHJ. (B) The synaptonemal complex (SC). Meiotic recombination occurs in the context of the SC, a meiosis-specific structure that binds the homologous chromosomes to one another. Several of the protein components of the SC are now known, including SYCP3 (which contributes to the outer, axial elements of the SC) and SYCP1 (which localizes to the central region, and helps to "zipper" the homologous chromosomes together). Sister chromatid cohesion proteins (e.g., SMC1β, REC8, STAG3, and SMC3) form an initial meiotic scaffold and complex with the axial element proteins as part of the mature SC.

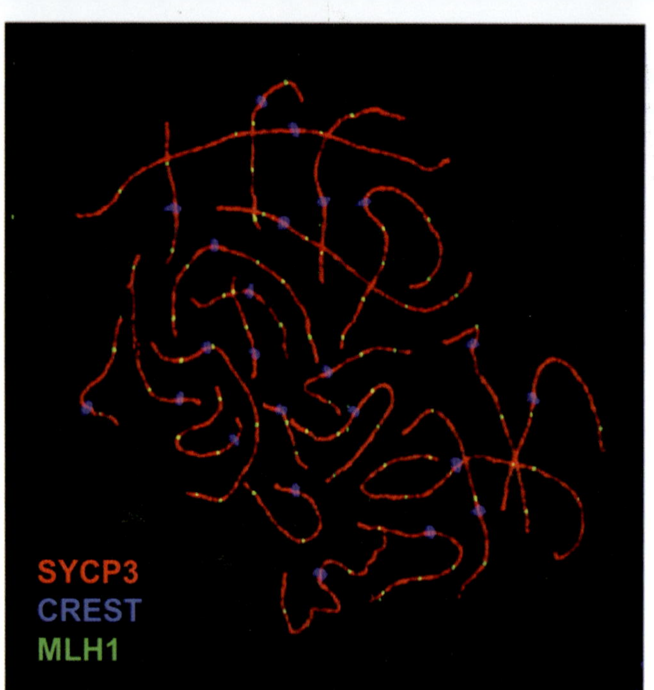

Figure 6.2 Representative image of a human pachytene stage oocyte. Antibodies against SYCP3 (in red) identify the synaptonemal complexes of the 23 pairs of homologs, antibodies against MLH1 (in green) the locations of crossovers, and CREST antisera (in blue) the centromeric regions.

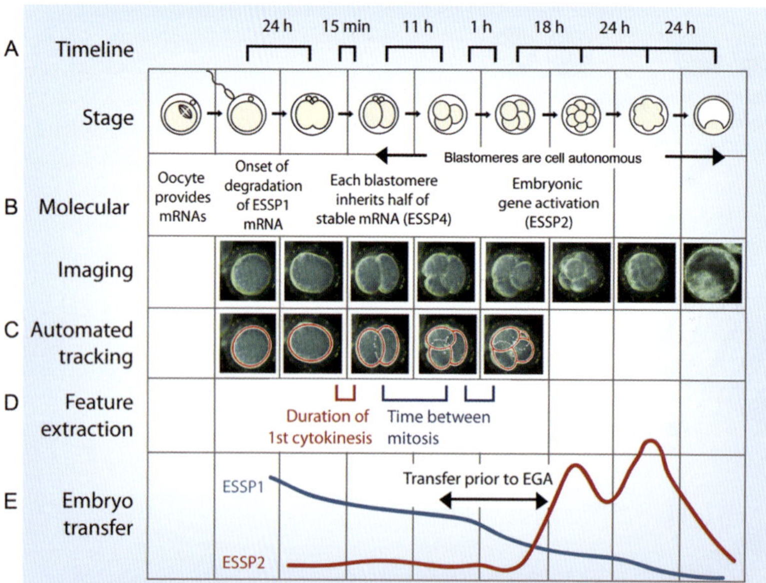

Figure 7.1 Imaging human embryo development and predicting developmental potential. (A) Timeline of human embryo development from the zygote to the blastocyst stage, highlighting critical times between stages that predict successful development. (B) Time-lapse images of human embryo development obtained. Essentially, imaging was performed on multiple systems that consisted of custom-built three-channel miniature microscope arrays that were accommodated in standard incubators, equipped with white-light Luxeon LEDs and apertures for darkfield illumination. Darkfield allowed optimal contrast of cell membranes for automated tracking and also decreased light intensity to a level significantly lower than the light typically used on an ART microscope due to the low power of the LEDs (relative to a typical 100W halogen bulb) and high sensitivity of camera sensors (estimated light exposure is equivalent to roughly 1 minute of exposure under a typical assisted-reproduction microscope). Images were captured at a 1 second exposure time every 5 minutes for up to 5 or 6 days, resulting in approximately 24 minutes of continuous light exposure. (C) Automated tracking demonstrates modeling via computer algorithms to predict success or failure. (D) Critical features that influence developmental success include the duration of first cytokinesis, the time between the first and second mitotic division, and the synchronicity of appearance of the third and fourth blastomeres. (E) Potential application in prediction of embryo developmental potential in ART. (From [6].)

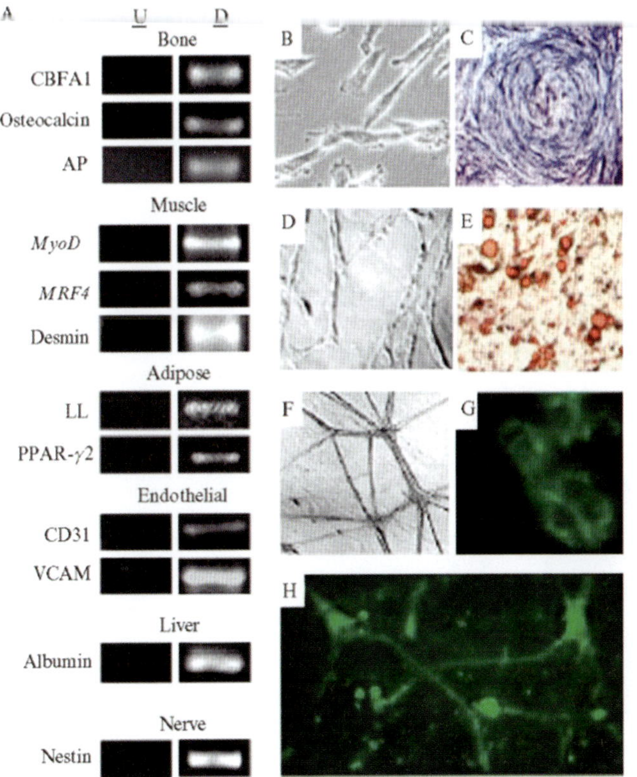

Figure 10.2 Multistage differentiation of AFSCs in vitro. (A) RT-PCR analysis of differentiation. U: Undifferentiated cells. D: Cells maintained under conditions for differentiation to: osteocytes (8 days), adipocytes (16 days), endothelial cells (8 days), hepatocytes (45 days), neurons (2 days). (B) Phase-contrast microscopy of undifferentiated AFSCs. (C) AFSC-derived osteocytes: histochemical staining for alkaline phosphatase. (D) AFSC-derived myocytes: multinucleated myotube-like cells. (E) AFSC-derived adipocytes: intracellular oil aggregation. (F) AFSC-derived endothelial cells: capillary-like structures. (G) AFSC-derived hepatocytes: immunofluorescent staining for albumin. (H) AFSC-derived neurons: immunofluorescent staining for nestin. From Delo D.M., De Coppi P., Bartsch G., Jr, Atala A. Amniotic fluid and palcental stem cells. *Methods Enzymol.* 2006; 419: 426–438.

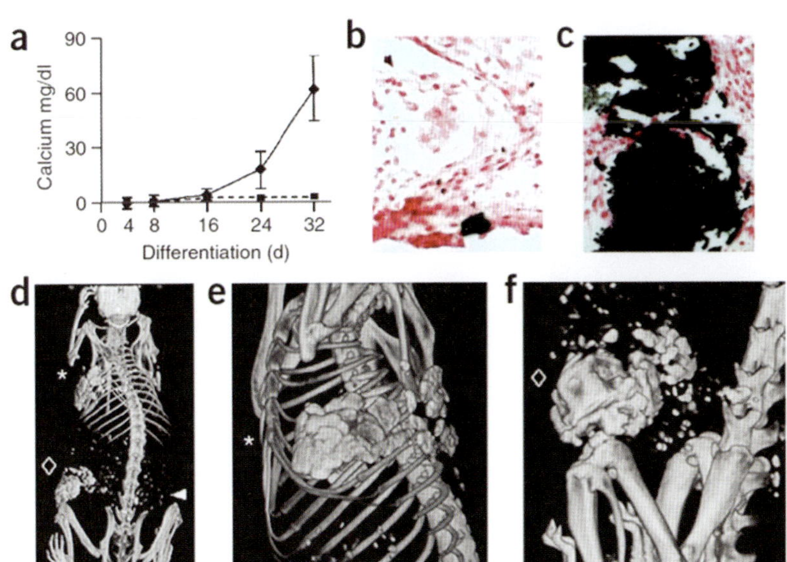

Figure 10.3 Tissue-engineered bone from AFSCs. (a) Measurement of calcium levels in AFSCs maintained in osteogenic differentiation medium (solid line) and undifferentiated AFSCs (broken line) in vitro. (b) Von Kossa staining of unseeded alginate/collagen scaffold recovered 8 weeks after implantation. (c) Von Kossa staining of AFSC seeded alginate/collagen scaffold recovered 8 weeks after implantation; black staining indicates strong mineralization. (d–f) Micro CT scan of mouse 18 weeks after implantation of printed constructs. Arrow: region of implantation of control scaffold without AFSCs. Asterisk and Diamond: scaffolds seeded with AFSCs. From De Coppi, P., Bartsch G., Jr., Siddiqui, M.M. *et al.* Isolation of amniotic stem cell lines with potential for therapy. Nature Medicine. 2007; 25: 100–106.

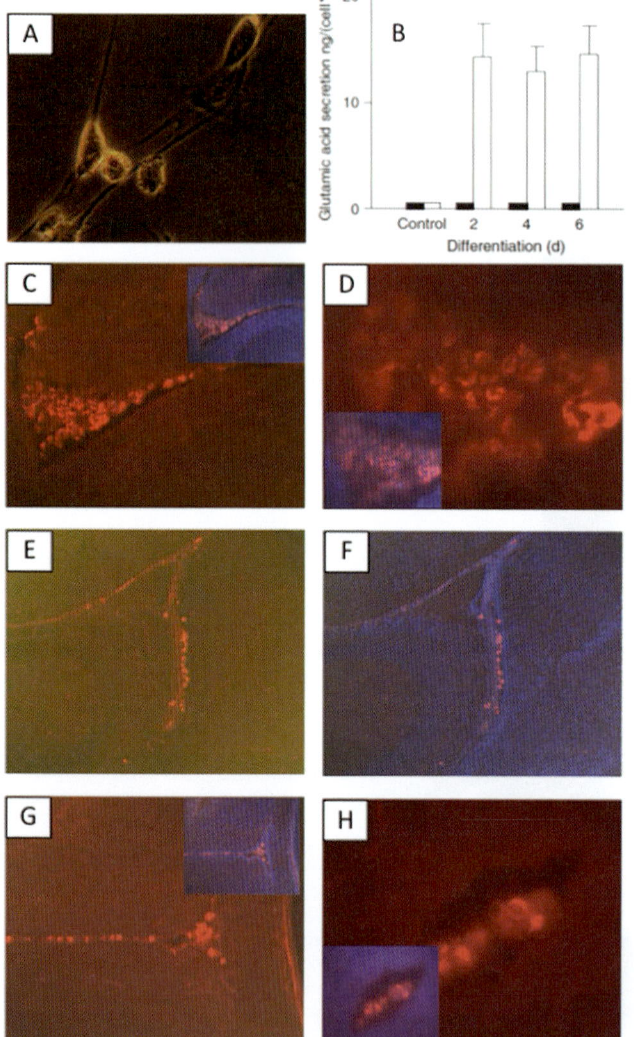

Figure 10.5 Neuronal differentiation and engraftment of AFSCs. (A) Phase contrast micrograph showing cells after second stage of neurogenic differentiation under conditions biasing for production of dopaminergic neurons. (B) Secretion of neurotransmitter glutamic acid in response to potassium ions in cells after neurogenic differentiation in the presence of NGF (open bars) and after maintenance of undifferentiated cells in standard growth medium (closed bars). (C–H) Engraftment of neurogenetically differentiated humn AFSCs 1 month after injection into the brain of newborn twitcher mice. Red staining (human mitochondrial protein) shows human cells. Blue staining (DAPI) shows cell nuclei. (C) Lateral ventricle. (D) Higher magnification view of lateral ventricle. (E) Periventricular area and hippocampus. (F) Same field as E, with DAPI staining superimposed. (G) Third ventricle. (H) Olfactory bulb. Modified from De Coppi, P., Bartsch, G., Jr., Siddiqui, M.M. *et al.* Isolation of amniotic stem cell lines with potential for therapy. *Nature Biotechnology.* 2007; 25: 100–106.

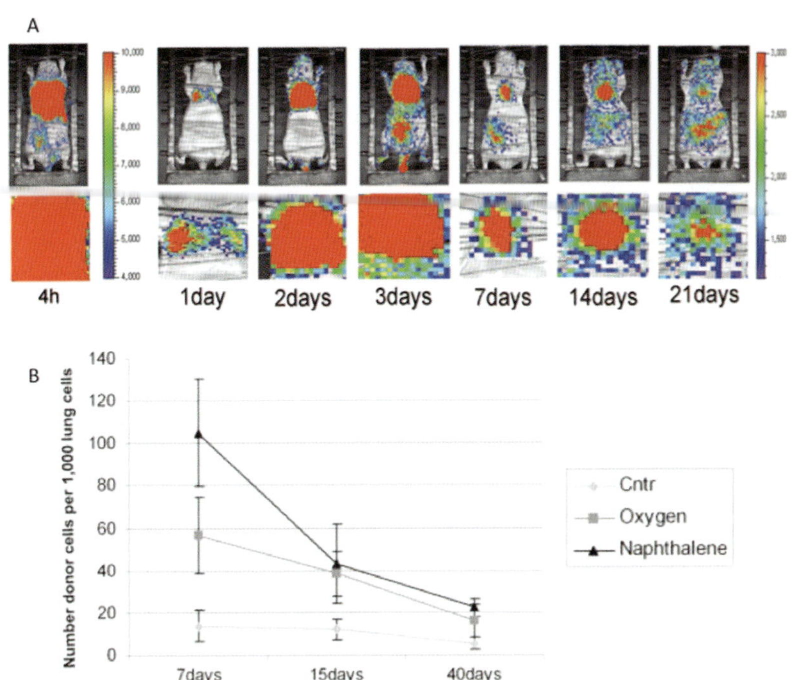

Figure 10.6 AFSCs integrate into adult mouse lung after tail vein injection. (A) Bioluminescence of mice injected with AFSCs expressing luciferase. Magnified views of the thorax are shown below each panel. Relatively intense AFSC luciferase bioluminescence was detected shortly after tail vein injection. After 21 days AFSCs were still detected at the lung position. (B) Lung injury increases the level of integration of AFSCs. Absolute quantification of Sry genes on the Y chromosome by real-time polymerase chain reaction. At 7 days the number of AFSCs was significantly elevated in naphthalene-injured trachea and oxygen-injured parenchyma compared with uninjured control lung. At 15 days naphthalene-injured and oxygen-injured mice reached similar numbers of AFSCs compared with uninjured control lung. Modified from Carraro, G., Perin, L., Sedrakyan, S. *et al.* Human amniotic fluid stem cells can integrate and differentiate into epithelial lung lineages. *Stem Cells.* 2008; 26: 2902–2911.

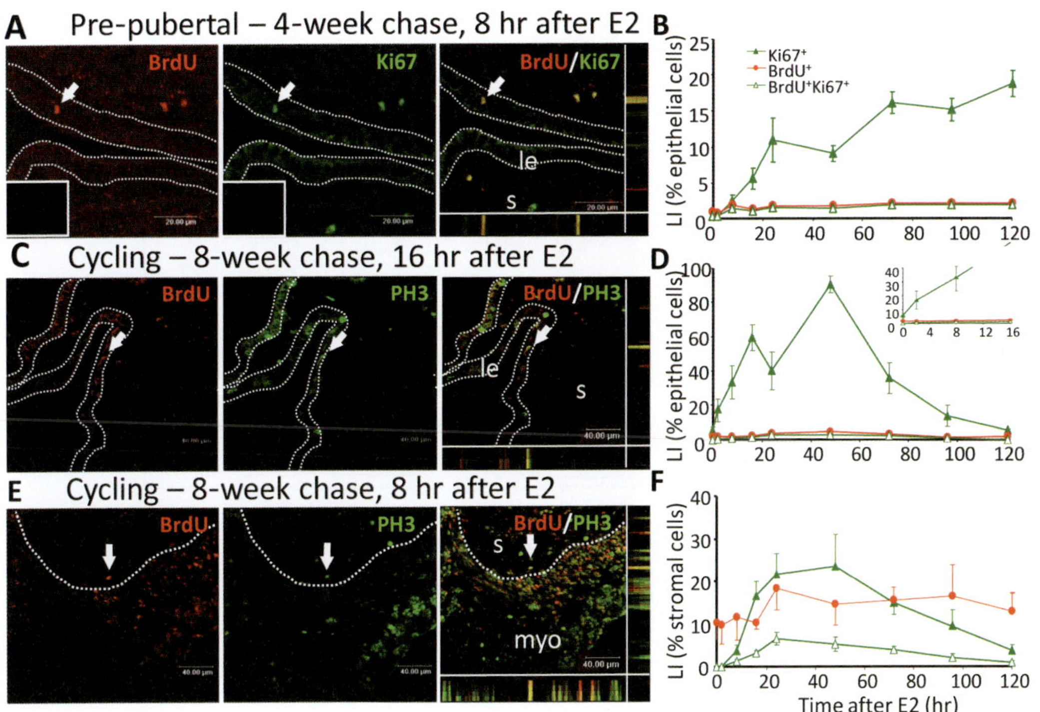

Figure 11.1 Label-retaining cell proliferation in estrogen-stimulated endometrial regeneration in ovariectomized mice. Post-natal day 3 mice were labelled with BrdU for three days and the label chased for (A, B) 4 weeks (pre-pubertal) or (C – F) 8 weeks (cycling). Mice were then ovariectomized and the endometrium allowed to regress for 14 days, after which a single injection of 17β-estradiol was given and uteri were collected from 2–120 h later (B, D, F). Sections were double immunofluorescently labeled with BrdU (A, C, E, left panels, red) and the (A) proliferation marker, Ki-67 (A, middle panel, green) or the (C, E) mitotic marker, phosphorylated histone H3 (PH3; C, E, middle panels, green) and examined by confocal microscopy. The right panels (A, C, E) show *x/z* and *y/z* planes obtained by optical sectioning on the far right and beneath the merged images and demonstrate true nuclear co-localisation of both markers. Insets in (A) negative control IgG. Arrows, (A) proliferating or (C) mitotic epithelial and (E) mitotic stromal LRC. Labeling indices (LIs) (B, D, E) of endometrial epithelial cells (D, E) for Ki-67 for 40-week chased pre-pubertal (B) and 8-week chased cycling (D) mice (inset first 8 h). LIs of stromal cells (F) for Ki-67 for 8-week chased cycling mice. E2, 17β-estradiol; le, luminal epithelium; myo, myometrium; s, stroma. Scale bars 40 μm. Adapted and reproduced with kind permission from SAGE, copyright 2012. Chan *et al.* Role of label-retaining cells in estrogen-induced endometrial regeneration. *Reproductive Sciences* 19: 102–114 [32].

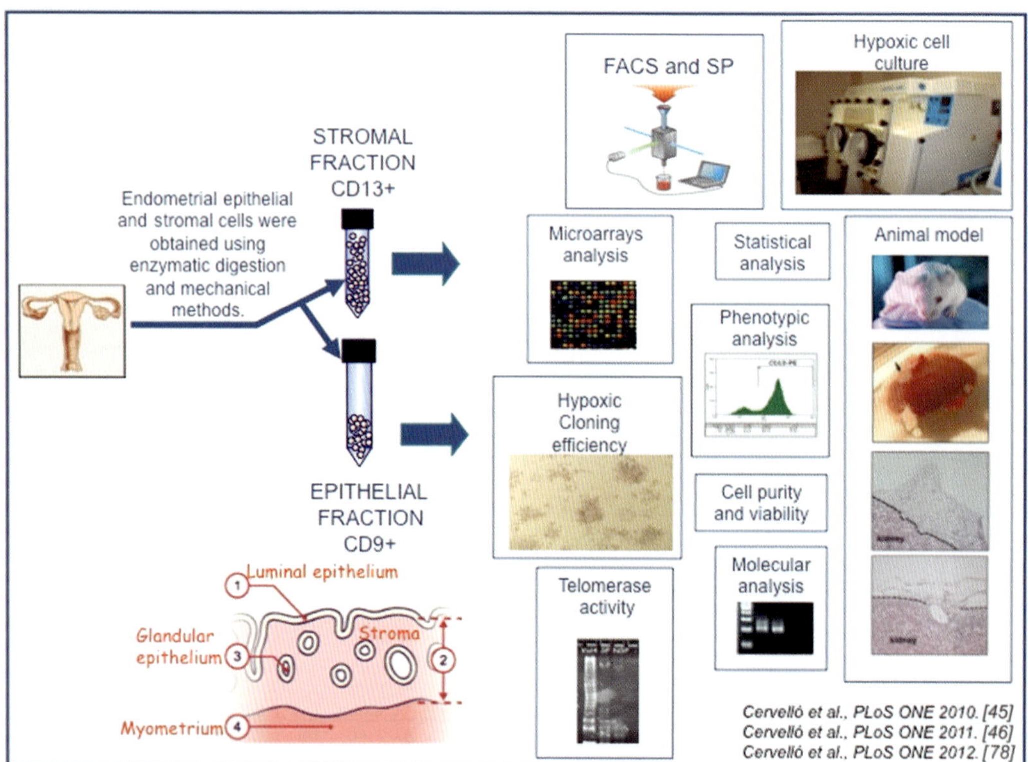

Figure 11.2 Schematic detailing the procedures used for the identification, characterization, and isolation of side population cells from human endometrium. After purification of human endometrial epithelial and stromal cells several assays were performed in order to confirm stem-cell features of this subset of cells, including molecular analysis (PCR, microarrays, telomerase activity), cell characterization (flow cytometry, hypoxic cell culture, cell cloning), in vitro differentiation (adipogenic and osteogenic lineages), and in vivo models (reconstruction in subcutaneous tissues and beneath the kidney capsule).

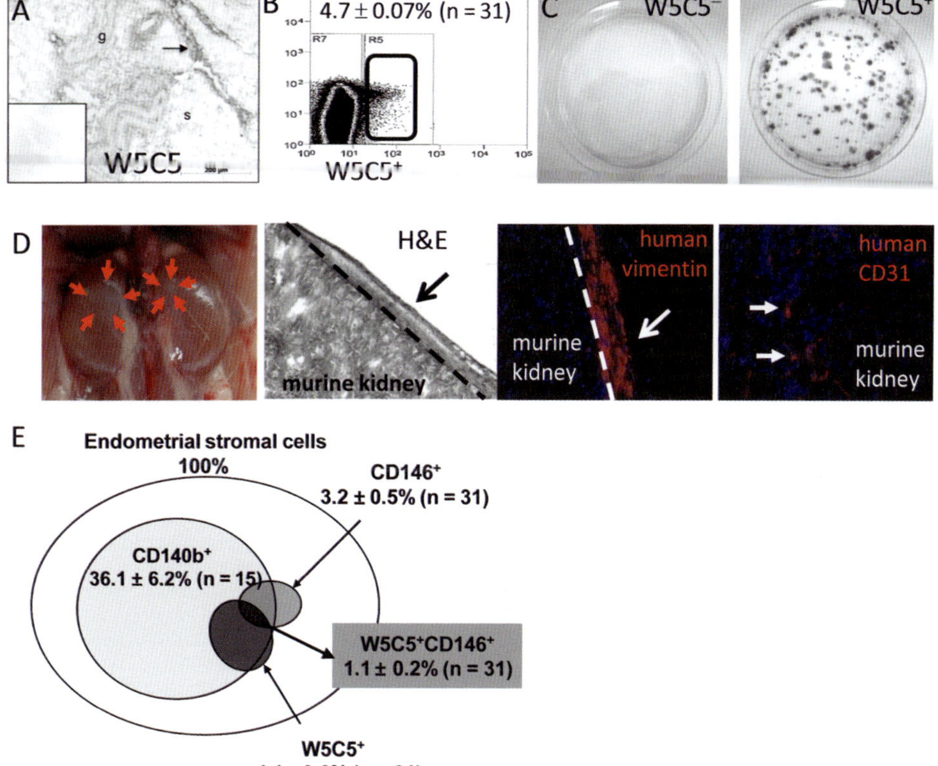

Figure 11.3 W5C5 is a novel marker of human endometrial mesenchymal stem/stromal cells (MSC). (A) Immunostained human endometrium showing perivascular W5C5 immunolocalization (arrow shows representative staining). (B) Representative flow cytometry histogram of W5C5 (n = 31) expression on human endometrial stromal cells. (C) Representative cloning plates of flow-cytometry-sorted W5C5− and W5C5+ cells showing that almost all cloning activity is in the W5C5+ population. (D) Xenografted W5C5+ cells under the kidney capsule of immunocompromised NSG mice resulted in reconstitution of endometrial vimentin+ stromal tissue under the capsule. Some transplanted cells differentiated into CD31+ (human) endothelial cells which migrated and incorporated into murine kidney blood vessels (arrows in right panels). (E) Schematic showing relationship between W5C5+ (n = 31), PDGF-Rβ+ (n = 15), and CD146+ (n = 31) cells. Adapted and reproduced with permission from Cognizant Communications Corporation, copyright 2012. Masuda, *et al*. A novel marker of human endometrial mesenchymal stem-like cells. *Cell Transplantation*. 2012; 21: 2201–2214 [58].

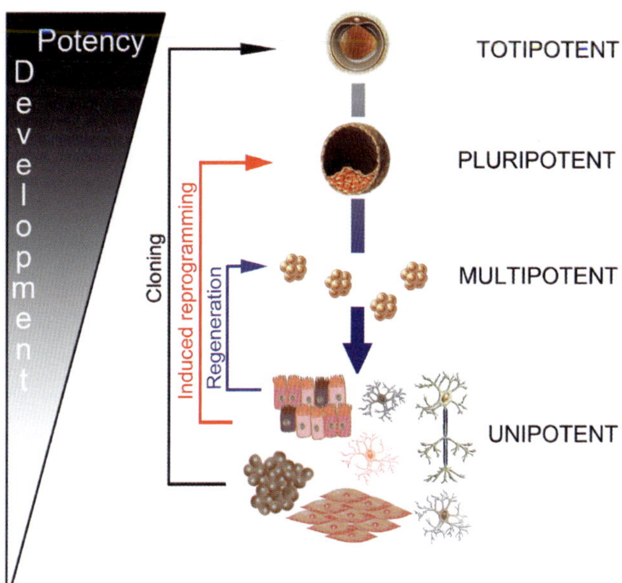

Figure 14.1 Cell potency loss during development. This model depicts the loss of cell potency during embryo development. Cells progressively lose their ability to differentiate into different cell types during development. The most potent cell type, the zygote is considering a totipotent entity. It has the capacity to generate the three germ layers (endoderm, mesoderm, and ectoderm), as well as extra-embryonic tissues. Before gastrulation, pluripotent cells of the inner cell mass of the blastocyst are able to generate cells of the three germ layers, but lose the structural organization capacity that is found in totipotent cells. In the adult organism, populations of multipotent stem or progenitor cells persist, which show a limited degree of differentiating options. Terminally differentiated cells and unipotent cell types build up the organs and tissues in the adult organism, and have lost all differentiation capacity. These cell types can, however, regain developmental potency and generate multipotent cells during regenerative processes in vivo, pluripotent cells by induced reprogramming in vitro, or even totipotent cells by using somatic-cell nuclear-transfer techniques.

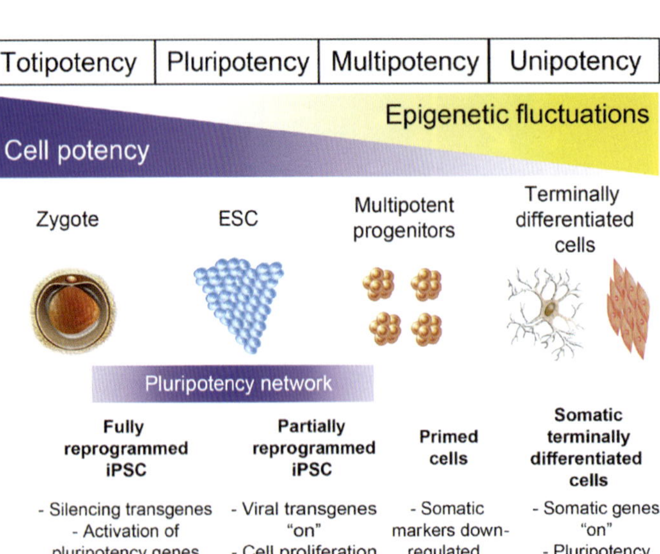

Figure 14.2 Cell potency transitions during reprogramming. Loss or gain of developmental potency is related with epigenetic fluctuations in the cell. Epigenetic marks characteristic of high-potency states are replaced in terminally differentiated cells during differentiation. This is related to specific gene expression changes that determine cell transitions. In a related process, forced expression of reprogramming factors used to generate pluripotent stem cells is related with the initial silencing of somatic programs in terminally differentiated cells. After this initiation event, primed cells start to express endogenous pluripotency-associated genes and activate cell proliferation programs. Partially reprogrammed cells begin to appear shortly afterward. These cells resemble pluripotent stem cells in some aspects, like teratoma formation ability, but still express viral transgenes and show aberrant expression of lineage genes, and thus fail to generate adult chimeras. Finally, transition to a fully reprogrammed state depends on the acquisition of a self-autonomous pluripotency network. This last step is marked by a series of events that include complete silencing of the viral transgenes, activation of endogenous pluripotency-associated markers, and complete epigenetic memory erasure.

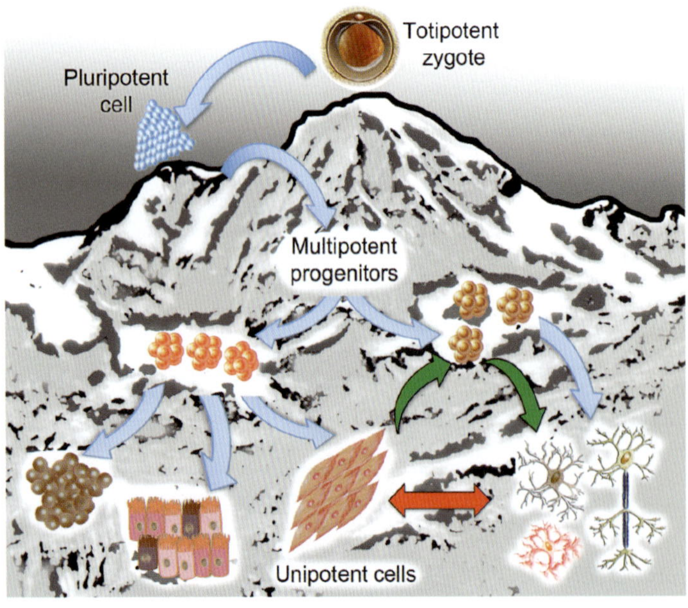

Figure 14.3 The epigenetic landscape of cell potency. This model depicts cells with different developmental potential according to their position in the "mountain of cell potency." The top of the mountain represents totipotent cells, just below these, pluripotent cells, and downstream multipotent progenitors with specific differentiation capacities. Cells, like marbles, roll down across the valleys of the mountain (blue arrows), progressively losing their developmental potency. Unipotent cells residing in the valleys can move uphill (green arrow) depicting dedifferentiation, or they can move directly to other valleys (red arrow) by transdifferentiation.

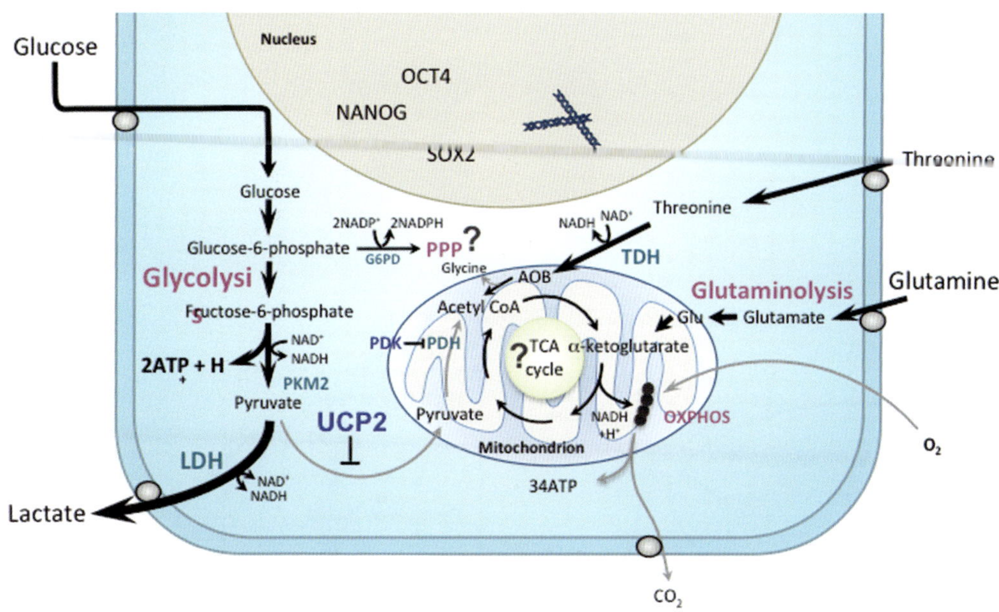

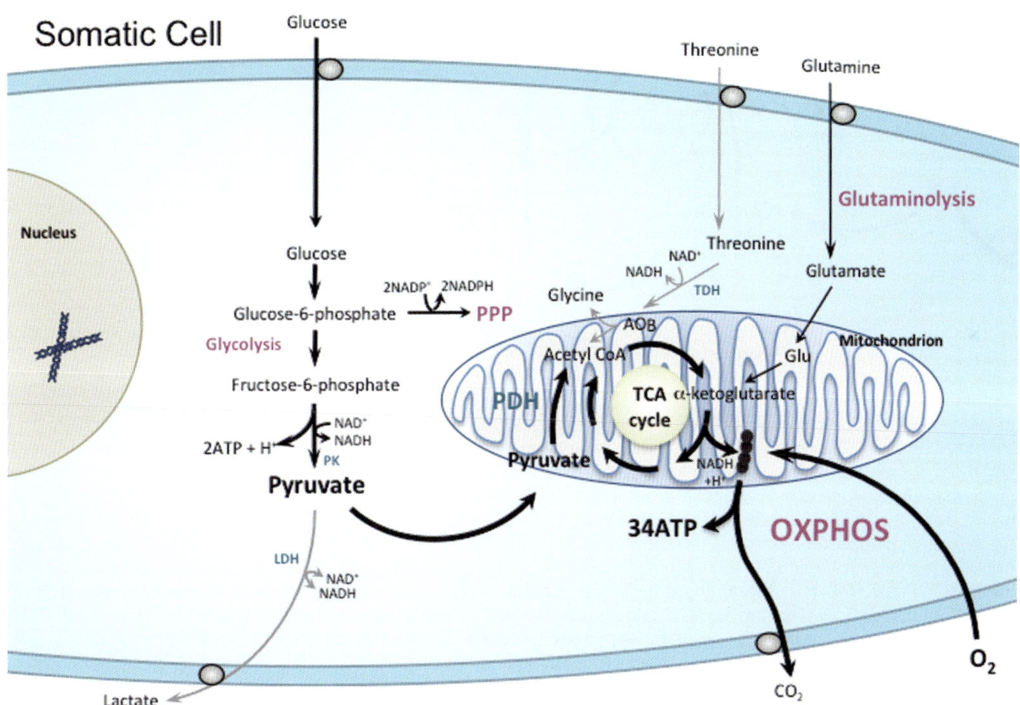

Figure 15.1 Schematic representation of differences between pluripotent stem cell and somatic cell metabolism. Pluripotent stem cells (PSCs) are characterized by spherical, electron-poor mitochondria which contain few cristae and rely heavily on glycolysis for ATP generation (black arrows), resulting in significant lactate production through the conversion of pyruvate to lactate by lactate dehydrogenase (LDH). Consequently, oxidative phosphorylation (OXPHOS) contributes minimally to total ATP in PSCs. In PSCs, uncoupling protein 2 (UCP2) functions to shunt pyruvate away from the tricarboxylic acid (TCA) cycle, facilitating lactate production [81]. Pyruvate dehydrogenase kinase (PDK) activity also prevents the conversion of pyruvate to acetyl coenzyme A (acetyl CoA) [6]. PSCs also use both glutamine [2] and threonine [5] metabolism in culture, while the role of the pentose phosphate pathway (PPP) in PSCs is less clear. Most somatic cells in culture rely primarily on mitochondrial metabolism to generate ATP under aerobic conditions, with limited lactate production. In contrast, somatic cells are characterized by long, electron-dense mitochondria that contain numerous cristae, producing ATP largely through OXPHOS (black arrows); glycolysis provides pyruvate for TCA activity, while lactate production is minimal (grey arrows). Abbreviations: ATP, adenosine triphosphate; CO_2, carbon dioxide; O_2, oxygen; NAD^+, nicotinamide adenine dinucleotide; NADH, reduced form of NAD+; TCA, tricarboxylic acid cycle; PKM2, pyruvate kinase M2; LDH, lactate dehydrogenase.

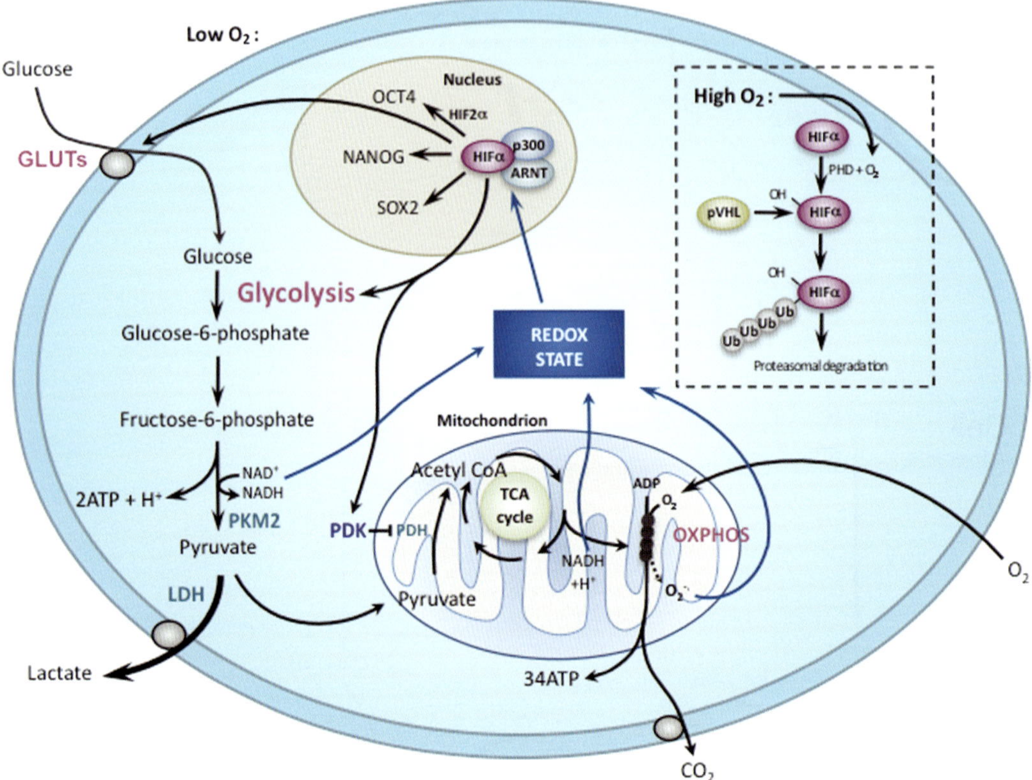

Figure 15.2 Schematic representation of oxygen and redox-regulated HIF modulation of ES cell metabolism. Under conditions of high oxygen concentrations (dashed box), HIFα proteins are targeted for proteasomal degradation through hydroxylation by proline hydroxylases (PHD) and recognition by pVHL (von Hippel Lindau tumor suppressor protein), leading to tagging of HIFα with polyubiquitin. In response to low oxygen concentrations, proline hydroxylation is inhibited, leading to stabilization and accumulation of HIFα protein, and translocation to the nucleus. This enables dimerization of HIFα with HIF1β (ARNT) and p300, and subsequent binding to hypoxia response elements within target genes. HIF targets include glucose transporters (GLUTs), glycolytic enzymes, and the pyruvate dehydrogenase kinase (PDK), resulting in increased glycolytic activity to maintain ATP [16]. Chemical inhibition of HIFα proteins reduces transcriptional and protein expression of *Oct4*, *Nanog*, and *Sox2* in mouse and rat ES cells [66], supporting a role for HIF in regulating pluripotency markers; HIF2α is known to activate *Oct4* directly in mouse ES cells [69], while HIF2α silencing results in reduced *OCT4*, *NANOG*, and *SOX2* protein expression in human ES cells [68]. More recently, activation of HIF1α has been shown to switch mouse ES cell metabolism from a reliance on both oxidative and glycolytic metabolism, to predominantly glycolytic, rendering ES cells morphologically and metabolically similar to EpiSCs [51]. Changes in redox state have also been shown to stabilize HIF1α. The cellular redox state relies on the rates of production and elimination of reactive oxygen species, and the production and oxidation of reducing equivalents from cytoplasmic and mitochondrial metabolism (blue arrows), and functions to modulate cellular signalling and homeostasis. Abbreviations: HIF, hypoxia-inducible factor; Ub, ubiquitin; ATP, adenosine triphosphate; O₂, oxygen; O₂·, hydroxyl radical; NAD⁺, nicotinamide adenine dinucleotide; NADH, reduced form of NAD⁺; TCA, tricarboxylic acid cycle; PKM2, pyruvate kinase M2; LDH, lactate dehydrogenase.

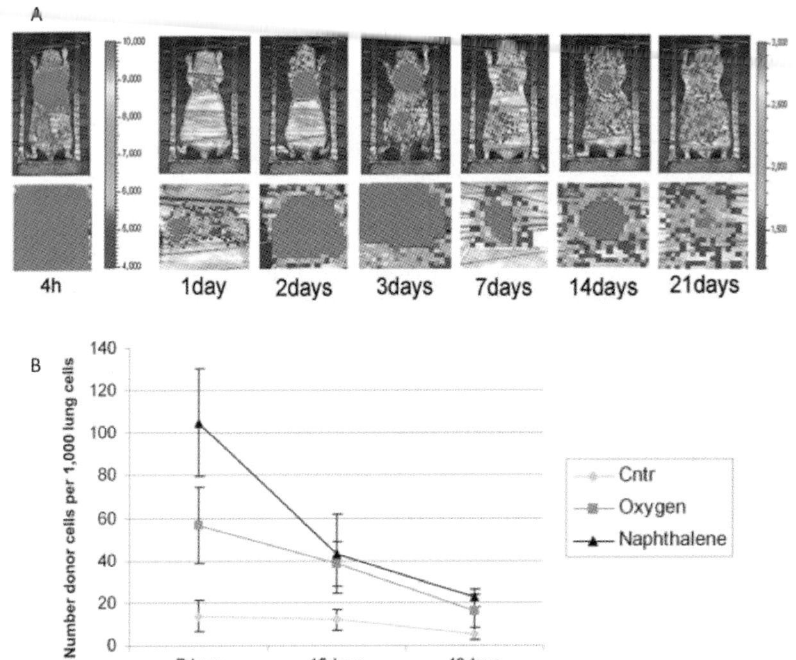

Figure 10.6 AFSCs integrate into adult mouse lung after tail vein injection. (A) Bioluminescence of mice injected with AFSCs expressing luciferase. Magnified views of the thorax are shown below each panel. Relatively intense AFSC luciferase bioluminescence was detected shortly after tail vein injection. After 21 days AFSCs were still detected at the lung position. (B) Lung injury increases the level of integration of AFSCs. Absolute quantification of Sry genes on the Y chromosome by real-time polymerase chain reaction. At 7 days the number of AFSCs was significantly elevated in naphthalene-injured trachea and oxygen-injured parenchyma compared with uninjured control lung. At 15 days naphthalene-injured and oxygen-injured mice reached similar numbers of AFSCs compared with uninjured control lung. (See also color plate.) Modified from Carraro, G., Perin, L., Sedrakyan, S. *et al.* Human amniotic fluid stem cells can integrate and differentiate into epithelial lung lineages. *Stem Cells.* 2008; 26: 2902–2911.

generating erythroid, myeloid, and lymphoid cells in vitro, suggesting that AFSCs may be an important source of cells to regenerate the hematopoietic system [47]. This study demonstrated that 4 months following AFSCs injection into immune-deficient RAG1$^{-/-}$ C57BL/6 (Ly5.1) mice, AFSC-derived macrophages, NK, B, and T cells (both CD4+ and CD8+ CD3+) were found in transplanted animals. Secondary transplantation was partially successful, suggesting the presence of a small number of hematopoietic progenitor cells within the multipotent AFSCs population. These transplantation experiments indicated that AFSCs possess long-term in vivo hematopoietic repopulating capacity and potential therapeutic applications for the treatment of blood and immune disorders.

Other clinical applications

An additional characteristic that makes AFSCs an ideal candidate for cell therapy is their ability to readily take up retroviral, lentiviral, adenoviral, and baculoviral vectors without altering the differentiation potential of the cells [48]. This aids in the ability to track cells both in vitro and in vivo by infecting cells with a viral vector carrying a GFP or luciferase tag, and it also suggests that the cells could eventually be used

in cell-based gene-therapy applications. AFSCs are also more rapidly, easily, and efficiently reprogrammed into induced pluripotent stem cells (iPS cells) than neonatal or adult cells, possibly due to their embryonic-like epigenetic background [5]. Thus AFSCs seem to be an abundant iPS cell source for various basic developmental studies and for future patient-specific cell therapies. AFSCs also possess potent immunosuppressive properties, a useful tool for the treatment of disease such as graft vs. host (GvH) and other inflammatory diseases. Mirebella *et al.* demonstrated that AFSCs display immunosuppressive effects on T-cell proliferation and lack of expression of HLA-DR and co-stimulatory molecules such as CD80 and CD86, suggesting that AFSCs may be immune-privileged, thus not rejected by the immune system [49]. These studies also highlighted the role of AFSCs in recruiting endogenous stem cells to contribute to wound repair and regeneration.

Conclusion

Transplantation of stem cells derived from gestational tissue has the potential to treat a variety of conditions ranging from battle wounds to neural degeneration. As gestational tissue is an abundant source of stem cells, with minimal ethical and legal considerations, stem cells such as AFSCs are a valuable tool for the field of regenerative medicine. While still in its infancy, research into AFSCs has demonstrated their potential to generate osteocytes, myocytes, adipocytes, endothelial cells, hepatocytes, chondrocytes, and neural cells in the laboratory. In pre-clinical studies, AFSCs have shown efficacy in the treatment of bone defects, heart disease, kidney disease, neural degeneration, lung disease, and blood disorders. Future applications of AFSCs include the treatment of diabetes, the generation of a living-skin equivalent, for muscle regeneration, as a novel drug delivery system, as well as anti-inflammatory applications for graft vs. host disease. Stem cells derived from gestational tissue remain an abundant, but valuable tool for regenerative therapy.

References

1. De Coppi, P., Bartsch, G., Jr., Siddiqui, M.M. *et al.* Isolation of amniotic stem cell lines with potential for therapy. *Nature Biotechnology.* 2007; 25: 100–106.

2. Murphy, S., Rosli, S., Acharya, R. *et al.* Amnion epithelial cell isolation and characterization for clinical use. *Current Protocols in Stem Cell Biology.* 2010; Chapter 1: Unit 1E 6.

3. Serikov, V., Hounshell, C., Larkin, S. *et al.* Human term placenta as a source of hematopoietic cells. *Experimental Biology and Medicine (Maywood).* 2009; 234: 813–823.

4. Troyer, D.L., Weiss, M.L. Wharton's jelly-derived cells are a primitive stromal cell population. *Stem Cells.* 2008; 26: 591–599.

5. Galende, E., Karakikes, I., Edelmann, L. *et al.* Amniotic fluid cells are more efficiently reprogrammed to pluripotency than adult cells. *Cell Reprogramming.* 2010; 12: 117–125.

6. Ballen, K.K. New trends in umbilical cord blood transplantation. *Blood.* 2005; 105: 3786–3792.

7. Shaw, S.W., David, A.L., De Coppi, P. Clinical applications of prenatal and postnatal therapy using stem cells retrieved from amniotic fluid. *Current Opinion in Obstetrics and Gynecology.* 2011; 23: 109–116.

8. Murphy, S., Lim, R., Dickinson, H. *et al.* Human amnion epithelial cells prevent bleomycin-induced lung injury and preserve lung function. *Cell Transplantation.* 2011; 20: 909–923.

9. Furth, M.E., Atala, A. Stem cell sources to treat diabetes. *Journal of cellular biochemistry.* 2009; 106: 507–511.

10. Delo, D.M., Olson, J., Baptista, P.M. *et al.* Non-invasive longitudinal tracking of human amniotic fluid stem cells in the mouse heart. *Stem Cells and Development.* 2008; 17: 1185–1194.

11. Perin, L., Giuliani, S., Jin, D. *et al.* Renal differentiation of amniotic fluid stem cells. *Cell Proliferation.* 2007; 40: 936–948.

12. Swartz, W.J. Early mammalian embryonic development. *American Journal of Industrial Medicine.* 1983; 4: 51–61.

13. Luckett WP. The development of primordial and definitive amniotic cavities in early Rhesus monkey and human embryos. *American Journal of Anatomy.* 1975; 144: 149–167.

14. Robinson, W.P., McFadden, D.E., Barrett, I.J. *et al.* Origin of amnion and implications for evaluation of the fetal genotype in cases of mosaicism. *Prenatal Diagnosis.* 2002; 22: 1076–1085.

15. Sakuragawa, N., Elwan, M.A., Fujii, T. *et al.* Possible dynamic neurotransmitter metabolism surrounding the fetus. *Journal of Child Neurology.* 1999; 14: 265–266.

16. Baschat, A.A., Hecher, K. Fetal growth restriction due to placental disease. *Seminars in Perinatology.* 2004; 28: 67–80.

17. In 't Anker, P.S., Scherjon, S.A., Kleijburg-van der Keur, C. *et al.* Amniotic fluid as a novel source of mesenchymal stem cells for therapeutic transplantation. *Blood.* 2003; 102: 1548–1549.

18. Prusa, A.R., Hengstschlager, M. Amniotic fluid cells and human stem cell research: a new connection. *Medical Science Monitor.* 2002; 8: RA253–RA257.

19. Torricelli, F., Brizzi, L., Bernabei, P.A. *et al.* Identification of hematopoietic progenitor cells in human amniotic fluid before the 12th week of gestation. *Italian Journal of Anatomy and Embryology.* 1993; 98: 119–126.

20. Hoehn, H., Bryant, E.M., Karp, L.E. *et al.* Cultivated cells from diagnostic amniocentesis in second trimester pregnancies. II. Cytogenetic parameters as functions of clonal type and preparative technique. *Clinical Genetics.* 1975; 7: 29–36.

21. Tsai, M.S., Lee, J.L., Chang, Y.J. *et al.* Isolation of human multipotent mesenchymal stem cells from second-trimester amniotic fluid using a novel two-stage culture protocol. *Human Reproduction.* 2004; 19: 1450–1456.

22. Kaviani, A., Perry, T.E., Dzakovic, A. *et al.* The amniotic fluid as a source of cells for fetal tissue engineering. *Journal of Pediatric Surgery*. 2001; 36: 1662–1665.

23. Fleischman, R.A. From white spots to stem cells: the role of the Kit receptor in mammalian development. *Trends in Genetics*. 1993; 9: 285–290.

24. Hoffman, L.M., Carpenter, M.K. Characterization and culture of human embryonic stem cells. *Nature Biotechnology*. 2005; 23: 699–708.

25. Guo, C.S., Wehrle-Haller, B., Rossi, J. *et al.* Autocrine regulation of neural crest cell development by steel factor. *Developmental Biology*. 1997; 184: 61–69.

26. Maraldi, T., Riccio, M., Resca, E. *et al.* Human amniotic fluid stem cells seeded in fibroin scaffold produce in vivo mineralized matrix. *Tissue Engineering Part A*. 2011; 17: 2833–2843.

27. Sun, H., Feng, K., Hu, J. *et al.* Osteogenic differentiation of human amniotic fluid-derived stem cells induced by bone morphogenetic protein-7 and enhanced by nanofibrous scaffolds. *Biomaterials*. 2010; 31: 1133–1139.

28. Higuchi, A., Shen, P.Y., Zhao, J.K. *et al.* Osteoblast differentiation of amniotic fluid-derived stem cells irradiated with visible light. *Tissue Engineering Part A*. 2011; 17: 2593–2602.

29. Rosenblatt, J.D., Lunt, A.I., Parry, D.J. *et al.* Culturing satellite cells from living single muscle fiber explants. *In Vitro Cellular and Developmental Biology Animal*. 1995; 31: 773–739.

30. Hinterberger, T.J., Sassoon, D.A., Rhodes, S.J. *et al.* Expression of the muscle regulatory factor MRF4 during somite and skeletal myofiber development. *Developmental Biology*. 1991; 147: 144–156.

31. Guan, X., Delo, D.M., Atala, A. *et al.* In vitro cardiomyogenic potential of human amniotic fluid stem cells. *Journal of Tissue Engineering and Regenerative Medicine*. 2011; 5: 220–228.

32. Chen, J., Lu, Z., Cheng, D. *et al.* Isolation and characterization of porcine amniotic fluid-derived multipotent stem cells. *PLoS One*. 2011; 6: e19964.

33. Zhang, P., Baxter, J., Vinod, K. *et al.* Endothelial differentiation of amniotic fluid-derived stem cells: synergism of biochemical and shear force stimuli. *Stem Cells and Development*. 2009; 18: 1299–1308.

34. Schwartz, R.E., Reyes, M., Koodie, L. *et al.* Multipotent adult progenitor cells from bone marrow differentiate into functional hepatocyte-like cells. *Journal of Clinical Investigation*. 2002; 109: 1291–1302.

35. Morris, S.M., Jr. Regulation of enzymes of the urea cycle and arginine metabolism. *Annual Review of Nutrition*. 2002; 22: 87–105.

36. Zheng, Y.B., Gao, Z.L., Xie, C. *et al.* Characterization and hepatogenic differentiation of mesenchymal stem cells from human amniotic fluid and human bone marrow: a comparative study. *Cell Biology International*. 2008; 32: 1439–1448.

37. Kolambkar, Y.M., Peister, A., Soker, S. *et al.* Chondrogenic differentiation of amniotic fluid-derived stem cells. *Journal of Molecular Histology*. 2007; 38: 405–413.

38. Park, J.S., Shim, M.S., Shim, S.H. *et al.* Chondrogenic potential of stem cells derived from amniotic fluid, adipose tissue, or bone marrow encapsulated in fibrin gels containing TGF-beta3. *Biomaterials*. 2011; 32: 8139–8149.

39. Mareschi, K., Rustichelli, D., Comunanza, V. *et al.* Multipotent mesenchymal stem cells from amniotic fluid originate neural precursors with functional voltage-gated sodium channels. *Cytotherapy*. 2009; 11: 534–547.

40. Bollini, S., Cheung, K.K., Riegler, J. *et al.* Amniotic fluid stem cells are cardioprotective following acute myocardial infarction. *Stem Cells and Development*. 2011; 20: 1985–1994.

41. Lee, W.Y., Wei, H.J., Lin, W.W. *et al.* Enhancement of cell retention and functional benefits in myocardial infarction using human amniotic-fluid stem-cell bodies enriched with endogenous ECM. *Biomaterials*. 2011; 32: 5558–5567.

42. Perin, L., Sedrakyan, S., Giuliani, S. *et al.* Protective effect of human amniotic fluid stem cells in an immunodeficient mouse model of acute tubular necrosis. *PLoS One*. 2010; 5: e9357.

43. Pan, H.C., Chen, C.J., Cheng, F.C. *et al.* Combination of G-CSF administration and human amniotic fluid mesenchymal stem cell transplantation promotes peripheral nerve regeneration. *Neurochemical Research*. 2009; 34: 518–527.

44. Rehni, A.K., Singh, N., Jaggi, A.S. *et al.* Amniotic fluid derived stem cells ameliorate focal cerebral ischaemia-reperfusion injury induced behavioural deficits in mice. *Behavioural Brain Research*. 2007; 183: 95–100.

45. Carraro, G., Perin, L., Sedrakyan, S. *et al.* Human amniotic fluid stem cells can integrate and differentiate into epithelial lung lineages. *Stem Cells*. 2008; 26: 2902–2911.

46. Buckley, S., Shi, W., Carraro, G. *et al.* The milieu of damaged AEC2 stimulates alveolar wound repair by endogenous and exogenous progenitors. *American*

Journal of Respiratory Cell and Molecular Biology. 2011; 45: 1212–1221.

47. Ditadi, A., de Coppi, P., Picone, O. *et al.* Human and murine amniotic fluid c-Kit+Lin- cells display hematopoietic activity. *Blood.* 2009; 113: 3953–3960.

48. Grisafi, D., Piccoli, M., Pozzobon, M. *et al.* High transduction efficiency of human amniotic fluid stem cells mediated by adenovirus vectors. *Stem Cells and Development.* 2008; 17: 953–962.

49. Mirebella, T., Poggi, A., Scaranari, M. *et al.* Recruitment of host's progenitor cells to sites of human amniotic fluid stem cells implantation. *Biomaterials.* 2011; 32: 4218–4227.

Chapter

11

Adult stem cells in the human endometrium

Caroline E. Gargett, Irene Cervelló, Hong P.T. Nguyen, and Carlos Simón

Introduction

The human endometrium is a dynamically remodeling tissue which undergoes more than 400 cycles of regeneration, differentiation, and shedding during a woman's reproductive years. The co-ordinated and sequential action of estrogen and progesterone direct these major remodeling events to prepare the endometrium for blastocyst implantation. Endometrial regeneration also occurs following parturition, almost complete curettage, and in post-menopausal women taking estrogen replacement therapy; adult stem/progenitor cells are likely responsible for this endometrial regeneration. This chapter will review the functional approaches that have been used to identify candidate endometrial epithelial and stromal stem/progenitor cells, in particular by cell cloning, bromodeoxyuridine (BrdU) label retention, side population (SP) identification, and in vivo reconstruction of endometrial tissues from isolated SP cell populations. The rapid progress made in identifying markers that distinguish endometrial epithelial and mesenchymal stem/progenitor cells from their more differentiated progeny will also be described. In particular the co-expression of CD146 and PDGF Receptor-β (PDGF-Rβ), and the single novel W5C5 marker that purify human endometrial mesenchymal stem/progenitor cells will be examined. Both CD146$^+$PDGF-Rβ$^+$ and W5C5$^+$ populations have a surface phenotype similar to bone marrow and fat mesenchymal stem cells, demonstrate multipotency by undergoing multilineage differentiation into fat, cartilage, bone, and smooth muscle cells, and reside in a perivascular location in the functionalis and basalis layers of the endometrium. Moreover, stem/progenitor cells present in menstrual blood will also be examined. Application of these fundamental studies to the current knowledge of the pathophysiology of a variety of common gynecological diseases associated with abnormal endometrial proliferation, including endometrial cancer, endometriosis, and adenomyosis will also be explored. Additionally, the possible uses of endometrial stem/progenitor cells in autologous tissue-engineering applications relevant to urogynaecology will be discussed. Finally, future directions for human endometrial stem/progenitor cell research will be suggested.

Regenerative capacity of human endometrium

The human endometrium is a dynamically remodeling tissue that undergoes more than 400 cycles of regeneration, differentiation, and shedding during a woman's reproductive years [1,2]. Its main function is to support embryo implantation and to provide nutrients or the developing embryo until the placenta develops [3]. However, in the absence of an embryo, the functional layer of the endometrial lining is sloughed off and regenerates in the next menstrual cycle.

The first stage of endometrial regeneration is the repair of the surface epithelium which occurs in a focal manner and simultaneously with menstrual breakdown [4]. This process is initiated within 48 hours of shedding and involves migration of epithelial cells, from the foot of basal gland "stumps" over the denuded surface [5,6]. Endometrial repair does not require estrogen as re-epithelialization occurs while circulating estrogen levels are very low, and at a time when epithelial cells lack estrogen receptor-α (ERα) expression [6]. However, this dogma has recently been questioned. From histological analyses it has been

---

Stem Cells in Reproductive Medicine 3rd edition, ed. Carlos Simón, Antonio Pellicer and Renee Reijo Pera.
Published by Cambridge University Press. © Cambridge University Press 2013.

suggested that re-epithelialization of the denuded basalis results from the differentiation of small stromal cells into epithelial cells through interaction with a fibrinous matrix [7], or from the deposition of sloughed endometrial fragments that remain within the uterus [4]. Endometrial regeneration then follows from the re-epithelialized basalis layer of the endometrium, which acts as a germinal compartment providing a source of endometrial cells [8]. The basalis is relatively insensitive to sex steroid hormones and undergoes little proliferation or differentiation [9–11], whereas the regenerating functionalis mucosa grows rapidly; 4–7 mm within 4–10 days during the proliferative stage [12], with extensive proliferation of glandular and luminal epithelial cells, and to a lesser extent, stromal cells [8,11,13,14]. Recently, Wnt7a expression was demonstrated in the luminal epithelium and upper region of the uterine glands during estrogen-regulated endometrial regeneration in human and primate endometrium, which correlated with the proliferation of epithelial cells [14]. Following ovulation, proliferation gradually ceases and the estrogen-primed functionalis commences differentiation under the influence of progesterone. Luminal and upper glandular epithelial expression of Wnt7a was down-regulated in the secretory phase, indicating the importance of the Wnt signaling pathway in endometrial growth and differentiation [14]. Hence, endometrial regeneration and differentiation are accompanied by dramatic changes in gene expression profiles [15,16].

Endometrial regeneration also occurs following parturition, extensive resection, and when endometrial ablation therapies are not successful [2]. When menstrual cycles cease at menopause, the endometrium becomes very thin and atrophic, containing few glands in a stroma which resembles the basalis, both morphologically and in gene expression profile, particularly with genes involved in the Wnt signaling pathway [17]. Women taking oral contraceptive pills (OCP) do not exhibit cyclic changes in circulating sex steroid hormones and their endometrium does not undergo cyclical growth, differentiation, and regression. Histologically, OCP-affected endometrium appears inactive, with a similar morphology to post-menopausal endometrium; however, when post-menopausal women take estrogen replacement therapy or women cease OCP medication, their endometrium regenerates [2,18].

Endometrial stem/progenitor cell hypothesis

The monthly regeneration of the human endometrium and its reconstruction following parturition is at least equivalent to the level of cellular turnover that occurs in other highly regenerative organs such as the blood-forming tissue of the bone marrow, epidermis, and intestinal epithelium [2]. In these regenerative tissues, adult stem cells, responsible for providing replacement cells to maintain tissue homeostasis, have been identified. The concept that basalis endometrium harbours adult stem/progenitor cells responsible for the remarkable regenerative capacity of endometrium was first proposed many years ago and indirect evidence for their existence has accumulated in the intervening years (reviewed in [2]). Attempts to isolate, characterize, and locate endometrial stem/progenitor cells have recently been undertaken by applying techniques used to isolate adult stem cells in other tissues (reviewed in [2]). Indeed these approaches have resulted in the identification of rare populations of epithelial stem/progenitor cells and mesenchymal stem-like cells in human endometrium (reviewed in Gargett and Masuda [19]).

Adult stem cells and their properties

Adult stem cells are undifferentiated cells present in most adult tissues. However, their rarity, lack of distinguishing morphological features, and the difficulty in identifying specific markers for them has hampered their identification in many tissues. Adult stem cells are defined by their functional properties: high proliferative potential, self-renewal, and capacity to differentiate into one or more lineages [20]. The retention of a DNA synthesis label (BrdU) for prolonged periods of time is another property of adult stem cells, which proliferate less frequently than their daughter cell progeny [21]. Adult stem cells maintain tissue homeostasis by providing replacement cells in regenerating tissues and in routine cellular turnover, and are responsible for tissue repair after acute injury [22,23]. The balance between self-renewal and differentiation in adult stem cells is regulated by the stem-cell niche, comprising the adult stem cell, surrounding niche cell(s), and extracellular matrix. The niche ensures an appropriate balance between stem-cell replenishment and sufficient differentiation of daughter cells to maintain tissue homeostasis for proper organ function [22].

Endometrial epithelial stem/progenitor cells

Cell cloning studies

The first published evidence for the existence of human endometrial epithelial stem/progenitor cells came from cell cloning studies. Freshly isolated single endometrial epithelial cell suspensions (EpCAM$^+$) were seeded at cloning density in culture [24]; rare clonogenic epithelial cells were identified in normal cycling and inactive perimenopausal endometrium, as well as in endometrium from women on oral contraceptives [24,25]. This indicates that clonogenic epithelial cells may be responsible for regenerating endometrial glands in cycling and non-cycling endometrium [26]. These studies found that 0.22% of human endometrial epithelial cells had colony-forming unit (CFU) activity, of which 0.09% initiated large CFUs and 0.14% small CFUs. Further studies showed that individual large, but not small, CFUs exhibited self-renewal activity, high proliferative potential, and differentiated into cytokeratin-expressing gland-like structures in 3D culture [27]. These studies suggest that large epithelial CFUs are initiated by progenitor cells, possibly located at the base of the glands in the basalis, and that small epithelial CFUs are initiated by more differentiated transit-amplifying cells, likely located in the functionalis layer and which are responsible for the extensive proliferation observed in the proliferative stage of the menstrual cycle [2,24,28]. The percentage of endometrial epithelial CFUs was highly variable between subjects and did not differ during the menstrual cycle, indicating their continued presence in human endometrium [25].

Label-retaining cells

Label-retaining cells (LRCs) have been identified as candidate adult stem cells in vivo in mouse endometrium [29–31]. The LRC approach identifies adult stem cells by their quiescent, slowly cycling nature, since they only undergo cell division during tissue turnover in order to initiate the replacement of lost cells. It is based on pulse labeling the majority of tissue cells with a DNA synthesis label (bromodeoxyuridine;

BrdU), during a time when adult stem cells are proliferating, and subsequently chasing the label over long periods of time. Slowly cycling stem cells retain the label, while rapidly dividing transit-amplifying cells dilute the label to undetectable levels. Immunohistochemistry is used to localize bromodeoxyuridine (BrdU$^+$) LRCs, revealing both their location and the stem-cell niche. Endometrial epithelial LRCs have been difficult to detect in mouse endometrium due to complete loss of label over the 8–12-week chase periods following neonatal labeling. This loss is even more rapid when adult mice are labeled [29]. Rapid BrdU label dilution results from extensive luminal epithelium proliferation, as nascent glands develop during neonatal and pre-pubertal endometrial growth, and during subsequent estrus cycles. Nevertheless, epithelial LRCs, comprising 3% of mouse endometrial epithelial cells, were observed as separate cells in the luminal but not glandular epithelium during an 8-week chase period, suggesting that luminal epithelial stem/progenitor cells are responsible for the growth of glands during development and in cycling adult mice [29]. These epithelial LRCs did not express ERα and yet responded to estrogen by undergoing rapid proliferation [29,32]. In a pre-pubertal mouse model of estrogen-induced growth during endometrial development, mice were labeled with BrdU on post-natal days 3–6, chased for 4 weeks, then ovariectomised to regress the endometrium for 2 weeks, and given a single estradiol injection. The first cells to proliferate were the luminal epithelial LRCs, 8 hours after the estrogen injection, as detected by co-localization of BrdU with the proliferation marker Ki-67, and a mitosis marker, phosphorylated histone H3 (PH3) [32]. In pre-pubertal mice, all epithelial LRCs were in cell cycle at 8 hours, behaving like adult stem cells by driving the estrogen-induced proliferative response during the final stages of endometrial development (Figure 11.1A, B). In contrast, in a cycling mouse model of estrogen-induced endometrial regeneration, when BrdU-labeled mice were ovariectomised at 8 weeks, within 2 hours of a single estrogen injection, not only were all epithelial LRCs proliferating, but 16% of unlabeled epithelial cells had also proliferated [32] (Figure 11.1C, D). Thus in cycling mice, the epithelial proliferative response to estrogen is rapid and is initiated by both LRCs and non-LRCs, suggesting that mature epithelial cells may undergo self-replication. However, lineage-tracing studies will be required to

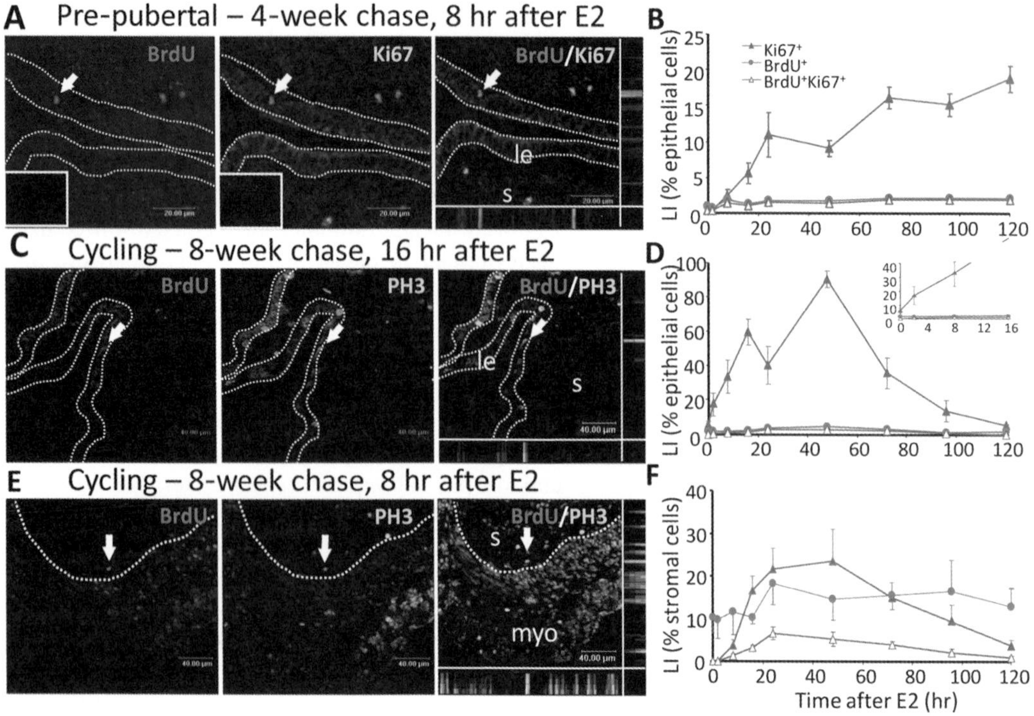

Figure 11.1 Label-retaining cell proliferation in estrogen-stimulated endometrial regeneration in ovariectomized mice. Post-natal day 3 mice were labelled with BrdU for three days and the label chased for (A, B) 4 weeks (pre-pubertal) or (C – F) 8 weeks (cycling). Mice were then ovariectomized and the endometrium allowed to regress for 14 days, after which a single injection of 17β-estradiol was given and uteri were collected from 2–120 h later (B, D, F). Sections were double immunofluorescently labeled with BrdU (A, C, E, left panels, red) and the (A) proliferation marker, Ki-67 (A, middle panel, green) or the (C, E) mitotic marker, phosphorylated histone H3 (PH3; C, E, middle panels, green) and examined by confocal microscopy. The right panels (A, C, E) show x/z and y/z planes obtained by optical sectioning on the far right and beneath the merged images and demonstrate true nuclear co-localisation of both markers. Insets in (A) negative control IgG. Arrows, (A) proliferating or (C) mitotic epithelial and (E) mitotic stromal LRC. Labeling indices (LIs) (B, D, E) of endometrial epithelial cells (D, E) for Ki-67 for 40-week chased pre-pubertal (B) and 8-week chased cycling (D) mice (inset first 8 h). LIs of stromal cells (F) for Ki-67 for 8-week chased cycling mice. E2, 17β-estradiol; le, luminal epithelium; myo, myometrium; s, stroma. Scale bars 40 μm. Adapted and reproduced with kind permission from SAGE, copyright 2012. Chan *et al.* Role of label-retaining cells in estrogen-induced endometrial regeneration. *Reproductive Sciences* 19: 102–114 [32]. (See also color plate.)

determine the relative roles of LRCs and mature cells in regenerating murine endometrial epithelium, and this requires a definitive marker of endometrial epithelial progenitor cells.

Endometrial mesenchymal stromal/stem cells

Cell cloning studies

Human endometrial mesenchymal stromal/stem cells were first demonstrated by cell cloning freshly isolated, single-cell suspensions of stromal cells depleted of epithelial cells (EpCAM⁻) [24]; 1.25% possessed colony-forming ability [24]. Stromal CFUs are retained in these cultures and their proportion increases to 15% after prior expansion in culture at normal seeding densities [33]. Both large and small stromal CFU types formed from freshly isolated cells, but only 0.02% of stromal cells initiated large CFUs, supporting the concept of a stromal cellular hierarchy, hypothesized to exist in human endometrium [2]. Large individual stromal CFUs underwent self-renewal in vitro, persisting through 3–5 rounds of serial cloning, and exhibiting high proliferative potential by undergoing 30 population doublings [27]. Large stromal CFUs also expressed a typical MSC surface phenotype. Both epithelial and stromal CFU growth was supported by EGF, TGFα and PDGF-BB growth factors in serum-free culture, but only stromal CFUs formed in FGF2-containing medium [24,25], indicating that stromal and epithelial CFUs differ, and that there are distinct epithelial and stromal adult stem cells in human endometrium.

Multilineage differentiation

A key adult stem-cell property is the ability to undergo multilineage differentiation. Mesenchymal stem/stromal cells (MSCs) have been identified in bone marrow and adipose tissue and these cells differentiate into at least three mesodermal lineages in vitro under appropriate induction conditions [34]. Large self-renewing stromal CFUs differentiate into four mesodermal lineages; adipose, smooth muscle, bone, and cartilage, indicating their multipotency, given that the CFUs themselves originate from a single cell [27]. Cultured human endometrial stromal cells also differentiate into fat or chondrocyte lineages [33,35], and lineages of ectodermal and endodermal origin [36,37], indicating that stromal cells have considerable plasticity.

Label-retaining cells

Candidate stromal stem/progenitor cells have been identified in mouse endometrium as stromal LRCs [29–31]. Between 6–9% of the stromal cells were identified as LRCs after BrdU pulse-labeling neonatal mice and chasing for at least 12 weeks. A large proportion of these were located near blood vessels, close to the endometrial–myometrial junction [29,30], correlating with their postulated basalis location in human endometrium. Stromal LRCs were further characterized for expression of various markers. These cells were not leukocytes or of bone marrow origin as they did not express CD45 [29]. Some expressed ERα [29] and others expressed typical markers of undifferentiated cells, c-kit and Oct4 [30], although in another study c-kit was not expressed by endometrial stromal LRCs [31]. The continued decline in the percentage of LRCs as the chase period lengthened indicates that LRC also undergo symmetric cell divisions in adulthood, or do not necessarily retain template DNA strands, as has been demonstrated for intestinal LRCs [38]. In the estrogen-induced endometrial regeneration model, only 12% of the stromal LRCs initiated stromal proliferation in 8-week pulse-chased LRC cycling, ovariectomized mice (Figure 11.1F). These proliferating stromal LRCs were located near the endometrial–myometrial junction or directly beneath

the luminal epithelium (Figure 11.1E). In a mouse model of endometrial decidualization, breakdown, and repair, where BrdU labeling was performed in adult mice, stromal LRCs were also associated with blood vessels, particularly in the non-decidualized "basalis" regions [39]. These stromal LRCs proliferated during estrogen priming of the endometrium prior to progesterone-induced decidualization, rather than during re-epithelialization of the luminal epithelium. Collectively these functional studies in several LRC mouse models suggest that a small proportion of stromal LRCs function as stem/progenitor cells in generating stromal tissue to support the rapidly growing glands and luminal epithelium upon estrogen replenishment, but not during the initial repair phase [32,39].

Side population (SP) cells

In the absence of known specific markers to identify and isolate adult stem cells in tissues and/or organs, an alternative approach is to use the Hoechst dye exclusion method. Using this method, a specific side population (SP) displaying low red and low blue fluorescence can be identified by dual-wavelength flow cytometry after incubating the target cells with the DNA-binding dye Hoechst 33342 [40] (Figure 11.2). Although SP cells represent only a small fraction of the whole cell population, their adult stem-cell properties have been demonstrated in several organs and tissues. SP cells express high levels of various ABC transporter family members, such as multidrug resistance protein (MDR1) and breast cancer resistance protein (BCRP). Although the exact physiological role of these transporters is not fully understood, it is likely that cellular protection against exogenous chemicals by their active exclusion is their best-characterized function. This protective role is associated with the survival and maintenance of adult stem cells in several adult tissues/organs [41]. In this context, the SP phenotype is thought to be a universal marker of adult stem cells and has been used to isolate them from many adult tissues [42].

In the last 5 years, several papers have confirmed the existence of SP cells in human endometrium, and indeed, have demonstrated that it is possible to reconstruct human endometrium in vivo, reinforcing the concept that the SP technique could be a putative tool for the isolation of human endometrial adult stem cells (Table 11.1) [43–48]. This SP population

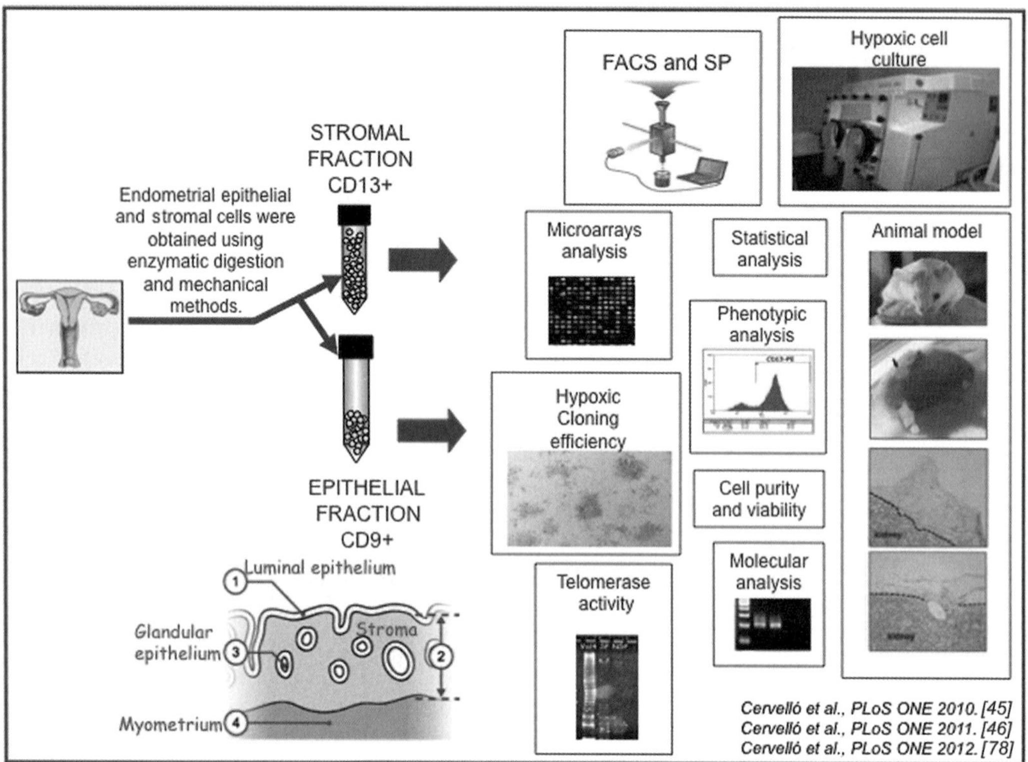

Figure 11.2 Schematic detailing the procedures used for the identification, characterization, and isolation of side population cells from human endometrium. After purification of human endometrial epithelial and stromal cells several assays were performed in order to confirm stem-cell features of this subset of cells, including molecular analysis (PCR, microarrays, telomerase activity), cell characterization (flow cytometry, hypoxic cell culture, cell cloning), in vitro differentiation (adipogenic and osteogenic lineages), and in vivo models (reconstruction in subcutaneous tissues and beneath the kidney capsule). (See also color plate.)

demonstrates high clonogenicity, expresses undifferentiation cell markers, has a mesenchymal stem-cell phenotype demonstrated by the expression of CD90, CD105, and CD73, and has the ability to differentiate in vitro to adipogenic, osteogenic, and chondrogenic lineages (Figure 11.2). However, the ultimate demonstration of the veracity of these candidate endometrial stem/progenitor cells was the reconstruction of human endometrium in an animal model, which has so far been accomplished by two independent groups (Table 11.1) [45–47].

A comparative genome-wide analysis of the epithelial and stromal SPs vs. their corresponding total endometrial counterparts revealed the existence of an endometrial SP gene signature [45]. Using pre-defined criteria, a total of 196 up- and 117 down-regulated genes were differentially expressed in the epithelial SP vs. the whole epithelium, and 121 up- and 73 down-regulated genes in the stromal SP vs. the

complete stromal compartment. The raw data files of these experiments have been uploaded to the NCBI Gene Expression Omnibus (GEO) database, accession number GSE21633. All the biological processes associated with the changes in gene regulation in SP cells suggest that this subset of cells is involved with cell fate and proliferation.

The SP method has also been used for the identification of progenitor candidates in the human myometrium [49]. Myometrial SP cells do not express CD34 or CD45, are relatively undifferentiated, and express lower levels of ERα, PR, and the smooth-muscle cell markers, calponin and smoothelin, compared with myometrial cells. They also spontaneously differentiate into mature myometrial cells expressing αSMA and calponin under hypoxic conditions [49]. Human myometrial SP cells transplanted into the uterine horns of estrogen-supplemented NOD/SCID/gc-null (NOG) mice [50] incorporated

Table 11.1 Summary of the scientific publications found when searching for endometrial stem cells using the side population (SP) method, and their take-home messages

Candidate endometrial stem/ progenitor cells	Number of samples	Take-home message	Reference
Isolated epithelial and stromal side population cells	34	Differentiation of endometrial SP cells to epithelial glands and stroma in vitro.	[43]
Isolation of endometrial side population cells	17	SP cells are highly clonogenic, express mesenchymal stem-cell markers, and decidualize in vitro. BCRP-1$^+$ cells are located in the basalis layer.	[48]
Isolation of epithelial and stromal side population cells	53	The % of SP cells remains constant throughout menstrual cycle; express undifferentiated markers such as c-kit and OCT4. Phenotypic analysis (CD90$^+$) confirmed their mesenchymal origin.	[44]
Isolation of epithelial and stromal side population cells	128	SP cells possess a mesenchymal phenotype, express markers of undifferentiated cells, and show an intermediate telomerase activity pattern, with a high cloning efficiency in hypoxic environments. Differentiated in vitro to adipocytes and osteocytes, and reconstructed human endometrium in an animal model.	[45]
Isolation of epithelial and stromal side population cells	78	SP cells differentiate into multiple types of endometrial cells in vitro and regenerated functional endometrium in vivo. Predominantly endothelial cells.	[47]
Generation of epithelial and stromal side population cell Lines (ICE)	7	SP endometrial stem-cell lines were generated with a mesenchymal phenotype (CD90, CD105, and CD73 positive); expressed markers of undifferentiated cells and show telomerase activity; differentiated in vitro into mesenchymal lineages and reconstructed human endometrium after cell-line injection as a xenograft.	[46]

into the myometrium and co-expressed vimentin and αSMA. Recently this SP methodology has been used to isolate and identify putative tumor-initiating leiomyoma stem cells. In this context, the Simón group has isolated and characterized SPs from human leiomyomas, analyzing their clonogenic activity under hypoxic conditions, and establishing two leiomyoma SP cell lines (LeioSP1 and LeioSP2), thus demonstrating their ability to differentiate into different mesenchymal lineages, and form leiomyoma-like tissues in an animal model [51].

Endometrial reconstitution in vivo

The functional proof of concept for a putative endometrial stem/progenitor cell population is the in vivo reconstitution of the original tissue [2]. Functional endometrium has been regenerated from unfractionated human endometrial single-cell suspensions xenotransplanted beneath the kidney capsule of ovariectomized and estrogen-supplemented NOG mice (lacking T, B, and natural killer cells) [52]. Well-organized endometrial tissue, comprising glandular structures expressing typical epithelial markers such as cytokeratin and CD9, stroma-positive for CD10 and CD13, and myometrial layers was reproduced [52]. In this animal model, both compartments underwent typical hormone-dependent changes characteristic of the secretory phase, such as production of tortuous glands and stromal decidualization, upon simulation of the menstrual cycle by cyclic administration of estrogen and progesterone [52]. Grafts collected after hormonal withdrawal contained large blood-filled cysts similar to the red-spot lesions of active endometriosis. Additionally, immunohistochemichal staining of cystic lesions revealed that the glandular structures were partly destroyed and that hemorrhage had occurred in the degenerated stroma [52]. Therefore this animal model provides an excellent in vivo assay system to test whether candidate human or mouse endometrial stem/progenitor cell populations, such as SP cells or CD146$^+$PDGF-Rβ$^+$ stromal cells, can reconstitute endometrial tissue [21].

Following this line of investigation, recent publications by two independent groups give further support to the regenerative ability of human endometrial SPs [45–47]. In the first study subcutaneous injection of the endometrial stromal SP fraction produced a vascularized structure in the subcutaneous fat at the injection site. The human origin of these structures was assessed by RT-PCR using primer sequences specifically designed to distinguish human from mouse cells and by immunohistochemical analysis of the human PR [45]. In the second study single-cell suspensions derived from human endometrial stem/progenitor cell lines obtained by the SP isolation method, were injected under the kidney capsule and animals were treated hormonally with estrogen alone and/or estrogen plus progesterone [46]. In all cases endometrial-like tissues were generated, but animals injected with a combination of epithelial and stromal cell lines and treated with both estrogen and progesterone showed a higher endometrial regenerative ability. This finding indicates the importance of epithelial–stromal interactions for SP cells as they reconstitute endometrial tissue in vivo and suggests that these interacting cells types may form the endometrial stem-cell niche.

Endometrial stem/progenitor cell markers

Currently there are no publications identifying specific markers for endometrial epithelial stem/progenitor cells, although several candidates are under investigation in our and other laboratories. In these ongoing studies candidate markers are being assessed in rigorous adult stem-cell functional assays to verify their utility.

Human endometrial MSC markers

MSC-like cells have been isolated from human endometrium using co-expression of two perivascular cell markers, CD146 and PDGF receptor-β (PDGF-Rβ) [53]. The flow-cytometry-sorted CD146$^+$PDGF-Rβ^+ subpopulation was enriched eightfold for CFUs compared to unfractionated stromal cells. These CD146$^+$PDGF-Rβ^+ cells expressed the typical MSC surface markers, CD29, CD44, CD73, CD90, and CD105, and were negative for haematopoietic and endothelial markers (CD31, CD34, and CD45) [53]. STRO-1, the classic marker used to prospectively isolate bone marrow MSCs

was not expressed by these cells nor by clonogenic stromal CFUs [54]. CD146$^+$PDGF-Rβ^+ cells were multipotent and were able to differentiate into adipogenic, myogenic, chondrogenic, and osteoblastic lineages. Moreover, confocal microscopy showed that CD146 and PDGF-Rβ co-expressing cells were located perivascularly in the functionalis and basalis, and appeared to be pericytes [53]. Subsequent gene profiling of the CD146 and PDGF-Rβ sorted populations showed that CD146$^+$PDGF-Rβ^+ cells express signaling pathway markers relevant to stem-cell self-renewal and multipotency [55]. This double-positive population clustered with endometrial fibroblasts and was distinct from endothelial cells, indicating its genetic program was predictive of its differentiated lineage, the stromal fibroblast [55]. The gene profile of endometrial CD146$^+$PDGF-Rβ^+ cells suggested they have immunomodulatory potential and low immunogenicity (low MHC class I gene expression), similar to menstrual blood-derived MSC-like cells [56] and other sources of MSCs [57].

Screening endometrial tissues and cells with perivascular markers has identified W5C5 as a single novel marker (Figure 11.3A, B), which purifies endometrial MSCs with all the in vitro properties of MSCs [58]. W5C5$^+$ cells reconstruct human stromal tissue when transplanted under the kidney capsule of immunocompromised NSG mice (Figure 11.3D). Purification of endometrial MSCs has been greatly simplified using W5C5 as a single marker by allowing magnetic bead sorting, thereby significantly increasing the yield [58]. As for CD146$^+$PDGF-Rβ^+ cells, W5C5$^+$ cells are located in the functionalis and basalis, indicating they will be shed in menstrual effluent. Together these data suggest that the CD146$^+$PDGF-Rβ^+ or W5C5$^+$ subpopulation of endometrial stromal cells contains MSC-like cells (Figure 11.3E) similar to bone marrow and adipose tissue MSCs.

A number of studies have examined stem-cell marker expression in human and mouse endometrium by immunotechniques. These studies, while valuable, require further analysis to validate whether the cells expressing these markers indeed function as endometrial stem/progenitor cells [21]. Nevertheless, Oct4 (POU5F1), a transcription factor and marker of pluripotent human embryonic stem cells [61], and more recently of adult stem cells [62], was expressed in some human endometrial samples in the

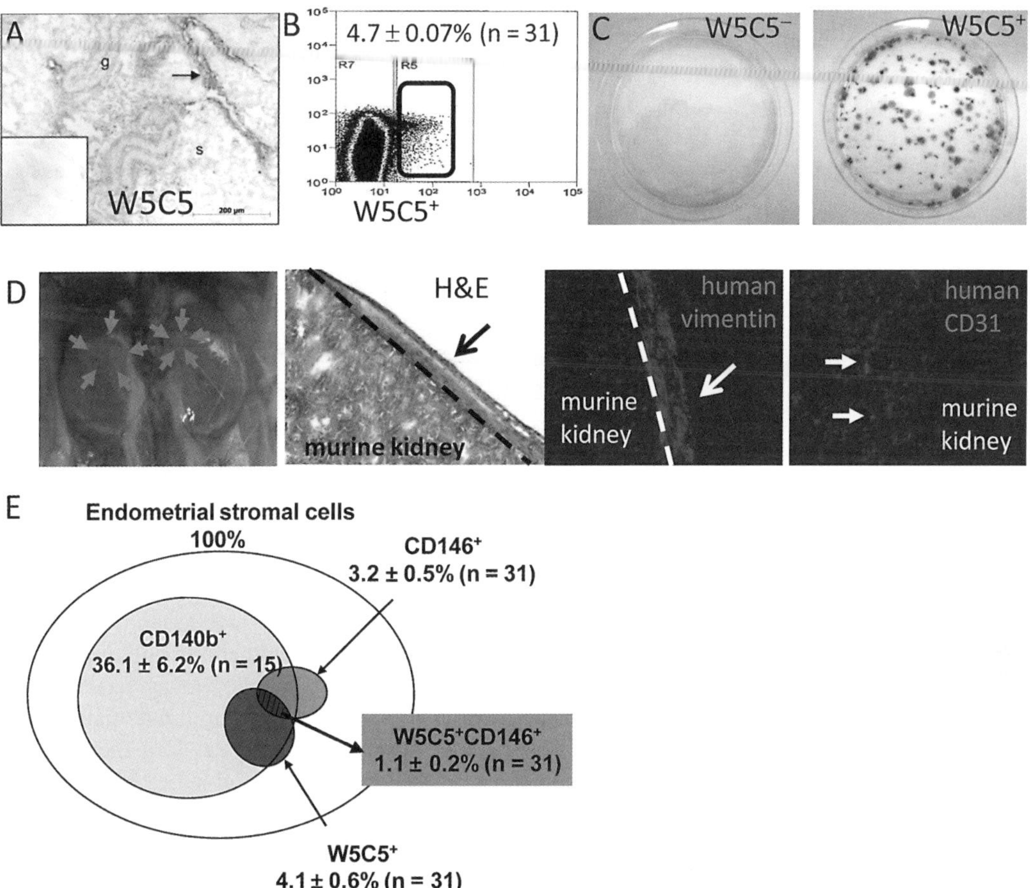

Figure 11.3 W5C5 is a novel marker of human endometrial mesenchymal stem/stromal cells (MSC). (A) Immunostained human endometrium showing perivascular W5C5 immunolocalization (arrow shows representative staining). (B) Representative flow cytometry histogram of W5C5 (n = 31) expression on human endometrial stromal cells. (C) Representative cloning plates of flow-cytometry-sorted W5C5− and W5C5+ cells showing that almost all cloning activity is in the W5C5+ population. (D) Xenografted W5C5+ cells under the kidney capsule of immunocompromised NSG mice resulted in reconstitution of endometrial vimentin+ stromal tissue under the capsule. Some transplanted cells differentiated into CD31+ (human) endothelial cells which migrated and incorporated into murine kidney blood vessels (arrows in right panels). (E) Schematic showing relationship between W5C5+ (n = 31), PDGF-Rβ+ (n = 15), and CD146+ (n = 31) cells. Adapted and reproduced with permission from Cognizant Communications Corporation, copyright 2012. Masuda, *et al.* A novel marker of human endometrial mesenchymal stem-like cells. *Cell Transplantation.* 2012; 21: 2201–2214 [58]. (See also color plate.)

proliferative stage of the menstrual cycle [63]. However this study did not quantify or determine the identity or location of the Oct4+ cells. POU5F1 was co-localized with 0.19% of stromal LRCs in the lower region of the murine endometrial stroma, suggesting that this specific subset of LRCs is highly undifferentiated [30]. Furthermore, nested-PCR confirmed the presence of POU5F1 mRNA in mouse uteri during the pre-pubertal period (day 21) and in adulthood (day 50) [30]. Together, these studies indicate that Oct4 could be a candidate endometrial stem-cell marker.

Musashi-1, an RNA-binding protein in neural stem cells, and an epithelial progenitor cell marker that regulates stem-cell self-renewal signaling pathways, was recently localized to single epithelial and stromal cells, as well as small clusters of stromal cells in the human endometrium [64]. Musashi-1-expressing cells were greater in number in the basalis compared to the functionalis in the proliferative stage of the menstrual cycle, suggesting their possible stem/progenitor cell function. Moreover, Notch-1 and telomerase, key downstream targets of Musashi-1, co-localized with Musashi-1+ endometrial cells. Interestingly the stromal Musashi-1[+] cells were not found in a perivascular location [53], although some were found in a peri-glandular region, similar to some stromal LRCs in mouse endometrium [29]. It is now an important task to determine whether Musashi-1 is expressed in endometrial stromal CFUs and in CD146[+]PDGF-Rβ[+] or W5C5[+] cells, although the latter would appear unlikely given their different localizations.

A recent flow-cytometric analysis identified cells with a haematopoietic stem-cell phenotype (CD34[+]CD45[+]) in human endometrial cell suspensions that co-expressed CD7 and CD56 and appeared to be lymphoid progenitors [65]. Whether these cells function as haematopoietic stem cells and generate endometrial leukocytes in the endometrium or contribute to the SP remains unknown. A principal haematopoietic stem-cell marker is the proto-oncogene c-*KIT* (CD117), which encodes a 145-kDa trans-membrane tyrosine kinase receptor specific for its ligand, stem-cell factor [66]. While c-kit co-localized to 0.32% of stromal LRCs in the lower region of murine endometrium [30] in one study, it was not detected in endometrial stromal LRCs in another [31]. Neither human endometrial epithelial nor stromal CFUs responded to stem-cell factor in CFU assays, suggesting that c-KIT may not be important in the function of human endometrial stem/progenitor cell function [24,25].

Menstrual blood stem/progenitor cells

Stromal cells have been cultured from menstrual blood in a manner similar to bone marrow-derived MSCs [67–69], indicating that endometrial MSCs are shed during menstruation. This concurs with the idea that they are located in the functionalis, as identified by the presence of CD146[+]PDGF-Rβ[+] and W5C5[+] markers [19]. Cultured menstrual blood cells appear fibroblastic and have substantial proliferative capacity [68,69]. In addition, they show telomerase activity and express hTERT as well as similar phenotypic markers to endometrial MSCs [67–70]. They also have a broad differentiation capacity, producing all meso-dermal lineages including skeletal and cardiac muscle cells [67,68], and neural lineages [69]. Menstrual blood MSCs express HLA-class I but not class II molecules [67,69], are of low immunogenicity when transplanted into immunocompetent mice and may

have immunomodulatory properties [56]. Our own unpublished studies have also demonstrated that menstrual blood contains clonogenic, multipotent MSCs and subpopulations of W5C5[+] cells [71]. Shedding of endometrial MSCs during menstruation suggests they may play a key role in initiating endometriotic lesions [2,72,73].

Sources of endometrial stem/progenitor cells

Remnant fetal stem cells

The human embryonic female reproductive tract has its origins in the intermediate mesoderm, which begins to form soon after gastrulation. As this embryonic tissue proliferates, it is thought that some cells undergo mesenchymal-to-epithelial transition to give rise to the coelomic epithelium that later invaginates to form the paramesonephric or Müllerian ducts. These ducts comprise surface epithelium and underlying urogenital ridge mesenchyme. During fetal life the glands start to develop as the undifferentiated uterine surface epithelium invaginates into the underlying mesenchyme and the inner myometrium begins to form, at the same time that smooth muscle cells differentiate from the mesenchyme [74].

A small number of fetal epithelial and mesenchymal stem cells are thought to remain in the adult endometrium and contribute to tissue replacement during its cyclic regeneration [2]. Whether there is an ultimate uterine stem cell that has the capacity to replace all endometrial and myometrial cells, including epithelial, stromal, vascular, and smooth muscle cells, or whether there are separate epithelial and mesenchymal stem cells is unknown. The different phenotypes, growth factor dependence, and frequency of clonogenic endometrial epithelial and stromal cells suggest that there are at least two endometrial progenitor cells. However, this does not exclude the possibility that an unidentified, more primitive precursor resides in human endometrium.

Circulating stem cells from the bone marrow

There is increasing evidence that bone-marrow-derived cells may also be a potential source of cells for endometrial regeneration [75–77]. Significant chimerism, ranging from 0.2–52%, was detected in the endometrial glands and stroma of four women who received single antigen HLA-mismatched bone-marrow transplants, suggesting that bone-marrow stem cells contributed, at least in part, to endometrial regeneration in a setting of cellular turnover and inflammatory stimuli [75]. It is not known whether bone-marrow donor cells contributing to the chimeric endometrial tissue are haemopoietic or mesenchymal in origin. Further evidence for bone-marrow stem-cell contribution to endometrial repair comes from gender-mismatch bone-marrow transplant studies in mice, where <0.01% of cytokeratin-positive endometrial epithelial cells and <0.1% of stromal cells contained a Y chromosome [77]. Nevertheless, a recent study from the Simón group, demonstrated that bone-marrow donor-derived cells did not contribute to the endometrial SP population of recipients. Using a clinical model of female bone-marrow transplant recipients who received bone marrow from human leukocyte antigen (HLA)-identical male donors, the presence of XY donor-derived cells in the recipient endometrium was confirmed, and ranged from 1.7% to 2.62% [78]. From these it was determined that 0.45% to 0.85% of the donor-derived cells in the epithelial compartment displaying the CD9 marker, and 1.0% to 1.83% vimentin-positive XY donor-derived cells segregated to the stromal cell compartment. However, XY donor-derived cells were not found in the SP population, suggesting that they could be a limited exogenous source of transdifferentiated endometrial cells rather than a cycling endogenous source [78]. Therefore, bone-marrow cell contribution to endometrial repair is modest, and engraftment of the endometrium seems more likely to occur during repair after injury or regeneration that occurs during pregnancy and after parturition.

In a mouse model, circulating $CD45^+$ bone-marrow cells were shown to contribute to 82% of mouse uterine epithelium during pregnancy in a novel double-reporter *CD45/Cre-Z/EG* transgenic mouse used to track the fate of $CD45^+$ green fluorescent protein (GFP) cells in female mice [76]. However, these results must be interpreted with caution as data was only obtained from a single pregnant reporter mouse. Endometrial epithelial and stromal LRCs did not express CD45 [29], but expression of this haematopoietic marker may be lost if bone-marrow cells incorporate and transdifferentiate into endometrial epithelium. The role of estrogen and progesterone in recruiting bone-marrow cells has not been examined, although progesterone may have a role during pregnancy.

Endometrial stem/progenitor cells: clinical perspective

Since adult stem cells regulate tissue homeostasis, it is expected that abnormal functioning of endometrial stem/progenitor cells, and/or their surrounding niche cells, may also be involved in the initiation and progression of gynecological diseases associated with abnormal endometrial proliferation, such as endometriosis, adenomyosis, endometrial hyperplasia, and endometrial cancer [2]. Furthermore, epithelial and stromal CFUs are present in non-cycling and perimenopausal endometrium [25] and may be responsible for the regeneration of endometrium in women given estrogen replacement therapy [2].

Cancer stem cells in endometrial cancer

The cellular composition of any cancer is heterogeneous. Individual cancer cells vary in their ability to initiate tumors, in marker expression, gene expression profiles, proliferation, differentiation potential, and lifespan. Like their normal tissue counterparts, there is a cellular hierarchy in tumors, with the rare stem cells or cancer stem cells (CSCs) at the apex. CSCs are thought to give rise to more-differentiated daughter tumor cells [79]. CSCs have been extensively characterized in leukemia and many other solid human tumors including breast, glioblastoma, colon, pancreas, prostate, and ovary (reviewed by Lobo *et al.* [80]). However, the origin of CSCs remains questionable. It has been suggested that CSCs could arise from the transformation of normal adult stem or progenitor cells, or even from mature cells after acquiring genetic changes conferring the ability to self-renew [81]. CSCs are defined as self-renewing cells present within a tumor that have the capacity to regenerate the phenotypic diversity of the original tumor [80]. Thus CSCs initiate, maintain, and propagate tumors in vivo, producing heterogeneous tumor cell progeny. CSCs can initiate clones in vitro, undergo self-renewal, and exhibit high proliferative potential. In cancers where

CSCs have been identified, they comprise <1% of the total cancer-cell population.

Endometrial cancer is characterized by abnormal endometrial epithelial cell proliferation. It affects around 6430 women each year in the UK, resulting in approximately 1630 deaths [82], making endometrial cancer the most common gynecological malignancy in the Western world. There are two types of endometrial adenocarcinoma. Type I generally affects pre- and perimenopausal women, is estrogen dependent, and is associated with mutations in Pten, K-ras, and β-catenin genes or with microsatellite instability (MSI) [83]. Type II normally affects post-menopausal women, is estrogen independent, and is associated with mutations in p53 and HER-2/neu [83].

Evidence for endometrial CSCs has recently been obtained from studies in human endometrial-cancer cell lines and isolated primary endometrial cancer cells [84,85]. A small population (<1%) of freshly isolated endometrial cancer cells demonstrated clonogenic activity and self-renewal ability in vitro and in vivo [85]. In this study clonally derived endometrial-cancer cells expressed several stem-cell self-renewal genes, including *BMI-1*, *NANOG*, and *SOX2*. When these cells were transplanted into immunocompromised mice, they recapitulated parent tumor histoarchitecture and marker expression, including cytokeratin, vimentin, and estrogen and progesterone receptors. Side populations, another key property of adult stem cells, have been identified in endometrial cancer and in several endometrial-cancer cell lines [84,86]. In particular, a small SP population (0.22%) detected in the AN3CA cell line exhibited typical stem-cell properties of relative quiescence, self-renewal, and chemoresistance [84], although it remains to be seen if these properties are present in tumor cells isolated from primary human endometrial carcinomas. Tumor-initiating cells were also demonstrated in the SP, but not in the non-SP cell fraction, when both of these cell subsets were injected subcutaneously into male NOD/SCID mice with estrogen implants [84]. Similarly, SP cells in the Hec1 cell line were also clonogenic, underwent self-renewal, and produced large tumors in vivo [86].

CD133 has also been examined as a marker of endometrial CSCs, using the CD133/1 epitope in an attempt to isolate this population [87]; in an extensive study of 113 endometrial cancer samples, CD133+ cells were shown to have a higher cloning efficiency, proliferation rates, and chemoresistance. While this study showed that both the CD133+ and CD133− fractions contained clonogenic cells, only xenograft-derived, but not freshly dissociated CD133+ cells, were capable of tumor formation in vivo. Another recent report demonstrated that CD133+ cells more readily formed tumors when compared with CD133− cells [88]. Moreover, the percentage of CD133+ cells increased with serial transplantation of human endometrial cancer cells. Overall, both studies demonstrated that CD133+ and CD133− cells exhibit tumor-forming ability, thus further research is required to confirm that CD133 is indeed a marker of endometrial CSCs. Similarly, an immunohistochemical study showed that Musashi-1 is expressed in small clusters of endometrial cancer tissue, suggesting a potential cancer stem- or progenitor-cell origin [64]. However, the stem-cell activity of Musashi-1-expressing cells was not investigated, and until functional studies are undertaken, it is not known if Musashi-1 enriches endometrial CSCs.

Endometriosis

Endometriosis is characterized by the growth of ectopic endometrial tissue on pelvic organs and the peritoneum [89]. It is thought that retrograde menstruation, which occurs in most menstruating women, deposits menstrual debris into the peritoneal cavity. However, it is not known why only 6–10% of women develop endometriosis and its associated symptoms of inflammation, pain, and infertility. It has been postulated that in women who develop endometriosis, endometrial stem/progenitor cells are inappropriately shed during menstruation and reach the peritoneal cavity where they adhere and establish endometriotic implants [2,19]. Recently, MSC-like cells were identified in cultures of ectopic endometrial stromal cells [90]. These MSC-like cells had a typical MSC surface phenotype, were multipotent, as they differentiated into mesodermal and ectodermal lineages, and were invasive in an in vivo model. Clonogenic epithelial and stromal CFUs have also been identified in ovarian endometrioma [91]. These CFUs underwent self-renewal in serial cloning assays and the stromal CFUs were multipotent. Together these studies indicate that endometrial stem/progenitor cells are present in ectopic endometrial lesions, but they do not provide evidence for their direct role in initiating endometriosis or whether they reach the peritoneal cavity by retrograde menstruation. Bone-marrow stem cells may also contribute to the progression of endometrial lesion development, as demonstrated recently in a mouse model [77]. Some forms of endometriosis may arise from remnant fetal Müllerian cells, which may behave like stem cells to establish ectopic growth of endometrial tissue. Clearly the role of endometrial stem/progenitor cells or bone-marrow stem cells in the development of endometriosis will require extensive further research.

Adenomyosis

Adenomyosis, a condition affecting 1% of women, results from extensive myometrial invasion by the basal endometrium. It is associated with smooth muscle hyperplasia, and is also considered to arise from fetal Müllerian cells [92]. In a study designed to examine stem/progenitor cell activity in adenomyosis tissue, cells were cultured at normal seeding densities and shown to have MSC-like properties similar to cultured eutopic endometrial cells [93]. These adenomyosis cells had a surface-marker phenotype similar to endometrial MSCs and were multipotent. No epithelial progenitor-cell activity was reported. In gene profiling, the adenomyosis MSC-like cells, principal-component analysis showed that while endometrial MSC-like cells clustered near bone-marrow MSCs, their profiles were distant from the adenomyosis MSC-like populations [93]. Clearly more research is required to determine if there is a role for endometrial stem/progenitor cells in adenomyosis, particularly for the epithelial progenitor population, in the development of the ectopic glands. Furthermore, the possible role of endometrial MSC populations or myometrial SP cells in the development of excessive smooth muscle differentiation associated with myometrial hyperplasia has not yet been examined.

Tissue-engineering applications

There is great interest in the use of both embryonic and adult stem cells in tissue-engineering applications for restoring function to aging or diseased tissues and organs. Medical advances have ensured increasing longevity and the aging population has many tissues in need of repair [94]. The failure of artificial implants to last longer than 10–15 years and the problems associated with non-degradable synthetic materials make cell-based therapies for tissue replacement

an attractive prospect [95]. There is now a focus on using tissue-engineering approaches, combining temporary biological scaffold materials to provide initial support, and stem cells to promote appropriate tissue genesis and regeneration of functional tissue. This is particularly important for the provision of supportive tissues and could be adapted to tissue-engineer support for the female reproductive tract. Pelvic-floor prolapse is a major problem which results in 19% of women requiring surgery, and approximately 15% of these requiring repeat surgery [96]. The use of artificial and biological scaffolds for pelvic-floor-prolapse surgery has improved outcomes to a limited degree, but has also introduced a new set of problems. Thus the use of tissue-engineering constructs comprising scaffolds and autologous endometrial mesenchymal stem/progenitor cells may provide a possible solution for treatment of pelvic-floor prolapse in the future [26].

Conclusions and future directions for human endometrial stem/progenitor cell research

Adult stem cells have been identified in human and mouse endometrium on the basis of their functional attributes. The identification of specific markers for endometrial MSCs has demonstrated their perivascular location in the basalis and functionalis. Once candidate markers for epithelial progenitors are verified, the opportunity for investigating endometrial stem/progenitor cells and their potential roles in endometrial proliferative disorders are likely to become a reality. Endometrial stem-cell research continues to gain momentum and the knowledge generated may be translated into the clinic within the next decade. However, there are still many unresolved issues in endometrial stem-cell biology; these include the exact relationship between cultured endometrial stromal cells, clonogenic stromal cells, and SP cells. Whether there is a single more primitive endometrial stem cell that produces all cell types in the uterus remains unknown, and the identification of definitive markers for endometrial epithelial stem/progenitor cells will certainly advance the field. Furthermore, characterization of the endometrial stem-cell niches and the signaling pathways involved in the regulation of the resident stem/progenitor cells is also required. Investigation into the possible roles of developmental pathways involving bone morphogenetic protein, Hedgehog, Notch, and Wnt signaling in endometrial stem/progenitor cell self-renewal and cell-fate differentiation decisions would be a valuable starting point. These molecules or pathways have already been detected in endometrium or have important roles during endometrial development and decidualization when stromal cells undergo terminal differentiation. More extensive studies examining how estrogen, progesterone, and the growth factors EGF, TGFα, PDGF, and bFGF interact with endometrial stem/progenitor cells and their niche cells would also be useful. Further investigation into the mechanisms by which estrogen interacts with endometrial stem/progenitor cells or their neighboring niche cells needs to be explored. Obtaining such additional knowledge will assist the investigation into the role of endometrial stem/progenitor cells in gynecological disorders associated with abnormal endometrial proliferation, and will not only increase our understanding of the pathophysiology of endometriosis, adenomyosis, endometrial hyperplasia, and endometrial cancer, but also has the potential to change the way these hormone-dependent diseases are treated in the future.

Acknowledgments

The authors' work described in this review was supported by project grants from the National Health and Medical Research Council (NHMRC) of Australia (545992, 1021127) and an NHMRC RD Wright Career Development Award (465121) (to CEG), and was supported by the Victorian Government's Operational Infrastructure Support Program, as well as grants funded SAF (Plan Nacional de Biomedicina) 2008–02048 supported by the Spanish Ministry of Science and Innovation (PI: C.S.), Fundacion Gent per Gent 08/09 (PI: C.S.), and PROMETEO/2008/163 (PI: C.S.) (HPTN was supported by an Australian Postgraduate Award and Postgraduate Publication Award.)

References

1. Jabbour, H.N., Kelly, R.W., Fraser, H.M., Critchley, H.O.D. Endocrine regulation of menstruation. *Endocrine Reviews.* 2006; 27: 17–46.

2. Gargett, C.E. Uterine stem cells: what is the evidence? *Human Reproduction Update.* 2007; 13: 87–101.

3. Burton, G.J., Watson, A.L., Hempstock, J., Skepper, J.N., Jauniaux, E. Uterine glands provide histiotrophic nutrition for the human fetus during the first trimester of pregnancy. *Journal of Clinical Endocrinology and Metabolism.* 2002; 87: 2954–2959.

4. Henriet, P., Gaide Chevronnay, H.P., Marbaix, E. The endocrine and paracrine control of menstruation. *Molecular Cell Endocrinology.* 2011; 358: 197–207.

5. Ludwig, H., Metzger, H., Frauli, M. Endometrium: tissue remodelling and regeneration. In: D'Arcangues, C., Fraser, I.S., Newton, J.R., and Odlind, V., eds. *Contraception and Mechanisms of Endometrial Bleeding.* Cambridge: Cambridge University Press. 1990; 441–446.

6. Okulicz, W.C., Scarrell, R. Estrogen receptor a and progesterone receptor in the rhesus endometrium during the late secretory phase and menses. *Proceedings of the Society for Experimental Biology and Medicine.* 1998; 218: 316–321.

7. Garry, R., Hart, R., Karthigasu, K.A, Burke, C. A re-appraisal of the morphological changes within the endometrium during menstruation: a hysteroscopic, histological and scanning electron microscopic study. *Human Reproduction.* 2009; 24: 1393–1401.

8. Padykula, H.A., Coles, L.G., Okulicz, W.C. *et al.* Kaiserman–Abramof IR. The basalis of the primate endometrium: a bifunctional germinal compartment. *Biology of Reproduction.* 1989; 40: 681–690.

9. Slayden, O.D., Brenner, R.M. Hormonal regulation and localization of estrogen, progestin and androgen receptors in the endometrium of nonhuman primates: effects of progesterone receptor antagonists. *Archives of Histology and Cytology.* 2004; 67: 393–409.

10. Padykula, H.A. Regeneration of the primate uterus: the role of stem cells. *Annals of the New York Academy of Science.* 1991; 622: 47–56.

11. Ferenczy, A., Bertrand, G., Gelfand, M.M. Proliferation kinetics of human endometrium during the normal menstrual cycle. *American Journal of Obstetrics and Gynecology.* 1979; 133: 859–867.

12. McLennan, C.E., Rydell, A.H. Extent of endometrial shedding during normal menstruation. *Obstetrics and Gynecology.* 1965; 26: 605–621.

13. Brenner, R.M., Slayden, O.D., Rodgers, W.H. *et al.* Immunocytochemical assessment of mitotic activity with an antibody to phosphorylated histone H3 in the macaque and human endometrium. *Human Reproduction.* 2003; 18: 1185–1193.

14. Fan, X., Krieg, S., Hwang, J.Y. *et al.* Dynamic regulation of Wnt7a expression in the primate endometrium: implications for postmenstrual regeneration and secretory transformation. *Endocrinology.* 2012; 153: 1063–1069.

15. Ponnampalam, A.P., Weston, G.C., Trajstman, A.C., Susil, B., Rogers, P.A. Molecular classification of

human endometrial cycle stages by transcriptional profiling. *Molecular Human Reproduction*. 2004; 10: 879–893.

16. Talbi, S., Hamilton, A.E., Vo, K.C. *et al.* Molecular phenotyping of human endometrium distinguishes menstrual cycle phases and underlying biological processes in normo-ovulatory women. *Endocrinology*. 2006; 147: 1097–1121.

17. Nguyen, H.P.T., Sprung, C.N., Gargett, C.E. Differential expression of Wnt signaling molecules between pre- and postmenopausal endometrial epithelial cells suggests a population of putative epithelial stem/progenitor cells reside in the basalis layer. *Endocrinology*. 2012; 153: 2870–2883.

18. Paulson, R.J., Boostanfar, R., Saadat, P. *et al.* Pregnancy in the sixth decade of life: obstetric outcomes in women of advanced reproductive age. *Journal of the American Medical Association*. 2002; 288: 2320–2323.

19. Gargett, C.E., Masuda, H. Adult stem cells in the endometrium. *Molecular Human Reproduction*. 2010; 16: 818–834.

20. Eckfeldt, C.E., Mendenhall, E.M., Verfaillie, C.M. The molecular repertoire of the "almighty" stem cell. *Nature Reviews Molecular Cell Biology*. 2005; 6: 726–737.

21. Gargett, C.E., Chan, R.W., Schwab, K.E. Endometrial stem cells. *Current Opinion in Obstetrics and Gynecology*. 2007; 19: 377–383.

22. Li, L., Xie, T. Stem cell niche: structure and function. *Annual Review of Cell Developmental Biology*. 2005; 21: 605–631.

23. Snyder, E.Y., Loring, J.F. A role for stem cell biology in the physiological and pathological aspects of aging. *Journal of the American Geriatrics Society*. 2005; 53: S287–S291.

24. Chan, R.W.S., Schwab, K.E., Gargett, C.E. Clonogenicity of human endometrial epithelial and stromal cells. *Biology of Reproduction*. 2004; 70: 1738–1750.

25. Schwab, K.E., Chan, R.W., Gargett, C.E. Putative stem cell activity of human endometrial epithelial and stromal cells during the menstrual cycle. *Fertility and Sterility*. 2005; 84 Suppl 2: 1124–1130.

26. Gargett, C.E., Chan, R.W. Endometrial stem/progenitor cells and proliferative disorders of the endometrium. *Minerva Ginecologica*. 2006; 58: 511–526.

27. Gargett, C.E., Schwab, K.E., Zillwood, R.M., Nguyen, H.P.T., Wu, D. Isolation and culture of epithelial progenitors and mesenchymal stem cells from human endometrium. *Biology of Reproduction*. 2009; 80: 1136–1145.

28. Gargett, C.E. Identification and characterisation of human endometrial stem/progenitor cells. *Australian and New Zealand Journal of Obstetrics and Gynaecology*. 2006; 46: 250–253.

29. Chan, R.W., Gargett, C.E. Identification of label-retaining cells in mouse endometrium. *Stem Cells*. 2006; 24: 1529–1538.

30. Cervelló, I., Martinez-Conejero, J.A., Horcajadas, J.A., Pellicer, A., Simón, C. Identification, characterization and co-localization of label-retaining cell population in mouse endometrium with typical undifferentiated markers. *Human Reproduction*. 2007; 22: 45–51.

31. Szotek, P.P., Chang, H.L., Zhang, L. *et al.* Adult mouse myometrial label-retaining cells divide in response to gonadotropin stimulation. *Stem Cells*. 2007; 25: 1317–1325.

32. Chan, R.W.S, Kaitu'u-Lino, T., Gargett, C.E. Role of label-retaining cells in estrogen-induced endometrial regeneration. *Reproductive Sciences*. 2012; 19: 102–114.

33. Dimitrov, R., Timeva, T., Kyurkchiev, D. *et al.* Characterisation of clonogenic stromal cells isolated from human endometrium. *Reproduction*. 2008; 135: 551–558.

34. Vaananen, H.K. Mesenchymal stem cells. *Annals of Medicine*. 2005; 37: 469–479.

35. Wolff, E.F., Wolff, A.B., Du, H., Taylor, H.S. Demonstration of multipotent stem cells in the adult human endometrium by in vitro chondrogenesis. *Reproductive Sciences*. 2007; 14: 524–533.

36. Santamaria, X., Massasa, E.E., Feng, Y., Wolff, E., Taylor, H.S. Derivation of insulin producing cells from human endometrial stromal stem cells and use in the treatment of murine diabetes. *Molecular Therapies*. 2011; 19: 2065–2071.

37. Wolff, E.F., Gao, X.B., Yao, K.V. *et al.* Endometrial stem cell transplantation restores dopamine production in a Parkinson's disease model. *Journal of Cell and Molecular Medicine*. 2010; 15: 747–755.

38. Potten, C.S., Owen, G., Booth, D. Intestinal stem cells protect their genome by selective segregation of template DNA strands. *Journal of Cell Science*. 2002; 115: 2381–2388.

39. Kaitu'u-Lino, T.J., Ye, L., Salamonsen, L.A., Girling, J.E., Gargett, C.E. Identification of label-retaining perivascular cells in a mouse model of endometrial decidualization, breakdown, and repair. *Biology of Reproduction*. 2012; 86: 184.

40. Goodell, M.A., Brose, K., Paradis, G., Conner, A.S., Mulligan, R.C. Isolation and functional properties of murine hematopoietic stem cells that are replicating in vivo. *Journal of Experimental Medicine*. 1997; 183: 1797–1806.

41. Zhou, S., Schuetz, J.D., Bunting, K.D. *et al*. The ABC transporter Bcrp1/ABCG2 is expressed in a wide variety of stem cells and is a molecular determinant of the side-population phenotype. *Nature Medicine*. 2001; 7: 1028–1034.

42. Smalley, M.J., Clarke, R.B. The mammary gland "side population": a putative stem/progenitor cell marker? *Journal of Mammary Gland Biology and Neoplasia*. 2005; 10: 37–47.

43. Kato, K., Yoshimoto, M., Kato, K. *et al*. Characterization of side-population cells in human normal endometrium. *Human Reproduction*. 2007; 22: 1214–1223.

44. Cervelló, I., Martinez-Conejero, J.A., Horcajadas, J.A., Pellicier, A., Simón, C. Side population phenotype: an essential characteristic for the somatic stem cells in the human endometrium? *Reproductive Sciences*. 2008; 15 Suppl 2-72A.

45. Cervelló, I., Gil-Sanchis, C., Mas, A. *et al*. Human endometrial side population cells exhibit genotypic, phenotypic and functional features of somatic stem cells. *PLoS One*. 2010; 5: e10964.

46. Cervelló, I., Mas, A., Gil-Sanchis, C. *et al*. Reconstruction of endometrium from human endometrial side population cell lines. *Plos One*. 2011; 6: e21221.

47. Masuda, H., Matsuzaki, Y., Hiratsu, E. *et al*. Stem cell-like properties of the endometrial side population: Implication in endometrial regeneration. *PLoS One*. 2010; 5: e10387.

48. Tsuji, S., Yoshimoto, M., Takahashi, K. *et al*. Side population cells contribute to the genesis of human endometrium. *Fertility and Sterility*. 2008; 90: 1528–1537.

49. Ono, M., Maruyama, T., Masuda, H. *et al*. Side population in human uterine myometrium displays phenotypic and functional characteristics of myometrial stem cells. *Proceedings of the National Academy of Sciences of the United States of America*. 2007; 104: 18700–18705.

50. Ito, M., Hiramatsu, H., Kobayashi, K. *et al*. NOD/SCID/g_c^null mouse: an excellent recipient mouse model for engraftment of human cells. *Blood*. 2002; 100: 3175–3182.

51. Mas, A., Cervelló, I., Gil-Sanchis, C. *et al*. Identification and characterization of the human leiomyoma side population as putative tumor-initiating cells. *Fertility and Sterility*. 2012; 98: 741–751.

52. Masuda, H., Maruyama, T., Hiratsu, E. *et al*. Noninvasive and real-time assessment of reconstructed functional human endometrium in NOD/SCID/g_c^null immunodeficient mice. *Proceedings of the National Academy of Sciences of the United States of America*. 2007; 104: 1925–1930.

53. Schwab, K.E., Gargett, C.E. Co-expression of two perivascular cell markers isolates mesenchymal stem-like cells from human endometrium. *Human Reproduction*. 2007; 22: 2903–2911.

54. Schwab, K.E., Hutchinson, P., Gargett, C.E. Identification of surface markers for prospective isolation of human endometrial stromal colony-forming cells. *Human Reproduction*. 2008; 23: 934–943.

55. Spitzer, T.L., Rojas, A., Zelenko, Z. *et al*. Perivascular human endometrial mesenchymal stem cells express pathways relevant to self-renewal, lineage specification, and functional phenotype. *Biology of Reproduction*. 2012; 86: 58.

56. Murphy, M.P., Wang, H., Patel, A.N. *et al*. Allogeneic endometrial regenerative cells: an "off the shelf solution" for critical limb ischemia? *Journal of Translational Medicine*. 2008; 6: 45.

57. Caplan, A.I. Why are MSCs therapeutic? New data: new insight. *Journal of Pathology*. 2009; 217: 318–324.

58. Masuda, H., Anwar, S.S., Buhring, H.J., Rao, J.R., Gargett, C.E. A novel marker of human endometrial mesenchymal stem-like cells. *Cell Transplantation*. 2012; 21: 2201–2214.

59. Pittenger, M.F., Mackay, A.M., Beck, S.C. *et al*. Multilineage potential of adult human mesenchymal stem cells. *Science*. 1999; 284: 143–147.

60. Zuk, P.A., Zhu, M., Ashjian, P. *et al*. Human adipose tissue is a source of multipotent stem cells. *Molecular Biology of the Cell*. 2002; 13: 4279–4295.

61. Hansis, C., Tang, Y.X., Grifo, J.A., Krey, L.C. Analysis of Oct-4 expression and ploidy in individual human blastomeres. *Molecular Human Reproduction*. 2001; 7: 155–161.

62. Tai, M.H., Chang, C.C., Kiupel, M. *et al*. Oct4 expression in adult human stem cells: evidence in support of the stem cell theory of carcinogenesis. *Carcinogenesis*. 2005; 26: 495–502.

63. Matthai, C., Horvat, R., Noe, M. *et al*. Oct-4 expression in human endometrium. *Molecular Human Reproduction*. 2006; 12: 7–10.

64. Götte, M., Wolf, M., Staebler, A. *et al*. Increased experssion of the adult stem cell marker Musashi-1 in endometriosis and endometrial carcinoma. *Journal of Pathology*. 2008; 215: 317–329.

65. Lynch, L., Golden-Mason, L., Eogan, M. *et al*. Cells with haematopoietic stem cell phenotype in adult human endometrium: relevance to infertility? *Human Reproduction*. 2007; 22: 919–926.

66. Lev, S., Blechman, J.M., Givol, D., Yarden, Y. Steel factor and c kit protooncogene: genetic lessons in signal transduction. *Critical Reviews in Oncogenesis.* 1994; 5: 141–168.

67. Cui, C.H., Uyama, T., Miyado, K. *et al.* Menstrual blood-derived cells confer human dystrophin expression in the murine model of Duchenne muscular dystrophy via cell fusion and myogenic transdifferentiation. *Molecular Biology of the Cell.* 2007; 18: 1586–1594.

68. Hida, N., Nishiyama, N., Miyoshi, S. *et al.* Novel cardiac precursor-like cells from human menstrual blood-derived mesenchymal cells. *Stem Cells.* 2008; 26: 1695–1704.

69. Patel, A.N., Park, E., Kuzman, M. *et al.* Multipotent menstrual blood stromal stem cells: isolation, characterization, and differentiation. *Cell Transplantation.* 2008; 17: 303–311.

70. Meng, X., Ichim, T.E., Zhong, J. *et al.* Endometrial regenerative cells: a novel stem cell population. *Journal of Translational Medicine.* 2007; 5: 57.

71. Anwar, S., Buhring, H.J., Gargett, C.E. A single perivascular marker identifies MSC in human endometrium and menstrual blood. *Australian Health and Medical Research Congress.* 2008; 4: P700.

72. Sasson, I.E., Taylor, H.S. Stem cells and the pathogenesis of endometriosis. *Annals of the New York Academy of Science.* 2008; 1127: 106–115.

73. Starzinski-Powitz, A., Zeitvogel, A., Schreiner, A., Baumann, R. In search of pathogenic mechanims in endometriosis: the challenge for molecular cell biology. *Current Molecular Medicine.* 2001; 1: 655–664.

74. Spencer, T.E., Hayashi, K., Hu, J., Carpenter, K.D. Comparative developmental biology of the mammalian uterus. *Current Topics in Developmental Biology.* 2005; 68: 85–122.

75. Taylor, H.S. Endometrial cells derived from donor stem cells in bone marrow transplant recipients. *Journal of the American Medical Association.* 2004; 292: 81–85.

76. Bratincsak, A., Brownstein, M.J., Cassiani-Ingoni, R. *et al.* CD45-positive blood cells give rise to uterine epithelial cells in mice. *Stem Cells.* 2007; 25: 2820–2826.

77. Du, H., Taylor, H.S. Contribution of bone marrow-derived stem cells to endometrium and endometriosis. *Stem Cells.* 2007; 25: 2082–2086.

78. Cervelló, I., Gil-Sanchis, C., Mas, A. *et al.* Bone marrow-derived cells from male donors do not contribute to the endometrial side population of the recipient. *Plos One.* 2012; 7: e30260.

79. Pardal, R., Clarke, M.F., Morrison, S.J. Applying the principles of stem-cell biology to cancer. *Nature Reviews Cancer.* 2003; 3: 895–902.

80. Lobo, N.A., Shimono, Y., Qian, D., Clarke, M.F. The biology of cancer stem cells. *Annual Review of Cell Developmental Biology.* 2007; 23: 675–699.

81. Jordan, C.T. Searching for leukemia stem cells: not yet the end of the road? *Cancer Cell.* 2006; 10: 253–254.

82. Cancer Research UK. http://infocancerresearchuk org/cancerstats/types/uterus/incidence/?a=5541. 2008; accessed 06/30/08.

83 Di Cristofano, A., Ellenson, L.H. Endometrial carcinoma. *Annual Reviews of Pathology: Mechanisms of Disease.* 2007; 2: 57–85.

84. Friel, A.M., Sergent, P.A., Patnaude, C. *et al.* Functional analyses of the cancer stem cell-like properties of human endometrial tumor initiating cells. *Cell Cycle.* 2008; 7: 242–249.

85. Hubbard, S.A., Friel, A.M., Kumar, B. *et al.* Evidence for cancer stem cells in human endometrial carcinoma. *Cancer Research.* 2009; 69: 8241–8248.

86. Kato, K., Takao, T., Kuboyama, A. *et al.* Endometrial cancer side-population cells show prominent migration and have a potential to differentiate into the mesenchymal cell lineage. *American Journal of Pathology.* 2010; 176: 381–392.

87. Rutella, S., Bonanno, G., Procoli, A. *et al.* Cells with characteristics of cancer stem/progenitor cells express the CD133 antigen in human endometrial tumors. *Clinical Cancer Research.* 2009; 15: 4299–4311.

88. Friel, A.M., Zhang, L., Curley, M.D. *et al.* Epigenetic regulation of CD133 and tumorigenicity of CD133 positive and negative endometrial cancer cells. *Reproductive Biology and Endocrinology.* 2010; 8: 147.

89. Giudice, L.C., Kao, L.C. Endometriosis. *Lancet* 2004; 364: 1789–1799.

90. Kao, A.P., Wang, K.H., Chang, C.C. *et al.* Comparative study of human eutopic and ectopic endometrial mesenchymal stem cells and the development of an in vivo endometriotic invasion model. *Fertility and Sterility.* 2011; 95: 1308–1315.

91. Chan, R.W., Ng, E.H., Yeung, W.S. Identification of cells with colony-forming activity, self-renewal capacity, and multipotency in ovarian endometriosis. *American Journal of Pathology.* 2011; 178: 2832–2844.

92. Ferenczy, A. Pathophysiology of adenomyosis. *Human Reproduction Update.* 1998; 4: 312–322.

93. Chen, Y.J., Li, H.Y., Chang, Y.L. *et al.* Suppression of migratory/invasive ability and induction of apoptosis in adenomyosis-derived mesenchymal stem cells by cyclooxygenase-2 inhibitors. *Fertility and Sterility.* 2010; 94: 1972–1979.

94. Vats, A., Bielby, R.C., Tolley, N.S., Nerem, R., Polak, J.M. Stem cells. *Lancet.* 2005; 366: 592–602.

95. Rahaman, M.N., Mao, J.J. Stem cell-based composite tissue constructs for regenerative medicine. *Biotechnology and Bioengineering.* 2005; 91: 261–284.

96. Smith, F.J., Holman, C.D., Moorin, R.E., Tsokos, N. Lifetime risk of undergoing surgery for pelvic organ prolapse. *Obstetrics and Gynecology.* 2010; 116: 1096–1100.

Chapter

12

In utero hematopoietic cell transplantation

Amar Nijagal and Tippi C. MacKenzie

Introduction

Fetal surgery is a promising treatment strategy for patients with congenital anatomic anomalies. Since the first open fetal operation in 1982 [1], the field has expanded to treat multiple anomalies using both conventional and minimally invasive techniques [2]. In addition to the treatment of anatomic anomalies such as myelomeningocele [3], recent advances in stem-cell biology and pre-natal diagnosis have brought in utero stem-cell therapy closer to clinical reality.

Hematopoietic stem-cell disorders such as sickle cell disease, thalassemias, and immunodeficiencies may be the most amenable diseases to consider for in utero treatment, given the wide experience with post-natal bone-marrow (BM) transplantation for these conditions [4–7]. However, BM transplantation is limited by many factors, such as: graft vs. host disease (Gvhd) graft rejection, the availability of few HLA-matched donors, and the morbidity of host myeloablation preceding transplantation [7]. Stem-cell transplantation into the early gestation fetus may lead to the induction of donor-specific tolerance, thus avoiding the toxicity of myeloablation and allowing for post-natal transplantation of allogeneic stem cells or organs [8]. The fetal environment can also promote the proliferation and differentiation of transplanted cells to facilitate widespread engraftment. Despite the theoretical advantages of in utero hematopoietic cell transplantation (IUHCTx) and its success in animal models, its efficacy in humans has been limited, and current research efforts are focused on understanding and surmounting the barriers to engraftment in the fetus.

The potential to achieve donor-specific tolerance is one of the most compelling reasons to use IUHCTx. Introducing allogeneic cells during the period of thymic education to self-antigens can lead to deletion of allospecific T cells by negative selection [9]. The resulting antigen-specific tolerance that is established in utero can therefore minimize the need for myeloablation during post-natal cellular or organ transplantation[10–12]. In addition, there are several characteristics of fetal hematopoiesis and the fetal environment that support the use of IUHCTx (reviewed in [8]). The natural migration of hematopoietic stem cells (HSCs) between the aorta–gonad–mesonephros region, yolk sac, placenta, fetal liver, and bone marrow may support the homing and engraftment of stem cells that are transplanted into the fetus early in gestation.

Experiments in nature support the connection between the engraftment of foreign cells and antigen-specific tolerance. For example, dizygotic cattle share placental circulation and have secondary long-term engraftment of foreign cells from their siblings, resulting in donor-specific tolerance [13]. Similar observations have been made in human twins, where chimerism has led to a lack of alloreactivity between the two siblings [14], and other animals [15,16], where levels of engraftment are high enough to be potentially therapeutic for hematologic diseases [8]. These observations support the concept that hematopoietic chimerism established in utero induces immune tolerance.

Cellular trafficking between the mother and fetus leads to the presence of maternal cells in fetuses [17], which may induce tolerance to non-inherited maternal antigens (NIMAs), supporting the rationale for in utero transplantation for tolerance induction. Mold and colleagues provided insight into the mechanism by which NIMA exposure may lead to tolerance when they found that the natural trafficking of maternal cells into the fetus leads to the generation of regulatory T cells that prevent an anti-maternal

---

Stem Cells in Reproductive Medicine 3rd edition, ed. Carlos Simón, Antonio Pellicer and Renee Reijo Pera.
Published by Cambridge University Press. © Cambridge University Press 2013.

Table 12.1 Proof of concept: treatment of inherited disorders using animal models of IUHCTx (adapted from [32]).

Disease	Experimental animal model	Genetic defect	Reference
Anemia	Mouse	c-kit tyrosine kinase	[35,36,65]
Autosomal recessive osteoporosis	Mouse	Tcirg1	[66,67]
Leukocyte adhesion deficiency	Dog	Leukocyte integrin CD18	[24]
Osteogenesis imperfecta	Mouse	Col1a1	[68]
Severe combined immunodeficiency	Mouse	Scid	[34,58,69–71]
Sickle cell disease	Mouse	α-globin	[23]
Thalassemia	Mouse	β-globin	[23]

immune response by the fetus [18]. Although the levels of maternal cells in the fetus are low, the presence of microchimerism may have implications for the success of post-natal transplantation when maternal cells are used. For example, we recently reported that patients with biliary atresia, in whom there is a higher level of baseline maternal microchimerism [19], have less graft failure when they receive a liver from their mother [20]. These results are supported by similar findings that have been reported from living-related kidney transplantation [21] and BM transplantation [22]. These observations support the strategy of in utero transplantation to induce donor-specific tolerance, even if the levels of engraftment after the initial fetal transplantation are not high enough to treat the disease. Post-natal "booster" transplants may then be performed to achieve therapeutic levels of donor cells [10,23,24].

Human clinical experience

In humans, the theoretical success of IUHCTx has not been realized in practice, except in cases of immunodeficiencies (reviewed in [25]). Fetuses with bare lymphocyte syndrome [26] and severe combined immunodeficiency (SCID) [27–31] have been treated successfully with IUHCTx. In all cases, CD34$^+$ cells were transplanted between 16 and 26 weeks' gestation and resulted in engraftment of donor cells at birth. Follow-up for one of these patients showed continued cellular reconstitution and intact immune responses to vaccinations [25].

Attempts at using IUHCTx to treat diseases other than SCID, such as chronic granulomatous disease, beta thalassemia, and Rh-disease have been unsuccessful, and have led investigators to study the barriers that limit transplantation success (reviewed in [25]).

It is possible that these studies were limited by the number and type of HSCs transplanted, lack of space in hematopoietic niches, and rejection of transplanted cells. Thus, animal models have been used to identify solutions to these issues prior to performing clinical trials of IUHCTx in human fetuses.

Animal experience with IUHCTx

Animal models of IUHCTx have not only improved our understanding of the barriers involved in successful stem-cell engraftment, but also have provided proof of concept for the treatment of several inherited disorders (Table 12.1). Billingham, Brent, and Medawar [33] were the first to transplant allogeneic cells into fetal mice to demonstrate donor-specific tolerance to skin grafts in mice. Subsequently, it was shown that immunodeficient mice engraft more efficiently, likely secondary to a competitive advantage of the transplanted cells in such an environment [34–37].

The mouse model of IUHCTx has become an invaluable system for improving the strategy of IUHCTx and multiple inherited disorders have been treated in transgenic mouse models (Table 12.1). Current research using the mouse model has focused on the mechanisms by which donor-specific tolerance is achieved. Several investigators have demonstrated that there are fewer allospecific host T cells in chimeras compared to normal controls, suggesting that clonal deletion is an important mechanism in the establishment of chimerism [38,39]. Anergy may also contribute to tolerance after IUHCTx [40]. Furthermore, the induction of a specialized population of regulatory T cells may also be a critical mechanism of tolerance [38,41]. Remarkably, stable engraftment of even low levels of allogeneic HSCs (greater than 1–2% engraftment) in mice has uniformly led to post-natal tolerance to the donor antigen. These data support the notion that tolerance depends on achieving and maintaining a critical threshold level of engraftment [42].

Large animal models of IUHCTx have proven that delivering HSCs into the fetal environment is technically feasible and leads to multilineage engraftment of donor cells. Successful engraftment of allogeneic cells after fetal transplantation was first demonstrated in fetal lambs [43]. Sheep have been a particularly useful tool to study the engraftment of various populations of human HSCs, since fetal lambs do not reject the xenogeneic cells. Interestingly, engraftment levels may even be boosted using human G-CSF [44–46]. Beyond HSCs, the sheep model has also been used to study the engraftment and differentiation capacity of human stem cells such as embryonic [47] and mesenchymal stem cells [48], with the advantage that the host has not received any irradiation or conditioning, which may alter the characteristics of the transplanted cells. Transplantation of HSCs in the canine model has also yielded important information, and IUHCTx has been used to achieve multilineage engraftment, as well as treatment of the canine equivalent of human leukocyte adhesion deficiency [24]. In the pig model of IUHCTx, induction of immune tolerance in the fetus has been used to test the strategy of tolerance induction using IUHCTx followed by post-natal solid organ transplantation. Lee *et al.* demonstrated that IUHCTx in fetal swine led to prolonged survival of a kidney allograft [49], providing experimental support for the use of this strategy in fetuses with congenital anomalies requiring post-natal organ transplantation. IUHCTx has been attempted in non-human primates, but the levels of engraftment have been low [50–52].

Barriers to engraftment after IUHCTx

Since clinical applications to IUHCTx have been limited, research has focused on understanding the barriers to engraftment. These may be summarized as lack of competitive advantage to transplanted cells in an intact fetal host, lack of space in hematopoietic niches, and rejection of transplanted cells [25].

Competitive advantage

In adult animals, conferring a survival advantage to donor cells leads to higher rates of engraftment. For example, c-kit knockout mice (which have a deficiency of host HSC proliferation) achieve full immune reconstitution after the transplantation of only one or two donor HSCs [53]. Furthermore, engraftment after post-natal BM transplantation is maintained consistently despite a relatively lower number of transplanted cells in an irradiated host where host competition is eliminated [54]. Modifying the host hematopoietic environment to promote SDF1-α-induced migration [55] or inhibit fetal hematopoiesis [56] may improve donor-cell homing and engraftment, but clinical applications will need significant testing to ensure safety. In addition, it is likely that adult donor cells are at a disadvantage when placed in the fetal environment [57,58].

Space in hematopoietic niches

The observation that selective depletion of host HSCs prior to BM transplant results in high rates of engraftment in adult animals suggests that vacating host stem-cell niches may improve chimerism after IUHCTx [59]. Furthermore, increasing the dose of donor cells results in an eventual plateau of engraftment efficiency in an allogeneic and xenogeneic fetal lamb model [60], which supports the idea that there are a finite number of available hematopoietic niches for donor-cell engraftment. In our fetal mouse model, reliable engraftment is achieved only after transplantation of a large dose of fetal liver-derived hematopoietic cells (0.5 to 1 donor per fetal recipient [39]). A similar result has been shown after in utero transplantation of adult BM-derived cells in fetal mice [61].

Rejection of transplanted cells

The lack of reliable engraftment in the fetal environment has been a conundrum, since the fetus has been shown to become tolerant to even small numbers of allogeneic cells [18]. Two recent studies in mice have implicated the *maternal* immune system in rejecting the in utero transplanted cells, and have rekindled enthusiasm in this field. Merianos *et al.* demonstrated that allogeneic IUHCTx leads to the formation of maternal antibodies transmitted in breast milk, causing an adaptive alloimmune response in the pups, and resulting in donor cell loss [38]. We have also demonstrated the importance of the maternal immune response, but implicated maternal T cells as the main barrier [39]. We demonstrated that rates of engraftment are significantly higher if the mother (but not the fetus) lacks T cells. Furthermore, performing IUHCTx

Table 12.2 Diseases amenable to in utero hematopoietic cell transplantation.

Hematopoietic Diseases

Chediak–Higashi syndrome

Chronic granulomatous disease

Hemophilia

Severe combined immunodeficiency (SCID)

Sickle cell disease

Thalassemia

Non-hematopoietic Diseases

Muscular dystrophy

Metabolic disorders

Tolerance for post-natal cellular/organ transplant

with donor cells matched to the mother (but not the fetus) led to significantly improved rates of engraftment. These data are clinically relevant in that they suggest transplantation may be improved by using HSCs that are matched to the mother (or donated by the mother). However, the other barriers discussed above are still likely to affect successful engraftment and need to be considered in clinical applications.

Conclusions

Achieving donor-specific tolerance after IUHCTx has the potential to treat many hematopoietic disorders. This strategy may even lead to treatments for non-hematopoietic stem-cell disorders such as muscular dystrophy [62] or single-gene disorders such as hemophilia (Table 12.2) [63]. The convergence of progress in IUHCTx with progress in inducible pluripotent stem-cell (iPS) technology may allow for correction of genetic diseases in iPS cells grown from placental chorionic villus sampling [64]. In addition, the current limitations in obtaining large numbers of matched HSCs may be addressed by generating tissue banks containing HLA-matched embryonic stem cells. Obviously, any clinical application of such strategies must overcome the current bottleneck in the differentiation of these cells along the hematopoietic lineage in vivo. Recent studies by our group and others suggest that the maternal immune response should be considered in future attempts at IUHCTx.

References

1. Harrison, M.R., Golbus, M.S., Filly, R.A. *et al.* Fetal surgery for congenital hydronephrosis. *New England Journal of Medicine.* 1982; 306(10): 591–593.

2. Sydorak, R.M., Nijagal, A., Albanese, C.T. Endoscopic techniques in fetal surgery. *Yonsei Medical Journal.* 2001; 42(6): 695–710.

3. Adzick, N.S., Thom, E.A., Spong, C.Y. *et al.* A randomized trial of prenatal versus postnatal repair of myelomeningocele. *New England Journal of Medicine.* 2011; 364(11): 993–1004.

4. Johnson, F.L., Look, A.T., Gockerman, J. *et al.* Bone-marrow transplantation in a patient with sickle-cell anemia. *New England Journal of Medicine.* 1984; 311(12): 780–783.

5. Kamani, N., August, C.S., Douglas, S.D. *et al.* Bone marrow transplantation in chronic granulomatous disease. *Journal of Pediatrics.* 1984; 105(1): 42–46.

6. Lucarelli, G., Galimberti, M., Polchi, P. *et al.* Bone marrow transplantation in patients with thalassemia. *New England Journal of Medicine.* 1990; 322(7): 417–421.

7. Parkman, R. The application of bone marrow transplantation to the treatment of genetic diseases. *Science.* 1986; 232(4756): 1373–1378.

8. Santore, M.T., Roybal, J.L., Flake, A.W. Prenatal stem cell transplantation and gene therapy. *Clinical Perinatology.* 2009; 36(2): 451–471, xi.

9. Palmer, E. Negative selection–clearing out the bad apples from the T-cell repertoire. *Nature Reviews Immunology.* 2003; 3(5): 383–391.

10. Ashizuka, S., Peranteau, W.H., Hayashi, S., Flake, A.W. Busulfan-conditioned bone marrow transplantation results in high-level allogeneic chimerism in mice made tolerant by *in utero* hematopoietic cell transplantation. *Experimental Hematology.* 2006; 34(3): 359–368.

11. Hayashi, S., Peranteau, W.H., Shaaban, A.F., Flake, A.W. Complete allogeneic hematopoietic chimerism achieved by a combined strategy of *in utero* hematopoietic stem cell transplantation and postnatal donor lymphocyte infusion. *Blood.* 2002; 100(3): 804–812.

12. Peranteau, W.H., Hayashi, S., Hsieh, M., Shaaban, A.F., Flake, A.W. High-level allogeneic chimerism achieved by prenatal tolerance induction and postnatal nonmyeloablative bone marrow transplantation. *Blood.* 2002; 100(6): 2225–2234.

13. Owen, R.D. Immunogenetic consequences of vascular anastomoses between bovine twins. *Science.* 1945; 102(2651): 400–401.

14. Thomsen, M., Hansen, H.E., Dickmeiss, E. MLC and CML studies in the family of a pair of HLA haploidentical chimeric twins. *Scandinavian Journal of Immunology.* 1977; 6(5): 523–528.

15 Picus, J., Aldrich, W.R., Letvin, N.L. A naturally occurring bone-marrow-chimeric primate. I. Integrity of its immune system. *Transplantation*. 1985; 39(3): 297–303.

16. Picus, J., Holley, K., Aldrich, W.R., Griffin, J.D., Letvin, N.L. A naturally occurring bone marrow-chimeric primate. II. Environment dictates restriction on cytolytic T lymphocyte-target cell interactions. *Journal of Experimental Medicine*. 1985; 162(6): 2035–2052.

17. Bianchi, D.W., Zickwolf, G.K., Weil, G.J., Sylvester, S., DeMaria, M.A. Male fetal progenitor cells persist in maternal blood for as long as 27 years postpartum. *Proceedings of the National Academy of Sciences of the United States of America*. 1996; 93(2): 705–708.

18. Mold, J.E., Michaelsson, J., Burt, T.D. *et al.* Maternal alloantigens promote the development of tolerogenic fetal regulatory T cells *in utero*. *Science*. 2008; 322(5907): 1562–1565.

19. Suskind, D.L., Rosenthal, P., Heyman, M.B. *et al.* Maternal microchimerism in the livers of patients with biliary atresia. *BMC Gastroenterology*. 2004; 4: 14.

20. Nijagal, A., Fleck, S., Hills, N.K. *et al.* Decreased risk of graft failure with maternal liver transplantation in patients with biliary atresia. *American Journal of Transplantation*. 2012; 12(2): 409–419.

21. Burlingham, W.J., Grailer, A.P., Heisey, D.M. *et al.* The effect of tolerance to noninherited maternal HLA antigens on the survival of renal transplants from sibling donors. *New England Journal of Medicine*. 1998; 339(23): 1657–1664.

22. van Rood, J.J., Loberiza, F.R., Jr., Zhang, M.J. *et al.* Effect of tolerance to noninherited maternal antigens on the occurrence of graft-versus-host disease after bone marrow transplantation from a parent or an HLA-haploidentical sibling. *Blood*. 2002; 99(5): 1572–1577.

23. Hayashi, S., Abdulmalik, O., Peranteau, W.H. *et al.* Mixed chimerism following *in utero* hematopoietic stem cell transplantation in murine models of hemoglobinopathy. *Experimental Hematology*. 2003; 31(2): 176–184.

24. Peranteau, W.H., Heaton, T.E., Gu, Y.C. *et al.* Haploidentical *in utero* hematopoietic cell transplantation improves phenotype and can induce tolerance for postnatal same-donor transplants in the canine leukocyte adhesion deficiency model. *Biology of Blood and Marrow Transplantation*. 2009; 15(3): 293–305.

25. Flake, A.W., Zanjani, E.D. *In utero* hematopoietic stem cell transplantation: ontogenic opportunities and biologic barriers. *Blood*. 1999; 94(7): 2179–2191.

26. Touraine, J.L., Raudrant, D., Royo, C. *et al.* In-utero transplantation of stem cells in bare lymphocyte syndrome. *Lancet*. 1989; 1(8651): 1382.

27. Flake, A.W., Roncarolo, M.G., Puck, J.M. *et al.* Treatment of X-linked severe combined immunodeficiency by *in utero* transplantation of paternal bone marrow. *New England Journal of Medicine*. 1996; 335(24): 1806–1810.

28. Wengler, G.S., Lanfranchi, A., Frusca, T. *et al.* In-utero transplantation of parental CD34 haematopoietic progenitor cells in a patient with X-linked severe combined immunodeficiency (SCIDXI). *Lancet*. 1996; 348(9040): 1484–1487.

29. Touraine, J.L., Raudrant, D., Laplace, S. Transplantation of hemopoietic cells from the fetal liver to treat patients with congenital diseases postnatally or prenatally. *Transplantation Proceedings*. 1997; 29(1–2): 712–713.

30. Gil, J., Porta, F., Bartolome, J. *et al.* Immune reconstitution after *in utero* bone marrow transplantation in a fetus with severe combined immunodeficiency with natural killer cells. *Transplantation Proceedings*. 1999; 31(6): 2581.

31. Pirovano, S., Notarangelo, L.D., Malacarne, F. *et al.* Reconstitution of T-cell compartment after *in utero* stem cell transplantation: analysis of T-cell repertoire and thymic output. *Haematologica*. 2004; 89(4): 450–461.

32. Nijagal, A., Flake, A.W., MacKenzie, T.C. *In utero* hematopoietic cell transplantation for the treatment of congenital anomalies. *Clinical Perinatology*. 2012; 39: 301–310.

33. Billingham, R.E., Brent, L., Medawar, P.B. Actively acquired tolerance of foreign cells. *Nature*. 1953; 172(4379): 603–606.

34. Blazar, B.R., Taylor, P.A., Vallera, D.A. *In utero* transfer of adult bone marrow cells into recipients with severe combined immunodeficiency disorder yields lymphoid progeny with T- and B-cell functional capabilities. *Blood*. 1995; 86(11): 4353–4366.

35. Blazar, B.R., Taylor, P.A., Vallera, D.A. Adult bone marrow-derived pluripotent hematopoietic stem cells are engraftable when transferred *in utero* into moderately anemic fetal recipients. *Blood*. 1995; 85(3): 833–841.

36. Fleischman, R.A., Mintz, B. Prevention of genetic anemias in mice by microinjection of normal hematopoietic stem cells into the fetal placenta. *Proceedings of the National Academy of Sciences of the United States of America*. 1979; 76(11): 5736–5740.

37. Fleischman, R.A., Mintz, B. Development of adult bone marrow stem cells in H-2-compatible

and -incompatible mouse fetuses. *Journal of Experimental Medicine*. 1984; 159(3): 731–745.

38. Merianos, D.J., Tiblad, E., Santore, M.T. *et al.* Maternal alloantibodies induce a postnatal immune response that limits engraftment following *in utero* hematopoietic cell transplantation in mice. *Journal of Clinical Investigation*. 2009; 119(9): 2590–2600.

39. Nijagal, A., Wegorzewska, M., Jarvis, E. *et al.* Maternal T cells limit engraftment after *in utero* hematopoietic cell transplantation in mice. *Journal of Clinical Investigation*. 2011; 121(2): 582–592.

40. Kim, H.B., Shaaban, A.F., Milner, R., Fichter, C., Flake, A.W. *In utero* bone marrow transplantation induces donor-specific tolerance by a combination of clonal deletion and clonal anergy. *Journal of Pediatric Surgery*. 1999; 34(5): 726–729; discussion 9–30.

41. Hayashi, S., Hsieh, M., Peranteau, W.H., Ashizuka, S., Flake, A.W. Complete allogeneic hematopoietic chimerism achieved by *in utero* hematopoietic cell transplantation and cotransplantation of LLME-treated, MHC-sensitized donor lymphocytes. *Experimental Hematology*. 2004; 32(3): 290–299.

42. Durkin, E.T., Jones, K.A., Rajesh, D., Shaaban, A.F. Early chimerism threshold predicts sustained engraftment and NK-cell tolerance in prenatal allogeneic chimeras. *Blood*. 2008; 112(13): 5245–5253.

43. Flake, A.W., Harrison, M.R., Adzick, N.S., Zanjani, E.D. Transplantation of fetal hematopoietic stem cells *in utero*: the creation of hematopoietic chimeras. *Science*. 1986; 233(4765): 776–778.

44. Almeida-Porada, G., Porada, C., Gupta, N. *et al.* The human-sheep chimeras as a model for human stem cell mobilization and evaluation of hematopoietic grafts' potential. *Experimental Hematology*. 2007; 35(10): 1594–1600.

45. Zanjani, E.D., Flake, A.W., Rice, H., Hedrick, M., Tavassoli, M. Long-term repopulating ability of xenogeneic transplanted human fetal liver hematopoietic stem cells in sheep. *Journal of Clinical Investigation*. 1994; 93(3): 1051–1055.

46. Zanjani, E.D., Pallavicini, M.G., Ascensao, J.L. *et al.* Engraftment and long-term expression of human fetal hemopoietic stem cells in sheep following transplantation *in utero*. *Journal of Clinical Investigation*. 1992; 89(4): 1178–1188.

47. Narayan, A.D., Chase, J.L., Lewis, R.L. *et al.* Human embryonic stem cell-derived hematopoietic cells are capable of engrafting primary as well as secondary fetal sheep recipients. *Blood*. 2006; 107(5): 2180–2183.

48. Liechty, K.W., MacKenzie, T.C., Shaaban, A.F. *et al.* Human mesenchymal stem cells engraft and demonstrate site-specific differentiation after *in utero*

transplantation in sheep. *Nature Medicine*. 2000; 6(11): 1282–1286.

49. Lee, P.W., Cina, R.A., Randolph, M.A. *et al. In utero* bone marrow transplantation induces kidney allograft tolerance across a full major histocompatibility complex barrier in swine. *Transplantation*. 2005; 79(9): 1084–1090.

50. Shields, L.E., Gaur, L.K., Gough, M. *et al. In utero* hematopoietic stem cell transplantation in nonhuman primates: the role of T cells. *Stem Cells*. 2003; 21(3): 304–314.

51. Tarantal, A.F., Goldstein, O., Barley, F., Cowan, M.J. Transplantation of human peripheral blood stem cells into fetal rhesus monkeys (Macaca mulatta). *Transplantation*. 2000; 69(9): 1818–1823.

52. Asano, T., Ageyama, N., Takeuchi, K. *et al.* Engraftment and tumor formation after allogeneic *in utero* transplantation of primate embryonic stem cells. *Transplantation*. 2003; 76(7): 1061–1067.

53. Mintz, B., Anthony, K., Litwin, S. Monoclonal derivation of mouse myeloid and lymphoid lineages from totipotent hematopoietic stem cells experimentally engrafted in fetal hosts. *Proceedings of the National Academy of Sciences of the United States of America*. 1984; 81(24): 7835–7839.

54. Stewart, F.M., Zhong, S., Wuu, J. *et al.* Lymphohematopoietic engraftment in minimally myeloablated hosts. *Blood*. 1998; 91(10): 3681–3687.

55. Peranteau, W.H., Endo, M., Adibe, O.O. *et al.* CD26 inhibition enhances allogeneic donor-cell homing and engraftment after *in utero* hematopoietic-cell transplantation. *Blood*. 2006; 108(13): 4268–4274.

56. Lindton, B., Tolfvenstam, T., Norbeck, O. *et al.* Recombinant parvovirus B19 empty capsids inhibit fetal hematopoietic colony formation in vitro. *Fetal Diagnosis and Therapy*. 2001; 16(1): 26–31.

57. Shaaban, A.F., Kim, H.B., Milner, R., Flake, A.W. A kinetic model for the homing and migration of prenatally transplanted marrow. *Blood*. 1999; 94(9): 3251–3257.

58. Taylor, P.A., McElmurry, R.T., Lees, C.J., Harrison, D.E., Blazar, B.R. Allogenic fetal liver cells have a distinct competitive engraftment advantage over adult bone marrow cells when infused into fetal as compared with adult severe combined immunodeficient recipients. *Blood*. 2002; 99(5): 1870–1872.

59. Czechowicz, A., Kraft, D., Weissman, I.L., Bhattacharya, D. Efficient transplantation via antibody-based clearance of hematopoietic stem cell niches. *Science*. 2007; 318(5854): 1296–1299.

60. Flake, A.W., Zanjani, E.D. Cellular therapy. *Obstetrics and Gynecology Clinics of North America*. 1997; 24(1): 159–177.

61. Peranteau, W.H., Endo, M., Adibe, O.O., Flake, A.W. Evidence for an immune barrier after *in utero* hematopoietic-cell transplantation. *Blood*. 2007; 109(3): 1331–1333.

62. Mackenzie, T.C., Shaaban, A.F., Radu, A., Flake, A.W. Engraftment of bone marrow and fetal liver cells after *in utero* transplantation in MDX mice. *Journal of Pediatric Surgery*. 2002; 37(7): 1058–1064.

63. Sabatino, D.E., Mackenzie, T.C., Peranteau, W. *et al.* Persistent expression of hF. IX. After tolerance induction by *in utero* or neonatal administration of AAV-1-F.IX in hemophilia B mice. *Molecular Therapeutics*. 2007; 15(9): 1677–1685.

64. Ye, L., Chang, J.C., Lin, C. *et al.* Induced pluripotent stem cells offer new approach to therapy in thalassemia and sickle cell anemia and option in prenatal diagnosis in genetic diseases. *Proceedings of the National Academy of Sciences of the United States of America*. 2009; 106(24): 9826–9830.

65. Howson-Jan, K., Matloub, Y.H., Vallera, D.A., Blazar, B.R. *In utero* engraftment of fully H-2-incompatible versus congenic adult bone marrow transferred into nonanemic or anemic murine fetal recipients. *Transplantation*. 1993; 56(3): 709–716.

66. Frattini, A., Blair, H.C., Sacco, M.G. *et al.* Rescue of ATPa3-deficient murine malignant osteopetrosis by hematopoietic stem cell transplantation *in utero*. *Proceedings of the National Academy of Sciences of the United States of America*. 2005; 102(41): 14629–14634.

67. Tondelli, B., Blair, H.C., Guerrini, M. *et al.* Fetal liver cells transplanted *in utero* rescue the osteopetrotic phenotype in the oc/oc mouse. *American Journal of Pathology*. 2009; 174(3): 727–735.

68. Panaroni, C., Gioia, R., Lupi, A. *et al. In utero* transplantation of adult bone marrow decreases perinatal lethality and rescues the bone phenotype in the knockin murine model for classical, dominant osteogenesis imperfecta. *Blood*. 2009; 114(2): 459–468.

69. Archer, D.R., Turner, C.W., Yeager, A.M., Fleming, W.H. Sustained multilineage engraftment of allogeneic hematopoietic stem cells in NOD/SCID mice after *in utero* transplantation. *Blood*. 1997; 90(8): 3222–3229.

70. Liuba, K., Pronk, C.J., Stott, S.R., Jacobsen, S.E. Polyclonal T-cell reconstitution of X-SCID recipients after *in utero* transplantation of lymphoid-primed multipotent progenitors. *Blood*. 2009; 113(19): 4790–4798.

71. Waldschmidt, T.J., Panoskaltsis-Mortari, A., McElmurry, R.T. *et al.* Abnormal T cell-dependent B-cell responses in SCID mice receiving allogeneic bone marrow *in utero*. Severe combined immune deficiency. *Blood*. 2002; 100(13): 4557–4564.

Bone-marrow stroma: A source of mesenchymal stem cells for cell therapy

Agustín G. Zapata

The bone marrow is the main hematopoietic organ in adult mammals. It contains hematopoietic stem cells (HSCs) and committed blood-cell progenitors that mature in a network of reticular cells, adipocytes, and blood vessels that constitute the stroma. In a previous edition of the current book we described distinct non-hematopoietic stem cells reported to occur in the adult bone marrow (BM) that could be a source of cell progenitors for cell therapy [1]. Within this category we then reported the so-called "multipotent adult progenitor cells," the "bone-marrow-derived multipotent stem cells," the "multipotent adult stem cells," "SSEA-1-positive cells," "marrow-isolated adult multilineage inducible cells," "mesenchymal stem cells or multipotent mesenchymal stem cells (MSCs)," "very small embryonic-like stem cells," and "endothelial progenitor cells," which had been described in vitro as presumptive stem cells depending on their phenotypes and the results of some functional studies in diverse experimental models. However, it was already evident that: (1) several of these cell types represented a unique (or equivalent) cell population, (2) it was difficult to establish the correlations between these cell subsets found in in vitro cultures and the known cell components of in vivo bone-marrow stroma, and (3) MSCs appear to show properties and phenotypes similar to those reported in other non-hematopoietic stem-cell populations of the bone marrow. Accordingly, the present review summarizes current data on the origin, properties, and possible therapeutic use of MSCs, with special emphasis on their relationships with the cell components that constitute the bone-marrow microenvironment. Our election is based on the idea that the term MSC includes most cell types reported to be present in the stroma of bone marrow. They are also currently the most frequently used cell type in clinical trials on cell therapy.

Mesenchymal stem cells (MSCs): general properties

MSCs, initially called colony-forming-unit fibroblasts (CFU-Fs) were first described in the BM in 1976 [2] and later in the connective tissue of almost all tissues [3]. Nevertheless, MSCs are presumably unique in each tissue, which can explain certain reported functional differences [4]. Despite currently being considered to be the most promising stem cells for cell therapy, we have progressed little in our knowledge of their nature, mechanisms of functioning, and true capacity for differentiation in vivo.

MSCs are obtained from cell suspensions of total BM after culture. In these conditions, adhered cells that are easily separated, form clonogenic CFU-Fs that exhibit high, although limited, self-proliferative capacity. The cells obtained, however, are highly dependent on the culture conditions, showing a great variability in the requirements from one species to another. In addition, these findings presumably reflect the great heterogeneity found in these cultures and their derived colonies, as well as the different methodologies used to isolate MSCs.

MSC cultures show a variable degree of plasticity. All assayed colonies exhibit osteogenic capacities and the majority also produce adipocytes, but have a more limited capacity to differentiate to chondrocytes [5]. Importantly, these results suggest that all MSC colonies do not contain multipotent progenitors and/or that both in vivo and in vitro protocols critically determine the differentiation properties of MSCs.

Stem Cells in Reproductive Medicine 3rd edition, ed. Carlos Simón, Antonio Pellicer and Renee Reijo Pera.
Published by Cambridge University Press. © Cambridge University Press 2013.

MSC markers

Most MSCs express CD29 and CD105 or both, and other cell markers (i.e., CD133, SSEA-1, SSEA-4, CD271) have been used to isolate enriched MSC populations from different sources (reviewed in [6–8]), but are not specific markers for MSCs. In addition, the phenotypic analysis of BM-MSCs has been mainly carried out on MSCs expanded in vitro; the phenotype of cells initiating cultures that give rise to MSCs is therefore unclear, although some new data have been recently reported. On the other hand, various results-support, as mentioned above, that in vitro-expanded BM-MSCs constitute a heterogeneous cell population. BM-MSCs exhibit a multimodal expression of certain surface markers, such as CD146 and CD200 [9], and only one-third of MSC clones appear to be really multipotent [5]. In fact, some of the markers listed in the next paragraph have only been described in mouse, not in human MSC, or in cells isolated from some tissues but not from others, reflecting the heterogeneity of these cells.

Cells recognized as MSCs for their capacity to generate different connective tissue lineages express CD29, CD44, CD49a-f, CD51, CD73, CD90, CD105, CD106, CD146, CD166, CD133, CD271 (low affinity-nerve-growth-factor receptor), Stro-1, SSEA-1, SSEA-4, and 3G5, and are negative for hematopoietic markers such as CD11b, CD14, CD34, and CD45 [10]. Other new markers are: Nestin [11], CD140a (PDGFRα), CD140b (PDGF-Rβ) [12], CD56, and MSCA-1 [13]. Human MSCs showing CFU-F capacity have recently been isolated from BM by using the expression of both CD271 and CD146 (melanoma-cell adhesion molecule) cell markers. The combination of these markers has allowed the identification of two MSC subsets in adult BM: CD271+CD146–/lo cells and CD271+CD146+ cells. Both subsets apparently have a similar capacity for differentiation but are located in two different regions of the BM microenvironment; CD271+CD146–/lo cells occur in the so-called endosteal niche, whereas CD271+ CD146+ cells exhibit a perivascular location [14]. In addition, a third, CD271–CD146+ MSC subpopulation containing CFU-F activity has been found in human fetal BM [15]. CD271+CD146– cells are the most frequent MSCs in adult BM, whereas CD271+CD146+ cells are predominant in children. Furthermore, the CD271+CD146– cell fraction is significantly reduced in elderly adults (more than 55 years), a finding that correlates with the previous reported age-dependent decrease in BM CFU F [16]. These results suggest importantly that BM niches are dynamic and contain different MSC subsets in distinct periods of life.

MSCs, express receptors for numerous cytokines (IL1, IL3 IL4, IL6, IL7, IL15, IFNγ, TNFα) and chemokines (CCR1, CCR7, CCR9, CXCR4, CXCR5, CXCR6) [5] and their effects on some immune responses are discussed later. Other receptors, such as TLRs, are described below.

Immunological properties of MSCs

Although numerous studies have described the immunosuppressive properties of MSCs, these cells are really immunoregulatory or immunomodulatory rather than merely immunosuppressive. Furthermore, their properties are not constitutive, but acquired depending on the environment. In this respect, IFNγ appears to be critical to induce MSC-mediated immune suppression. High levels of IFNγ produced during immune responses by infiltrating macrophages and T lymphocytes induce immunosuppressive MSCs [17]. Other cytokines, such as TNFα or IL1β, can also induce MSC-mediated immunosuppression, making the system more complex [18]. In general, an inflammatory environment favors immunosuppression, but not all inflammatory situations result in a similar condition.

MSCs can negatively affect every step of the immune response from antigen presentation to the activation of T and B lymphocytes. These immuno-modulatory effects of MSCs have been employed for therapeutic purposes in the treatment of graft vs. host reactions and autoimmune diseases, as well as for improving HSC engraftment (see later).

Allogeneic MSCs inhibit the generation of mature dendritic cells (DCs) [19], reduce their immune capacities, including antigen presentation and migration ability, and induce their apoptosis [20]. MSCs direct mature DCs to a tolerogenic stage by impeding their cytokine production, in a process that could be governed by PGE2, but also by IL6 and M-CSF [21,22]. MSCs decrease TNFα secretion from myeloid DCs and increase IL10 production from plasmacytoid DCs, favoring the generation of TH2 and Treg cells rather than TH1 lymphocytes [21]. MSCs also inhibit the production of TNFα and IL12 by human macrophages, whereas they increase IL6 and IL10 production and their phagocytic activity [23]. In addition, at low ratios MSCs inhibit apoptosis of both resting and IL8-activated neutrophils [24]. On the other hand, IFNγ-stimulated MSCs can act as antigen-presenting cells, processing and presenting antigens, and activating Ag-specific cells in vivo and in vitro [21,25].

MSCs suppress both T- and B-cell proliferation [21]. The immunosuppression affects both CD4+ and CD8+ T cells, can be induced by allogeneic or autologous MSCs, and is not HLA-restricted [26,27]. Likewise, MSCs inhibit B-cell proliferation (as well as B-cell migration) by arresting their cell cycle at the G_0/G_1 phase and the production of IgM, IgA, and IgG [28]. Conversely, MSCs do not induce T-cell apoptosis, but promote survival of resting T cells and rescue T lymphocytes from activation-induced cell death by down-regulated surface expression of both Fas receptors and ligands [29]. Co-cultures of MSCs with DCs induce decreased IFNγ production by TH1 cells and increased IL4 production by TH2 cells, resulting in an anti-inflammatory condition. MSCs also suppress T-cell-mediated cytotoxicity, the proportion of Treg cells in MLR [30], and naïve and memory T-cell responses to their cognate antigens [31].

TH17 cells are an effector T-cell subset characterized by the synthesis of cytokine IL17A, but also of IL17F, IL21, IL22, and CCL20 [32]. They mediate tissue inflammation against infections and are involved in autoimmune processes [33,34]. MSCs modulate their activity and differentiation, which could explain their effects on autoimmune diseases [35–37]. In vivo and in vitro MSCs provoke suppression of TH17 differentiation from both naïve and memory T-cell precursors [38,39], at least in part through PGE2 and IDO (Indolamine-2,3-dioxygenase) [40], although other factors are also directly or indirectly involved. On the other hand, TH17 expansion has been reported in co-cultures of fetal bone-marrow MSCs with human peripheral blood mononuclear cells or CD4+ cells [41]. MSCs also suppress naïve and memory T cells in a process that is not mediated by CD4+CD25+ Treg cells [31]. Other immune responses are, however, inhibited by MSCs through activation and/or expansion of Treg cells, a subset crucial to regulate susceptibility to autoimmunity [29,37,42].

The effects of MSCs on NK cell activity are contradictory. Ex vivo MSCs suppress IL2- and IL15-induced proliferation of resting NK cells, but only partially that of pre-activated NK cells [21]. These inhibitory effects have been associated with cell-to-cell contacts, as well as with the production of soluble factors, such as PGE2, TGFβ, IDO, or soluble HLA-G [43–45]. MSCs can also modulate NK cytotoxicity by reducing their secretion of IFNγ, IL10, and TNFα [43,44]. Conversely, MSCs are remarkably sensitive to NK-mediated lysis. MSCs may be lysed by both autologous and allogeneic IL2-stimulated NK cells [26,44]. These effects could be associated with the fact that MSCs weakly express MHC class I antigens, but also NK receptor ligands [44]. In fact, IFNγ-stimulated BM MSCs are less susceptible to NK lysis due to the down-regulated expression of surface MHC class I molecules [44].

MSCs express high levels of TLRs, including TLR1, TLR3, TLR4, and TLR5. Furthermore, TLR ligation affects the immunomodulatory properties of MSCs, although the reported results are controversial. Stimulation of TLR3 and TLR4 results in the production of pre-inflammatory cytokines, such as IL1β, IL6, and IL8, through Notch/Jagged-1 signaling [46,47]. However, it has been reported that TLR stimulation enhances MSC-induced immunosuppression by increasing IDO production [48]. It is possible that, depending on the TLR stimulated, MSCs acquire different, even opposing properties [49]. Thus, by using low-level, short-term TLR priming, Waterman and colleagues observed opposite effects on human MSCs. TLR 4-primed MSCs exhibited largely proinflammatory profiles of cytokines, whereas stimulation through TLR3 resulted in immunosuppressive MSCs [50].

Although numerous studies have been devoted to determining the nature of factors involved in the immunomodulatory properties of MSCs [26,51,52], few conclusive results have been reached. Apart from cell-to-cell interactions, many soluble factors, including HGF (hepatocyte growth factor), PGE2, TFGβ, IDO, nitric oxide, IL10, BMP4, galactins, etc. produced by self-MSCs or by immune cells in response to MSCs have been described to be concerned with MSC-mediated immunomodulation.

In vivo MSCs form a part of the cell microenvironment of bone marrow

For many years, the term MSCs was applied to a more-or-less homogeneous cell population obtained in vitro after adherent cultures of the stromal (or total) fraction of connective tissues, largely bone marrow and fat. The origins of these cultured cells and their in vivo equivalents in the tissue donors remain elusive. Over the last few years, numerous studies, using different direct and indirect approaches, were devoted to the *in situ* identification of MSCs in different tissues, largely the BM. Currently, it is assumed that MSCs represent approximately 0.001 to 0.01% of BM-nucleated cells, 10-fold less than the proportion of HSCs [53].

For many years, the BM stroma was described only in morphological terms as a network of irregular reticular cells (RCs); a type called adventitial reticular (AdR) cells is intimately associated with the blood vessel walls, macrophages, adipocytes, sinusoidal blood vessels, bone-lining cells, and nerve endings. Mature and developing hematopoietic cells occupy the holes in this mesh. In the early seventies, it was proposed that HSCs and committed hematopoietic progenitor cells occupied specific places in the network in order to create a gradient of maturation from bone endosteum, in which HSCs apparently occur, to central blood vessels, through which almost all mature cells migrated into the blood circulation. These pioneering studies also emphasized the relevance of HSC–stromal cell interactions for the maturation of hematopoietic cells, but they did not conclusively identify the cells involved, nor the molecules governing these cell-to-cell interactions. Currently, two hematopoietic niches, one endosteal and another vascular, are considered to occur in the adult bone marrow, but their organization and the nature of the hematopoietic progenitors within are still unclear [54].

Many different cell types identified in the BM stroma could be the *in situ* equivalents of MSCs isolated from BM cultures and it is difficult to establish the concrete relationships that exist between them. In 2007, firstly Sachetti and colleagues [55] and later other authors [6,8,56] pointed out that MSCs could either be identical to, or derived from, pericytes, an origin that would explain the presence of MSCs in many connective tissues apart from bone marrow. In the bone marrow, a CD146+ subendothelial cell population has been identified that, after *ex vivo* culture, produces bone, adipocytes, and a stroma capable of supporting hematopoiesis. Morikawa *et al.* [57] also identified a perivascular cell subpopulation that does not express hematopoietic markers, but was positive for both PDGFRα and Sca-1 and, after intravenous injection, generated perivascular cells, but also osteoblasts and adipocytes.

In human bone marrow, Stro-1+ stromal cells support hematopoiesis and exhibit the capacity to differentiate into multiple mesenchymal lineages [58,59]. Most of these BM stromal cells cultured for a long time are presumptive vascular smooth muscle cells expressing asM-actin. In vivo asM-actin+ cells occur in both fetal and adult bone marrow, and exhibit long cell processes that intimately contact with HSCs [60], similar to the alkaline phosphatase adventitial reticular cells described previously [61]. The AdR cells express CD271 and appear in the fetal BM before the occurrence of HSCs [62]. Also, bone-marrow CD146+ cells, which constitute a MSC subset [14], are anatomically and phenotypically similar to AdR cells and, after *ex vivo* expansion, express alkaline phosphatase, asM-actin, and CXCL12 [55].

Other studies into the role played by the CXCL12/CXCR4 pair in HSC mobilization and the mechanisms governing the G-CSF-mediated mobilization of HSCs, have provided indirect evidence of the organization of BM microenvironments and the possible origins of MSCs. CXCL12 is a chemokine implicated in the retention of CXCR4 (the CXCL12 receptor)-positive HSCs in the bone marrow. Several different cell types of the BM microenvironment, including stromal RCs, secrete CXCL12. Reticular cells that form the network of the BM niche and produce CXCL12 have been named CAR cells (CXCL12-rich cells) [63]. On the other hand, it was demonstrated that G-CSF mobilizes HSCs from bone marrow by the direct or indirect stimulation of β_3-adrenergic receptors that results in decreased secretion of CXCL12 [64]. Although endosteal osteoblasts were first involved in this process, later CAR cells were identified to be the true target cells of G-CSF action, since they express β_3-adrenergic receptors and osteoblasts do not. In fact, apart from adrenergic mediators, other neurotransmitters also stimulate mobilization of HSCs. Thus, dopamine increases the GM-CSF-mediated mobilization of CD34+ cell progenitors via D3 and D5 receptors [65]. Furthermore, dopamine mobilizes MSCs to peripheral blood (J.G. Castro, personal communication). One important feature of CAR cells that remains to be conclusively determined is whether they represent a homogeneous or heterogeneous stromal cell population and their true relationships with RCs and MSCs.

More recently, nestin, a cell marker of neuroectoderm stem cells, was used to identify a new cell type in the BM stroma that could also correspond to *in situ* MSCs [11]. These cells, which are morphologically similar to pericytes, appear to be restricted to the perivascular areas, to be associated with HSCs, and to strongly express genes known to be involved in HSC maintenance, such as CXCL12, SCF, angiopoietin-1, IL7, VCAM-1, and osteopontin [11]. Nestin+ cells are innervated by the sympathetic nervous system, express β_3-adrenergic receptors, mediate G-CSF-induced HSC mobilization, and regenerate in vivo a BM stroma capable of supporting hematopoiesis. In addition, β_3-adrenergic stimulation reduces the expression of the above-mentioned HSC maintenance genes. Once again the relationships between nestin+ cells and CAR cells are not clear (previously discussed in [66]).

Apparently, nestin+ cells and CAR cells could be two overlapping BM stromal-cell populations, the former being more primitive because it is less abundant, contains all the CFU-F activity of bone marrow, exhibits autorenewal capacity, and is able to differentiate into osteoblasts, chondrocytes, and adipocytes. Nevertheless, we do not know if nestin+ cells represent a homogeneous population and all nestin+ cells are (or not) CAR cells. It has been proposed that nestin+ cells could organize BM niches for housing HSCs, whereas CAR cells would only contain committed hematopoietic progenitors [66].

Other results have provided new interesting information on the physiological role of these cells in governing the biology of HSCs through the production of CXCL12. Apparently, nestin+ cells and CAR cells could co-ordinately modulate CXCL12 secretion through cell junctions establishing a syncitium in the BM stromal network [67]. These authors have recently demonstrated that nestin+ cells strongly express connexin 43 (C×43) and connexin 45 (C×45), molecules involved in the organization of gap junctions, and that C×43 is associated with HSC development. Thus, G-CSF-dependent decreased secretion of CXCL12 courses with reduced expression of both C×43 and C×45, and the pharmacological blocking of gap junctions results in decreased CXCL12 production and blockade of hematopoietic progenitor homing into the bone marrow. In vitro confluent cultures of human BM-MSCs control CXCL12 production by regulating the established gap junctions,

and the adherence of CD34+ cells to BM-MSCs is impeded in non-confluent cultures that contain small amounts of CXCL12 [67].

On the other hand, the expression of both CXCL12 and CXCR4 follows circadian rhythms that regulate the migration of HSCs from the bone marrow to the peripheral blood [68]. In mice, a decrease in the levels of the CXCL12/CXCR4 pair, which occurs at daybreak, results in a peak of HSCs in peripheral blood. Conversely, at nightfall, high levels of CXCL12 retain HSCs in the BM niche. The opposite cycle occurs in humans.

Very recently, GFAP+integrin $\beta 8+$ (a marker of Schwann cells) non-myelinated Schwann cells, which surround sympathetic nerves in bone marrow, have been reported to produce important niche factors and to be in close contact with an important number of HSCs [69]. These cells appear to be the principal cell type processing latent TGFβ into active TGFβ in the bone marrow, a key factor for controlling the niche of HSCs. The relationships of these cells with the above-described nestin+ cells, CAR cells, etc. remain elusive, but they seem to play different roles in the hematopoietic niche. PDGFRα+ cells, nestin+ cells and GFAP+ cells respectively represent 0.05, 0.026, and 0.004% of the BM area. Moreover, all GFAP+ cells express nestin, but not PDGFRα, although nestin+ cells and PDFGRα+ cells largely overlap. Thus, BM GFAP+ cells seem to differ from PDGFRα MSCs, as further supported by the finding that they do not express smooth muscle actin, a marker of pericytes [69].

In summary, further studies are necessary to conclusively demonstrate the lineage relationships between all these bone-marrow components, an organ in which there is increasing evidence to suggest that there is not just one, but many, functionally different micro environments that could be composed of a heterogeneous population of non-hematopoietic, stromal cells.

Therapeutic applications of MSCs

In this section, we present some examples of the clinical use of MSCs in an attempt to summarize the problems and controversies that arise rather than to provide a complete scope of the cell therapy with MSCs. Although the presumptive capacities of MSCs to differentiate into distinct mesoderm-derived tissues are often remarked upon, the most successful clinical results are really those which profit from their trophic and immunological properties to resolve different inflammatory, haematological, or immune pathologies.

Capacity of MSCs to differentiate towards various cell lineages

Although MSCs are currently the most frequently used cell type in cell therapy [70], emphasizing their capacity to generate not only osteoblasts, adipocytes, and chondrocytes, but also vascular, skeletal, and cardiac muscle, endothelial cells, neural cells, and hepatocytes, it is important to take into account the following considerations:

(1) In all cases, the success of these trials has been very limited.
(2) The best results have been obtained with diseases such as skeletal problems [71] or osteoarthritis [72], which affect tissues and organs that share the same embryological origin as the MSCs; i.e. the mesoderm layer.
(3) Although, as mentioned above, underlying mechanisms involved in MSC-mediated effects are largely unknown, most authors agree that there is no conclusive evidence of MSC differentiation to non-mesoderm-related tissues and MSC effects are paracrinely mediated by the production of cytokines, growth factors, and anti-inflammatory mediators [70].

MSCs in the treatment of GvH disease

Apart from other possible therapeutic capacities of MSCs, one of the most important applications of these cells is their use in the treatment of GvH disease, the major complication of allogeneic bone-marrow transplantation.

On the basis of the reported immunoregulatory properties of MSCs, pre-clinical studies in different animal models have addressed their potential application in the treatment and/or prevention of GvH disease. Reported results are, however, conflicting; whereas some studies described that co-transplantation of BM-MSCs prevented murine lethal GvHD [73], others found no evidence for effects on GvHD incidence or severity [74]. Clinical trials have also provided controversial results with response rates that vary considerably, ranging from 15–55% [75–77]. These discrepancies could be attributed to the different GvHD characteristics of treated patients and/or to different schedules of MSC application. In this respect, the time of MSC application seems to be particularly important. MSCs cannot prevent GvHD if they are given at the beginning or too late in the course of the disease. However, GvHD symptoms totally reverted when MSCs were provided weekly in several doses [78]. Furthermore, MSCs injected in one single dose were only effective when given at days +2 or +20, when IFNγ levels are high and therefore promote immunosuppressive MSCs [79].

A Phase II multicenter trial with 55 patients who received *ex-vivo*-expanded BM-MSCs derived from either HLA-identical sibling donors or haploidentical donors of HLA-mismatched donors in a single infusion (27 patients) or in two or more (the remaining patients) obtained promising results, with 30 patients showing a complete response and 9 a partial one, independent of HLA-match [80]. Unfortunately, these results have not been reproduced in other studies [81,82]. In other preliminary assays a significant improvement has been found in patients with GvHD affecting liver and gut, but not in those suffering skin GvHD [83].

In patients suffering *de novo* rather than refractory GvHD, steroid GvHD MSC treatment also produced promising results [84]. However, in one small trial using MSC treatment for GvHD prevention, Ning and colleagues [85] reported increased relapse rates, raising the possibility that MSCs could have deleterious effects in disease recurrence, a finding that needs confirmation. Nevertheless, this group has not provided any new evidence for these deleterious effects.

MSCs for improving HSC engraftment and preventing GvHD

Some pre-clinical studies have provided evidence that BM-MSCs could improve HSC engraftment and repopulation. Co-culture of MSCs with HSCs provokes improved hematopoiesis [86–88] and leads to distinct haematopoietic cell lineages [89]. Intramedullary grafting of *ex-vivo*-expanded labeled hMSCS in NOD/SCID mice results in their incorporation into BM stroma in the form of pericytes, reticular cells, endothelial cells, osteocytes, and bone-lining osteoblasts [90]. However, intravenously injected MSCs do not reside in the bone marrow and are largely trapped in the lungs [90]. It is important to remark, however, that these in vivo protocols are difficult to reproduce and need further confirmation. On the other hand, in primary human BM cultures, MSCs intimately associated with megakariocyte precursors induce their differentiation in the absence of exogenous cytokines [91] and co-cultures with cord-blood CD34+ cells induce B lymphopoiesis [92].

Clinical studies are still few and reported results are again conflicting. In general, reported trials indicate that the co-infusion of MSCs with HSCs improves the engraftment of the latter and favors hematopoiesis, but the results are highly dependent on the conditions applied [70].

Role of MSCs in autoimmunity

The therapeutic effects of MSC in autoimmune disease were first reported in experimental autoimmune encephalomyelitis (EAE) [93], and later in numerous experimental models of autoimmunity [94–99], but results are conflicting. In a case of collagen-induced arthritis, MSCs effectively protected from disease [94], but in another case MSC administration actually made the clinical symptoms worse [100]. On the other hand, as reported above for GvHD, the time of MSC administration seems to be important for the results, although some controversy remains. Maximal efficiency has been reported when MSCs were administered at the onset of disease, but there were no effects after disease stabilization [93]. However, other authors have reported prevention of the onset of disease, as well as decreased severity after stabilization [101]. It is also very important to note that the beneficial effects of MSC on autoimmunity are not restricted to syngeneic conditions alone, since allogeneic cells are also efficient.

The immunosuppressive effects of MSCs on autoimmunity have been accounted for on the basis of their immunomodulatory properties on effector cells and Treg cells. In chemically induced autoimmune colitis, systemic injection of MSCs improved the course of disease in correlation with inhibition of TH1-type immune reactivity and expansion of Treg cells [98]. Likewise, MSCs induced improvement of multiorgan autoimmunity courses with recovery

of Treg cell deficiency [102]. In EAU (experimental autoimmune uveoretinitis), the administration of MSCs negatively regulates TH17 activity [37], a finding previously reported in EAE [103].

Clinical evidence for the benefits of MSC application on the course of autoimmune diseases is controversial and requires further confirmation. Autologous bone-marrow-derived MSCs given intrathecally in 10 patients with advanced multiple sclerosis produced a clinical improvement in nearly 50%, although these results do not correlate with radiological benefits [104]. In another study, results were even less promising [105]. Autologous application of MSCs in two patients with systemic lupus erythematosus (SLE) did not result in a clinical benefit, although there were increased numbers of Treg cells [106]. Conversely, both allogeneic bone-marrow- and cord-derived MSCs improved clinical and laboratory parameters in SLE patients [107,108].

Conclusions and further directions

It is difficult to reach definitive conclusions on the clinical manifestations and biology of MSCs. In general, available information is controversial and difficult to compare. The lack of specific cell markers to achieve a good phenotypic characterization, the possibility of obtaining enriched cell populations from different sources, and the contradictory results on the molecular mediators that support their modulatory and trophic properties make it difficult to fully understand the significance of these cells. From a therapeutic view, it is evident that only their anti-inflammatory and immunoregulatory properties guarantee certain success when they are used in immunohematologic diseases. It is also necessary to obtain a significant improvement in the in vivo differentiation of these cells into other cell lineages, even those derived from the mesoderm. Furthermore, multicenter trials must be designed in which the different laboratories involved use the same protocols.

Acknowledgments

The author would like to thank Dr Javier G. Castro (Instituto de Salud Carlos III, Madrid, Spain) for his critical reading of the manuscript. This work was supported in part by grants: S-B10–0204/2006 (Regional Government of Madrid), BFU 2010–16250 (Spanish Ministry of Science and Innovation), RD06/0010/0003

(Spanish Ministry of Health and Consumption), GR35/10A-910552 (Complutense University, Spanish Association for Cancer Research).

References

1. Zapata, A. Stem cell populations in adult bone marrow: phenotypes and biological relevance for production of somatic stem cells. In: Simón, C. and Pellicer, A., eds. *Stem Cells in Human Reproduction. Basic Science and Therapeutic Potential*, 2nd edn. New York: Informa Healthcare. 2009; 178–188.

2. Friedenstein, A.J., Gorskaja, J.F., Kulagina, N.N. Fibroblast precursors in normal and irradiated mouse hematopoietic organs. *Experimental Hematology.* 1976; 4: 267–274.

3. Young, H.E., Mancini, M.L., Wright, R.P. *et al.* Mesenchymal stem cells reside within the connective tissues of many organs. *Developmental Dynamics.* 1995; 202: 137–144.

4. Kern, S., Eichler, H., Stoeve, J. *et al.* Comparative analysis of mesenchymal stem cells from bone marrow, umbilical cord blood, or adipose tissue. *Stem Cells.* 2006; 24: 1294–1301.

5. Pittenger, M.F., Mackay, A.M., Beck, S.C. *et al.* Multilineage potential of adult human mesenchymal stem cells. *Science.* 1999; 284: 143–147.

6. da Silva Meirelles, L., Caplan, A.I., Nardi, N.B. In search of the in vivo identity of mesenchymal stem cells. *Stem Cells.* 2008; 26: 2287–2299.

7. Deschaseaux, F., Pontikoglou, C., Sensebe, L. Bone regeneration: the stem/progenitor cells point of view. *Journal of Cell and Molecular Medicine.* 2010; 14: 103–115.

8. Pontikoglou, C., Delorme, B., Charbord, P. Human bone marrow native mesenchymal stem cells. *Regenerative Medicine.* 2008; 3: 731–741.

9. Caplan, A.I. Mesenchymal stem cells. *Journal of Orthopaedic Research.* 1991; 9: 641–650.

10. Phinney, D.G., Prockop, D.J. Concise review: mesenchymal stem/multipotent stromal cells: the state of transdifferentiation and modes of tissue repair – current views. *Stem Cells.* 2007; 25: 2896–2902.

11. Mendez-Ferrer, S., Michurina, T.V., Ferraro, F. *et al.* Mesenchymal and haematopoietic stem cells form a unique bone marrow niche. *Nature.* 2010; 466: 829–834.

12. Buhring, H.J., Battula, V.L., Treml, S. *et al.* Novel markers for the prospective isolation of human MSC. *Annals of the New York Academy of Science.* 2007; 1106: 262–271.

13. Battula, V.L., Treml, S., Bareiss, P.M. *et al.* Isolation of functionally distinct mesenchymal stem cell subsets using antibodies against CD56, CD271, and mesenchymal stem cell antigen-1. *Haematologica.* 2009; 94: 173–184.

14. Tormin, A., Li, O., Brune, J.C. *et al.* CD146 expression on primary nonhematopoietic bone marrow stem cells is correlated with in situ localization. *Blood.* 2011; 117: 5067–5077.

15. Maijenburg, M.W., Kleijer, M., Vermeul, K. *et al.* The composition of the mesenchymal stromal cell compartment in human bone marrow changes during development and aging. *Haematologica.* 2011; 97: 179–183.

16. Kuznetsov, S.A., Mankani, M.H., Bianco, P. *et al.* Enumeration of the colony-forming units-fibroblast from mouse and human bone marrow in normal and pathological conditions. *Stem Cell Research.* 2009; 2: 83–94.

17. Dazzi, F., Marelli-Berg, F.M. Mesenchymal stem cells for graft-versus-host disease: close encounters with T cells. *European Journal of Immunology.* 2008; 38: 1479–1482.

18. Ren, G., Zhang, L., Zhao, X. *et al.* Mesenchymal stem cell-mediated immunosuppression occurs via concerted action of chemokines and nitric oxide. *Cell Stem Cell.* 2008; 2: 141–150.

19. Chan, J.L., Tang, K.C., Patel, A.P. *et al.* Antigen-presenting property of mesenchymal stem cells occurs during a narrow window at low levels of interferon-gamma. *Blood.* 2006; 107: 4817–4824.

20. English, K., Barry, F.P., Mahon, B.P. Murine mesenchymal stem cells suppress dendritic cell migration, maturation and antigen presentation. *Immunology Letters.* 2008; 115: 50–58.

21. Aggarwal, S., Pittenger, M.F. Human mesenchymal stem cells modulate allogeneic immune cell responses. *Blood.* 2005; 105: 1815–1822.

22. Zhao, S., Wehner, R., Bornhauser, M. *et al.* Immunomodulatory properties of mesenchymal stromal cells and their therapeutic consequences for immune-mediated disorders. *Stem Cells and Development.* 2010; 19: 607–614.

23. Kim, J., Hematti, P. Mesenchymal stem cell-educated macrophages: a novel type of alternatively activated macrophages. *Experimental Hematology.* 2009; 37: 1445–1453.

24. Raffaghello, L., Bianchi, G., Bertolotto, M. *et al.* Human mesenchymal stem cells inhibit neutrophil apoptosis: a model for neutrophil preservation in the bone marrow niche. *Stem Cells.* 2008; 26: 151–162.

25. Stagg, J. Immune regulation by mesenchymal stem cells: two sides to the coin. *Tissue Antigens*. 2007; 69: 1–9.

26. Uccelli, A., Moretta, L., Pistoia, V. Mesenchymal stem cells in health and disease. *Nature Reviews Immunology*. 2008; 8: 726–736.

27. Siegel, G., Schafer, R., Dazzi, F. The immunosuppressive properties of mesenchymal stem cells. *Transplantation*. 2009; 87: S45–S49.

28. Corcione, A., Benvenuto, F., Ferretti, E. *et al.* Human mesenchymal stem cells modulate B-cell functions. *Blood*. 2006; 107: 367–372.

29. Benvenuto, F., Ferrari, S., Gerdoni, E. *et al.* Human mesenchymal stem cells promote survival of T cells in a quiescent state. *Stem Cells*. 2007; 25: 1753–1760.

30. Maccario, R., Podesta, M., Moretta, A. *et al.* Interaction of human mesenchymal stem cells with cells involved in alloantigen-specific immune response favors the differentiation of CD4+ T-cell subsets expressing a regulatory/suppressive phenotype. *Haematologica*. 2005; 90: 516–525.

31. Krampera, M., Glennie, S., Dyson, J. *et al.* Bone marrow mesenchymal stem cells inhibit the response of naive and memory antigen-specific T cells to their cognate peptide. *Blood*. 2003; 101: 3722–3729.

32. Mills, K.H. Induction, function and regulation of IL-17-producing T cells. *European Journal of Immunology*. 2008; 38: 2636–2649.

33. Bettelli, E., Oukka, M., Kuchroo, V.K. T(H)-17 cells in the circle of immunity and autoimmunity. *Nature Immunology*. 2007; 8: 345–350.

34. Turner, J.E., Paust, H.J., Steinmetz, O.M. *et al.* The Th17 immune response in renal inflammation. *Kidney International*. 2010; 77: 1070–1075.

35. Wang, J., Wang, G., Sun, B. *et al.* Interleukin-27 suppresses experimental autoimmune encephalomyelitis during bone marrow stromal cell treatment. *Journal of Autoimmunity*. 2008; 30: 222–229.

36. Zhao, W., Wang, Y., Wang, D. *et al.* TGF-beta expression by allogeneic bone marrow stromal cells ameliorates diabetes in NOD mice through modulating the distribution of CD4+ T cell subsets. *Cell Immunology*. 2008; 253: 23–30.

37. Zhang, X., Ren, X., Li, G. *et al.* Mesenchymal stem cells ameliorate experimental autoimmune uveoretinitis by comprehensive modulation of systemic autoimmunity. *Investigative Ophthalmology and Visual Science*. 2011; 52: 3143–3152.

38. Ghannam, S., Pene, J., Torcy-Moquet, G. *et al.* Mesenchymal stem cells inhibit human Th17 cell differentiation and function and induce a T regulatory cell phenotype. *Journal of Immunology*. 2010; 185: 302–312.

39. Duffy, M.M., Pindjakova, J., Hanley, S.A. *et al.* Mesenchymal stem cell inhibition of T-helper 17 cell-differentiation is triggered by cell-cell contact and mediated by prostaglandin E2 via the EP4 receptor. *European Journal of Immunology*. 2011; 41: 2840–2851.

40. Tatara, R., Ozaki, K., Kikuchi, Y. *et al.* Mesenchymal stromal cells inhibit Th17 but not regulatory T-cell differentiation. *Cytotherapy*. 2011; 13: 686–694.

41. Guo, Z., Zheng, C., Chen, Z. *et al.* Fetal BM-derived mesenchymal stem cells promote the expansion of human Th17 cells, but inhibit the production of Th1 cells. *European Journal of Immunology*. 2009; 39: 2840–2849.

42. Selmani, Z., Naji, A., Zidi, I. *et al.* Human leukocyte antigen-G5 secretion by human mesenchymal stem cells is required to suppress T lymphocyte and natural killer function and to induce CD4+ CD25highFOXP3+ regulatory T cells. *Stem Cells*. 2008; 26: 212–222.

43. Sotiropoulou, P.A., Perez, S.A., Gritzapis, A.D. *et al.* Interactions between human mesenchymal stem cells and natural killer cells. *Stem Cells*. 2006; 24: 74–85.

44. Spaggiari, G.M., Capobianco, A., Becchetti, S. *et al.* Mesenchymal stem cell-natural killer cell interactions: evidence that activated NK cells are capable of killing MSCs, whereas MSCs can inhibit IL-2-induced NK-cell proliferation. *Blood*. 2006; 107: 1484–1490.

45. Spaggiari, G.M., Capobianco, A., Abdelrazik, H. *et al.* Mesenchymal stem cells inhibit natural killer-cell proliferation, cytotoxicity, and cytokine production: role of indoleamine 2,3-dioxygenase and prostaglandin E2. *Blood*. 2008; 111: 1327–1333.

46. Tomchuck, S.L., Zwezdaryk, K.J., Coffelt, S.B. *et al.* Toll-like receptors on human mesenchymal stem cells drive their migration and immunomodulating responses. *Stem Cells*. 2008; 26: 99–107.

47. Romieu-Mourez, R., Francois, M., Boivin, M.N. *et al.* Cytokine modulation of TLR expression and activation in mesenchymal stromal cells leads to a proinflammatory phenotype. *Journal of Immunology*. 2009; 182: 7963–7973.

48. Liotta, F., Angeli, R., Cosmi, L. *et al.* Toll-like receptors 3 and 4 are expressed by human bone marrow-derived mesenchymal stem cells and can inhibit their T-cell modulatory activity by impairing Notch signaling. *Stem Cells*. 2008; 26: 279–289.

49. DelaRosa, O., Lombardo, E. Modulation of adult mesenchymal stem cells activity by toll-like receptors: implications on therapeutic potential. *Mediators of Inflammation*. 2010; 865601.

50. Waterman, R.S., Tomchuck, S.L., Henkle, S.L. *et al.* A new mesenchymal stem cell (MSC) paradigm: polarization into a pro-inflammatory MSC1 or an immunosuppressive MSC2 phenotype. *PLoS One.* 2010; 5: e10088.

51. Le Blanc, K., Ringden, O. Immunomodulation by mesenchymal stem cells and clinical experience. *Journal of Internal Medicine.* 2007; 262: 509–525.

52. Nauta, A.J., Fibbe, W.E. Immunomodulatory properties of mesenchymal stromal cells. *Blood.* 2007; 110: 3499–3506.

53. Pittenger, M.F., Martin, B.J. Mesenchymal stem cells and their potential as cardiac therapeutics. *Circulation Research.* 2004; 95: 9–20.

54. Trumpp, A., Essers, M., Wilson, A. Awakening dormant haematopoietic stem cells. *Nature Reviews Immunology.* 2010; 10: 201–209.

55. Sacchetti, B., Funari, A., Michienzi, S. *et al.* Self-renewing osteoprogenitors in bone marrow sinusoids can organize a hematopoietic microenvironment. *Cell.* 2007; 131: 324–336.

56. Crisan, M., Yap, S., Casteilla, L. *et al.* A perivascular origin for mesenchymal stem cells in multiple human organs. *Cell Stem Cell.* 2008; 3: 301–313.

57. Morikawa, S., Mabuchi, Y., Kubota, Y. *et al.* Prospective identification, isolation, and systemic transplantation of multipotent mesenchymal stem cells in murine bone marrow. *Journal of Experimental Medicine.* 2009; 206: 2483–2496.

58. Dennis, J.E., Carbillet, J.P., Caplan, A.I. *et al.* The STRO-1+ marrow cell population is multipotential. *Cells Tissues and Organs.* 2002; 170: 73–82.

59. Gang, E.J., Bosnakovski, D., Figueiredo, C.A. *et al.* SSEA-4 identifies mesenchymal stem cells from bone marrow. *Blood.* 2007; 109: 1743–1751.

60. Charbord, P., Tavian, M., Humeau, L. *et al.* Early ontogeny of the human marrow from long bones: an immunohistochemical study of hematopoiesis and its microenvironment. *Blood.* 1996; 87: 4109–4119.

61. Westen, H., Bainton, D.F. Association of alkaline-phosphatase-positive reticulum cells in bone marrow with granulocytic precursors. *Journal of Experimental Medicine.* 1979; 150: 919–937.

62. Quirici, N., Soligo, D., Bossolasco, P. *et al.* Isolation of bone marrow mesenchymal stem cells by anti-nerve growth factor receptor antibodies. *Experimental Hematology.* 2002; 30: 783–791.

63. Kiel, M.J., Morrison, S.J. Uncertainty in the niches that maintain haematopoietic stem cells. *Nature Reviews Immunology.* 2008; 8: 290–301.

64. Katayama, Y., Battista, M., Kao, W.M. *et al.* Signals from the sympathetic nervous system regulate hematopoietic stem cell egress from bone marrow. *Cell.* 2006; 124: 407–421.

65. Chakroborty, D., Chowdhury, U.R., Sarkar, C. *et al.* Dopamine regulates endothelial progenitor cell mobilization from mouse bone marrow in tumor vascularization. *Journal of Clinical Investigation.* 2008; 118: 1380–1389.

66. Ehninger, A., Trumpp, A. The bone marrow stem cell niche grows up: mesenchymal stem cells and macrophages move in. *Journal of Experimental Medicine.* 2011; 208: 421–428.

67. Schajnovitz, A., Itkin, T., D'Uva, G. *et al.* CXCL12 secretion by bone marrow stromal cells is dependent on cell contact and mediated by connexin-43 and connexin-45 gap junctions. *Nature Immunology.* 2011; 12: 391–398.

68. Lucas, D., Battista, M., Shi, P.A. *et al.* Mobilized hematopoietic stem cell yield depends on species-specific circadian timing. *Cell Stem Cell.* 2008; 3: 364–366.

69. Yamazaki, S., Ema, H., Karlsson, G. *et al.* Nonmyelinating Schwann cells maintain hematopoietic stem cell hibernation in the bone marrow niche. *Cell.* 2011; 147: 1146–1158.

70. Pontikoglou, C., Deschaseaux, F., Sensebe, L. *et al.* Bone marrow mesenchymal stem cells: biological properties and their role in hematopoiesis and hematopoietic stem cell transplantation. *Stem Cell in Review.* 2011; 7: 569–589.

71. Quarto, R., Mastrogiacomo, M., Cancedda, R. *et al.* Repair of large bone defects with the use of autologous bone marrow stromal cells. *New England Journal of Medicine.* 2001; 344: 385–386.

72. Wakitani, S., Imoto, K., Yamamoto, T. *et al.* Human autologous culture expanded bone marrow mesenchymal cell transplantation for repair of cartilage defects in osteoarthritic knees. *Osteoarthritis and Cartilage.* 2002; 10: 199–206.

73. Chung, N.G., Jeong, D.C., Park, S.J. *et al.* Cotransplantation of marrow stromal cells may prevent lethal graft-versus-host disease in major histocompatibility complex mismatched murine hematopoietic stem cell transplantation. *International Journal of Hematology.* 2004; 80: 370–376.

74. Sudres, M., Norol, F., Trenado, A. *et al.* Bone marrow mesenchymal stem cells suppress lymphocyte proliferation in vitro but fail to prevent graft-versus-host disease in mice. *Journal of Immunology.* 2006; 176: 7761–7767.

75. Ringden, O., Uzunel, M., Rasmusson, I. *et al.* Mesenchymal stem cells for treatment of therapy-resistant graft-versus-host disease. *Transplantation.* 2006; 81: 1390–1397.

76. Fang, B., Song, Y., Liao, L. *et al.* Favorable response to human adipose tissue-derived mesenchymal stem cells in steroid-refractory acute graft-versus-host disease. *Transplantation Proceedings*. 2007; 39: 3358–3362.

77. Muller, I., Kordowich, S., Holzwarth, C. *et al.* Application of multipotent mesenchymal stromal cells in pediatric patients following allogeneic stem cell transplantation. *Blood Cells, Molecules and Diseases*. 2008; 40: 25–32.

78. Tisato, V., Naresh, K., Girdlestone, J. *et al.* Mesenchymal stem cells of cord blood origin are effective at preventing but not treating graft-versus-host disease. *Leukemia*. 2007; 21: 1992–1999.

79. Polchert, D., Sobinsky, J., Douglas, G. *et al.* IFN-gamma activation of mesenchymal stem cells for treatment and prevention of graft versus host disease. *European Journal of Immunology*. 2008; 38: 1745–1755.

80. Le Blanc, K., Frassoni, F., Ball, L. *et al.* Mesenchymal stem cells for treatment of steroid-resistant, severe, acute graft-versus-host disease: a phase II study. *Lancet*. 2008; 371: 1579–1586.

81. von Bonin, M., Stolzel, F., Goedecke, A. *et al.* Treatment of refractory acute GVHD with third-party MSC expanded in platelet lysate-containing medium. *Bone Marrow Transplantation*. 2009; 43: 245–251.

82. Lucchini, G., Introna, M., Dander, E. *et al.* Platelet-lysate-expanded mesenchymal stromal cells as a salvage therapy for severe resistant graft-versus-host disease in a pediatric population. *Biology of Blood and Marrow Transplantation*. 2010; 16: 1293–1301.

83. Martin, P.J., Uberti, J.P., Soiffer, R.J. *et al.* Prochymal improves response rates in patients with steroid-refractory acute graft versus host disease (SR-GVHD) involving the liver and gut: results of a randomized placebo-controlled, multicenter phase III trial in GVHD. *Biology of Blood and Marrow Transplantation*. 2010; 16(2): 169–170.

84. Kebriaei, P., Isola, L., Bahceci, E. *et al.* Adult human mesenchymal stem cells added to corticosteroid therapy for the treatment of acute graft-versus-host disease. *Biology of Blood and Marrow Transplantation*. 2009; 15: 804–811.

85. Ning, H., Yang, F., Jiang, M. *et al.* The correlation between cotransplantation of mesenchymal stem cells and higher recurrence rate in hematologic malignancy patients: outcome of a pilot clinical study. *Leukemia*. 2008; 22: 593–599.

86. In 't Anker, P.S., Scherjon, S.A., Kleijburg-van der Keur, C. *et al.* Amniotic fluid as a novel source of mesenchymal stem cells for therapeutic transplantation. *Blood*. 2003; 102: 1548–1549.

87. Bensidhoum, M., Chapel, A., Francois, S. *et al.* Homing of in vitro expanded Stro-1- or Stro-1+ human mesenchymal stem cells into the NOD/SCID mouse and their role in supporting human CD34 cell engraftment. *Blood*. 2004; 103: 3313–3319.

88. Gottschling, S., Saffrich, R., Seckinger, A. *et al.* Human mesenchymal stromal cells regulate initial self-renewing divisions of hematopoietic progenitor cells by a beta1-integrin-dependent mechanism. *Stem Cells*. 2007; 25: 798–806.

89. Majumdar, M.K., Thiede, M.A., Mosca, J.D. *et al.* Phenotypic and functional comparison of cultures of marrow-derived mesenchymal stem cells (MSCs) and stromal cells. *Journal of Cell Physiology*. 1998; 176: 57–66.

90. Muguruma, Y., Yahata, T., Miyatake, H. *et al.* Reconstitution of the functional human hematopoietic microenvironment derived from human mesenchymal stem cells in the murine bone marrow compartment. *Blood*. 2006; 107: 1878–1887.

91. Cheng, L., Qasba, P., Vanguri, P. *et al.* Human mesenchymal stem cells support megakaryocyte and pro-platelet formation from CD34(+) hematopoietic progenitor cells. *Journal of Cell Physiology*. 2000; 184: 58–69.

92. Ichii, M., Oritani, K., Yokota, T. *et al.* Regulation of human B lymphopoiesis by the transforming growth factor-beta superfamily in a newly established coculture system using human mesenchymal stem cells as a supportive microenvironment. *Experimental Hematology*. 2008; 36: 587–597.

93. Zappia, E., Casazza, S., Pedemonte, E. *et al.* Mesenchymal stem cells ameliorate experimental autoimmune encephalomyelitis inducing T-cell anergy. *Blood*. 2005; 106: 1755–1761.

94. Augello, A., Tasso, R., Negrini, S.M. *et al.* Cell therapy using allogeneic bone marrow mesenchymal stem cells prevents tissue damage in collagen-induced arthritis. *Arthritis and Rheumatism*. 2007; 56: 1175–1186.

95. Zheng, Z.H., Li, X.Y., Ding, J. *et al.* Allogeneic mesenchymal stem cell and mesenchymal stem cell-differentiated chondrocyte suppress the responses of type II collagen-reactive T cells in rheumatoid arthritis. *Rheumatology (Oxford)*. 2008; 47: 22–30.

96. Fiorina, P., Jurewicz, M., Augello, A. *et al.* Immunomodulatory function of bone marrow-derived mesenchymal stem cells in experimental autoimmune type 1 diabetes. *Journal of Immunology*. 2009; 183: 993–1004.

97. Madec, A.M., Mallone, R., Afonso, G. *et al.* Mesenchymal stem cells protect NOD mice from diabetes by inducing regulatory T cells. *Diabetologia*. 2009; 52: 1391–1399.

98. Gonzalez, M.A., Gonzalez-Rey, E., Rico, L. *et al.* Adipose-derived mesenchymal stem cells alleviate experimental colitis by inhibiting inflammatory and autoimmune responses. *Gastroenterology.* 2009; 136: 978–989.

99. Sun, L., Akiyama, K., Zhang, H. *et al.* Mesenchymal stem cell transplantation reverses multiorgan dysfunction in systemic lupus erythematosus mice and humans. *Stem Cells.* 2009; 27: 1421–1432.

100. Djouad, F., Fritz, V., Apparailly, F. *et al.* Reversal of the immunosuppressive properties of mesenchymal stem cells by tumor necrosis factor alpha in collagen-induced arthritis. *Arthritis and Rheumatism.* 2005; 52: 1595–1603.

101. Constantin, G., Marconi, S., Rossi, B. *et al.* Adipose-derived mesenchymal stem cells ameliorate chronic experimental autoimmune encephalomyelitis. *Stem Cells.* 2009; 27: 2624–2635.

102. Parekkadan, B., Tilles, A.W., Yarmush, M.L. Bone marrow-derived mesenchymal stem cells ameliorate autoimmune enteropathy independently of regulatory T cells. *Stem Cells.* 2008; 26: 1913–1919.

103. Rafei, M., Campeau, P.M., Aguilar-Mahecha, A. *et al.* Mesenchymal stromal cells ameliorate experimental autoimmune encephalomyelitis by inhibiting CD4 Th17 T cells in a CC chemokine ligand 2-dependent manner. *Journal of Immunology.* 2009; 182: 5994–6002.

104. Yamout, B., Hourani, R., Salti, H. *et al.* Bone marrow mesenchymal stem cell transplantation in patients with multiple sclerosis: a pilot study. *Journal of Neuroimmunology.* 2010; 227: 185–189.

105. Mohyeddin Bonab, M., Yazdanbakhsh, S., Lotfi, J. *et al.* Does mesenchymal stem cell therapy help multiple sclerosis patients? Report of a pilot study. *Iranian Journal of Immunology.* 2007; 4: 50–57.

106. Carrion, F., Nova, E., Ruiz, C. *et al.* Autologous mesenchymal stem cell treatment increased T regulatory cells with no effect on disease activity in two systemic lupus erythematosus patients. *Lupus.* 2010; 19: 317–322.

107. Liang, J., Zhang, H., Hua, B. *et al.* Allogenic mesenchymal stem cells transplantation in refractory systemic lupus erythematosus: a pilot clinical study. *Annals of Rheumatic Diseases.* 2010; 69: 1423–1429.

108. Sun, L., Wang, D., Liang, J. *et al.* Umbilical cord mesenchymal stem cell transplantation in severe and refractory systemic lupus erythematosus. *Arthritis and Rheumatism.* 2010; 62: 2467–2475.

Chapter 14

Dedifferentiation, transdifferentiation, and reprogramming

Sergio Mora and Angel Raya

Introduction

Over the last 50 years, groundbreaking research on nuclear reprogramming has demonstrated that cell potency changes are possible in vivo and in vitro (recently reviewed in [1]). The capacity of differentiated cells to reacquire a totipotent state was first revealed in the 1950s when the nuclei of differentiated cells were reprogrammed in enucleated eggs to generate frogs. Elegant experiments in the early 1980s used cell fusion to produce stable heterokaryons, demonstrating that differentiated mammalian cells are plastic: their differentiated state can be reversed by fusing them to another cell to form a stable, non-dividing heterokaryon. The end of the 1980s witnessed the first demonstration that forced expression of a single transcription factor is enough to switch mammalian cell fate, with MyoD converting fibroblasts to myoblasts. Ten years later, two discoveries demonstrated dramatic changes in cell potency: on the one hand, cell fusion of mammalian embryonic germ cells with somatic cells provided evidence for epigenetic reprogramming at imprinted genes. On the other hand, the birth of Dolly the sheep provided the ultimate proof that mammalian cells can be reprogrammed to totipotency, and inaugurated a successful series of animal cloning experiments in other mammal species. In 2006, Kazutoshi Takahashi and Shinya Yamanaka showed that ectopic expression of just four transcription factors (Oct4, Klf4, c-Myc, and Sox2) was sufficient to reprogram mouse somatic cells to pluripotency [2], generating so-called induced pluripotent stem cells (iPSCs), which were also obtained from human somatic cells shortly afterward [3–5]. Fully reprogrammed iPSCs are similar to embryonic stem cells (ESCs) in terms of developmental potency, and can contribute extensively to the three embryo germ layers and to the germline.

The fertilized egg (or zygote) has the potential to differentiate and give rise to all the cell types in the organism, as well as to the embryo-derived portion of the placenta, and is thus considered a totipotent cell. At the blastocyst stage of the early embryo, the cells of the inner cell mass (from which ESC lines are derived), are pluripotent: they are able to form each of the three germ layers: endoderm, ectoderm, and mesoderm. During development, cells that are committed to each of these germ layers specialize to give rise to differentiated adult cells of the adult body. This process is accompanied by a loss of cell potency (Figure 14.1), so that differentiated adult somatic cells are unable to switch fates, at least under normal conditions in vivo. According to their degree of developmental potency, specific cell populations arising during development or generated experimentally are generally categorized as *totipotent* (zygote), *pluripotent* (cells in the inner cell mass, ESCs, embryonic germ (EG) cells, embryonic carcinoma (EC) cells, mouse epiblast stem cells (mEpiSCs), and iPSCs), *multipotent* (adult stem cells, partially reprogrammed cells), or *unipotent* (differentiated cell types). Cell populations showing different degrees of developmental potency are characterized by distinct transcriptional profiles, which, in turn, are thought to be maintained by specific epigenetic patterns. Therefore, reprogramming one cell type into another not only involves changing the subsets of genes that are on or off, but also their overall epigenetic landscape.

In this chapter, we present recent advances in the study of cell reprogramming within the broader context of regeneration research. In addition, we explore mechanisms of tissue regeneration in animal models as an example of how cells can regain developmental potency in vivo. Finally, we summarize current

---

Stem Cells in Reproductive Medicine 3ʳᵈ edition, ed. Carlos Simón, Antonio Pellicer and Renee Reijo Pera.
Published by Cambridge University Press. © Cambridge University Press 2013.

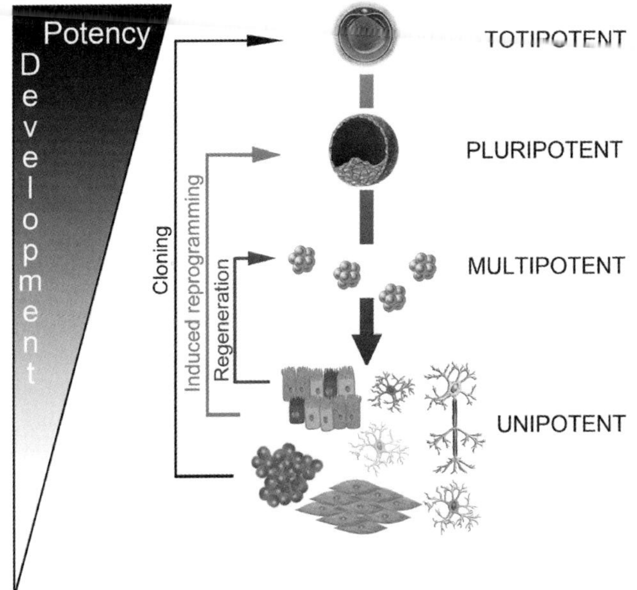

Figure 14.1 Cell potency loss during development. This model depicts the loss of cell potency during embryo development. Cells progressively lose their ability to differentiate into different cell types during development. The most potent cell type, the zygote is considering a totipotent entity. It has the capacity to generate the three germ layers (endoderm, mesoderm, and ectoderm), as well as extra-embryonic tissues. Before gastrulation, pluripotent cells of the inner cell mass of the blastocyst are able to generate cells of the three germ layers, but lose the structural organization capacity that is found in totipotent cells. In the adult organism, populations of multipotent stem or progenitor cells persist, which show a limited degree of differentiating options. Terminally differentiated cells and unipotent cell types build up the organs and tissues in the adult organism, and have lost all differentiation capacity. These cell types can, however, regain developmental potency and generate multipotent cells during regenerative processes in vivo, pluripotent cells by induced reprogramming in vitro, or even totipotent cells by using somatic-cell nuclear-transfer techniques. (See also color plate.)

approaches to investigate reprogramming, dedifferentiation, and transdifferentiation, and discuss the mechanisms that underlie the erasure of epigenetic memory during cellular reprogramming.

Different roads to changing cell potency

The ability of some animal species to completely regenerate parts of their body has fascinated researchers for centuries. Different mechanisms have been proposed to be responsible for this regenerative ability, some of them invoking a change in cells' identities. Humans and other mammalian vertebrates have a limited capacity to regenerate their organs and tissues. Instead, mammalian tissue restoration and maintenance appears to occur through the activation of multipotent stem or progenitor cells, or by the proliferation of the differentiated somatic cells themselves. In contrast, tissues and structures that do regenerate in some species may do so independently of stem or progenitor cells, by processes that involve dedifferentiation or transdifferentiation of specialized cell types. It has also been proposed that the aberrant activation of embryonic programs in differentiated cells, causing an imbalance between self-renewal and differentiation, could impair the preservation of the cell identity and eventually lead to tumorigenesis. Therefore, animals in which regeneration entails the

dedifferentiation or transdifferentiation of specialized cells must be endowed with robust mechanisms to accurately control the degree of developmental potency of somatic cells. By studying these regenerative capacities in animal models, researchers are uncovering molecular and cellular mechanisms that could be used to develop regenerative strategies for humans.

The ability of newts to regenerate their lens was one of the first noted examples of natural regeneration, but many other non-mammalian vertebrate species possess remarkable regenerating capacities. Zebrafish can regenerate their hearts after amputation of up to 20% of the ventricle. During this process, differentiated cardiomyocytes that are still present in the heart undergo limited dedifferentiation and proliferate to regenerate the missing tissue [6,7]. Recent studies have revealed that a similar mechanism operates in neonatal mice, which display robust heart regeneration ability during the first week of post-natal life [8]. Another example of limited dedifferentiation occurs during limb regeneration in urodeles. During limb regeneration, a progenitor cell zone known as a blastema is formed and regenerates the missing portion of the limb, maintaining cell memory of origin [9]. In mammals, some cases of cellular regeneration have been shown after stress conditions. For example, Schwann cells are regenerated in response to damage to the nerve with which they are associated [10]. Moreover, glucagon-producing cells can transdifferentiate into pancreatic insulin-producing ß-cells after ablation of α-cells [11]. The regeneration of pancreatic β-cells from pre-existing α-cells after massive α-cell loss in mice takes place through direct transdifferentiation, is independent of proliferation, and includes an intermediate stage in which cells co-express both the α-cell and β-cell programs. Taken together, these findings indicate that the regenerative process involves changes in gene expression related to the acquisition of cellular plasticity. Cells with a more permissive epigenetic context would be more prone to regenerate certain tissues through dedifferentiation or transdifferentiation, whereas important epigenetic restrictions may prevent the occurrence of cell identity transitions.

Over the last few years, many experiments have demonstrated that the identity of differentiated cells can be reversed to a large extent. Demonstration of nuclear reprogramming was adopted at first with some hesitation, but cumulative evidence over the last 15 years have conclusively disproved the prevailing view that the differentiated state of mammalian cells was fixed and irreversible. As a matter of fact, different experimental approaches have been used to change specific potency states in cells. In this respect, nuclear reprogramming describes either functional or molecular changes to cells undergoing fate changes. Specifically, nuclear reprogramming of adult somatic cells into pluripotent cells can be achieved by three different approaches: by somatic cell nuclear transfer (SCNT), by the fusion of somatic cells with pluripotent cells, or by the expression of a defined set of transcription factors in somatic cells. In the SCNT approach, the nucleus of a somatic cell (which is diploid) is introduced into an enucleated oocyte [12]. In the environment of the oocyte, the somatic cell nucleus is reprogrammed to a pluripotent state. From this diploid oocyte, a blastocyst is generated, from which ESC lines can be derived under specific cell-culture conditions. If development is allowed to proceed to completion, an entire cloned organism can be generated.

In the cell fusion approach, two or more distinct cell types are combined to form a single entity [13]. To induce nuclear reprogramming to pluripotency, one of the cell types is a pluripotent entity (ES, EG, or EC) and the other one is a somatic cell (reviewed in [1]). The resultant fused cells can be heterokaryons or hybrids, and can be established between cells from the same species or from different species. In the more recent approach of induced reprogramming to pluripotency,

the transient overexpression of a few factors in somatic cells determines a radical fate transition to generate iPSCs [2]. The development of this latter approach was preceded by a variety of experimental evidence in which overexpression of single transcription factors induced more limited, but still remarkable, changes in cell fate in the context of *Drosophila* embryo development [14] and mammalian cells in culture [15–17].

Nuclear reprogramming, from a functional point of view, also includes the stable conversion of one differentiated cell type into another. This induced transition leads to epigenetic fluctuations favorable to changes in cell potency (Figure 14.2). The terms "transdifferentiation" and "lineage conversion" refer to situations where reprogramming does not involve the generation of dedifferentiated progenitor cells, but rather the direct transition between differentiated somatic cell types. Dedifferentiation, in turn, implies the acquisition of a higher developmental potency, characteristic of less differentiated states, like a ball moving uphill in the valleys of Waddinton's epigenetic landscape model [18] (Figure 14.3). Reprogramming differentiated somatic cells to pluripotency, indeed, represents one of the most dramatic instances of dedifferentiation.

Cellular transitions open an exciting field of research aimed at understanding the molecular cues that determine cell fate changes in the same genetic background. Recent advances are focusing attention on cellular modeling and regenerative medicine using the background knowledge of stem-cell biology and cellular reprogramming.

Dedifferentiation

Dedifferentiation entails a stable change in cell fate (reprogramming) so that the resulting cell type represents earlier steps in the cell's developmental history, either molecularly or functionally. During cell dedifferentiation, cells climb up hills in the landscape of epigenetic reprogramming (Figure 14.3). Natural intermediate stages associated with dedifferentiation resemble a reversal of developmental differentiation. These transitions are accompanied by expression of genes typically expressed in multipotent progenitors and absent in differentiated cells. Processes of cell dedifferentiation have long been identified in a variety of experimental systems. Natural cell dedifferentiation phenomena could be readily analyzed both in

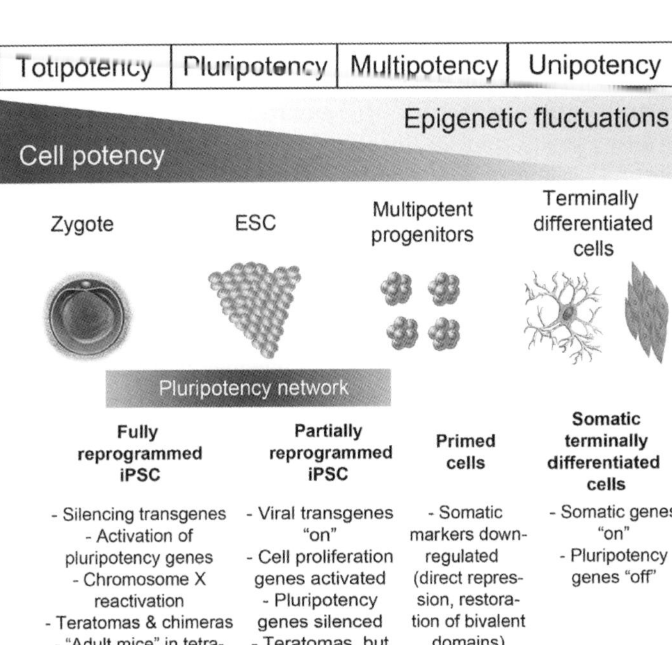

Figure 14.2 Cell potency transitions during reprogramming. Loss or gain of developmental potency is related with epigenetic fluctuations in the cell. Epigenetic marks characteristic of high-potency states are replaced in terminally differentiated cells during differentiation. This is related to specific gene expression changes that determine cell transitions. In a related process, forced expression of reprogramming factors used to generate pluripotent stem cells is related with the initial silencing of somatic programs in terminally differentiated cells. After this initiation event, primed cells start to express endogenous pluripotency-associated genes and activate cell proliferation programs. Partially reprogrammed cells begin to appear shortly afterward. These cells resemble pluripotent stem cells in some aspects, like teratoma formation ability, but still express viral transgenes and show aberrant expression of lineage genes, and thus fail to generate adult chimeras. Finally, transition to a fully reprogrammed state depends on the acquisition of a self-autonomous pluripotency network. This last step is marked by a series of events that include complete silencing of the viral transgenes, activation of endogenous pluripotency-associated markers, and complete epigenetic memory erasure. (See also color plate.)

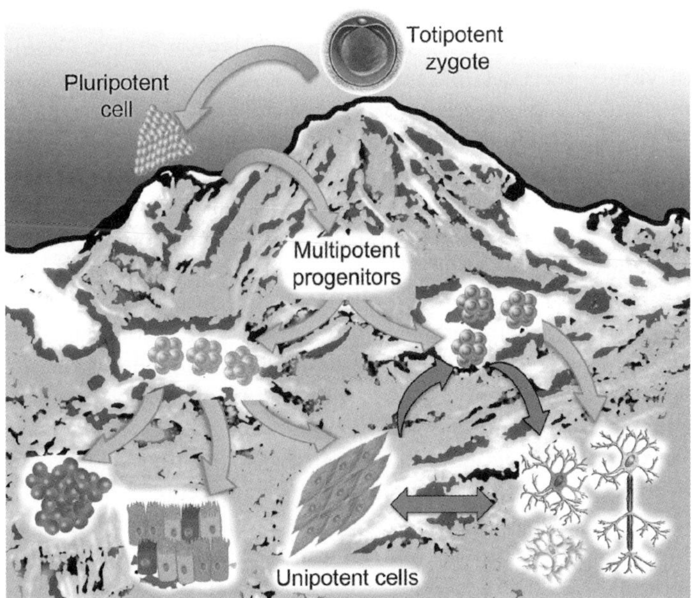

Figure 14.3 The epigenetic landscape of cell potency. This model depicts cells with different developmental potential according to their position in the "mountain of cell potency." The top of the mountain represents totipotent cells, just below these, pluripotent cells, and downstream multipotent progenitors with specific differentiation capacities. Cells, like marbles, roll down across the valleys of the mountain (blue arrows), progressively losing their developmental potency. Unipotent cells residing in the valleys can move uphill (green arrow) depicting dedifferentiation, or they can move directly to other valleys (red arrow) by transdifferentiation. (See also color plate.)

vivo and in vitro. During zebrafish heart regeneration, differentiated cardiomyocytes in the heart dedifferentiate and proliferate to regenerate the lost tissue [6,7]. This process is related to reorganization of the cell cytoskeleton and disassembly of the contractile apparatus, which coincide with up-regulation of cell-cycle regulators like *cdc2* and *polo-like kinase 1* and reactivation of embryonic cardiac gene *gata4* [6,7,19]. Another example of natural in vivo dedifferentiation occurs during limb regeneration in urodeles [9]. After limb amputation, cells adjacent to the wound de-differentiate, forming a blastema of proliferating cells that, while retaining memory of their origin, regenerate all the components of the lost limb, including muscle, dermis, epidermis, cartilage, nerves, skeleton, and blood vessels. Elegant experiments in mice demonstrated that *Pax5* deletion caused loss of B-cell lineage commitment and dedifferentiation in vivo [17]. In addition, loss of *Pax5* in late B cells could initiate lymphoma development in mice. All these data support the concept that in vivo dedifferentiation is markedly linked to cell-cycle regulation and involves the silencing of tissue-specific genes, as well as the induction of genes involved in embryonic programs, processes that are reminiscent of those taking place during reprogramming to pluripotency.

In vitro models of cell dedifferentiation have demonstrated that certain components of regenerating tissues may erase differentiation programs in somatic cells, and subsequently allow proliferation. Extracts of regenerating newt blastemas induce dedifferentiation of mouse myotubes in culture by suppressing the myoblast determination factor *MyoD* and *myogenin* [20]. MyoD had been previously shown to induce conversion of fibroblasts to myogenic cells [15], confirming the important role of this factor in cell fate decisions. Another example that illustrates in vitro transitions to multipotency during dedifferentiation comes from studies showing that suppression of *Pax5* induces loss of commitment in pro-B cells [21]. *Pax5*$^{-/-}$ pro-B cells regress in their lineage fate, and stimulation with appropriate cytokines induces them to differentiate into osteoclasts, macrophages, granulocytes, natural killer cells, and dendritic cells. In addition, ectopic expression of *Cebpα* leads to *Pax5* down-regulation and reprogramming of B cells into macrophages [16]. All these cases underscore the essential importance of certain factors in lineage commitment by suppressing alternative lineage choices. In fact, overexpressing *Cebpα* or knocking down *Pax5*, in addition to overexpressing the four Yamanaka factors (*Oct4*, *Sox2*, *Klf4*, and *c-Myc*, also known as O, S, K, M), enhance reprogramming efficiency to generate iPSCs from terminally differentiated B cells [22].

Mesenchymal-to-epithelial transitions (MET) are considered another type of transition to higher states of cell potency, and have been shown to occur both in vivo and in vitro. MET is a developmental process important for cell fate determination, and is characterized by a cell phenotypic change, involving epithelial intercellular contacts, accompanied by the loss of elongated (mesenchymal) shape, and decreased contractility and motility. MET occurs in many different biological contexts, including embryo development, pathological fibrogenesis, and metastasis. Moreover, MET has been shown to play an important role during the first steps of induced reprogramming to pluripotency [23]. All these data suggest that natural and experimentally induced dedifferentiation processes are well controlled from a genetic and microenvironmental perspective. Applications that may arise from the deciphering of the molecular basis of cell dedifferentiation could open new doors for implementing novel strategies in regenerative medicine.

Transdifferentiation

Directed reprogramming of differentiated cells can provide unexpected insights into development. In a similar way, lessons from studying embryo development may provide new insights into the molecular cues that control lineage conversions. The term "lineage conversion" or "transdifferentiation" is used to describe changes in cell fate that do not involve a gain in cell potency. In other words, transdifferentiation denotes the conversion between different cellular fates, like a ball moving across valleys in Waddington's epigenetic landscape model [18] (Figure 14.3). There are many examples that illustrate lineage conversions in vivo. One of the most elegant experiments in developmental biology comes from pioneering studies in homeotic transformations showing that misexpression of the Hox gene *Antennapedia* resulted in legs growing in place of antennae in *Drosophila* [14]. These experiments demonstrated the link between genetic factors and organogenesis in animal models and ushered in a new era for developmental biology. Reprogramming in vivo is most efficient in certain body regions and cell types, depending on the cellular context and developmental programs. This is the case for germ cells in *C. elegans* worm. Recent experiments have shown that knocking down the *lin53* histone chaperone gene in cells within the gonad of *C. elegans* resulted in loss of germline characteristics and their conversion into neural cells [24]. Moreover, the generation of specific neuron subtypes was shown to depend on the ectopic expression of terminal selector genes during larval development, with *che-1*, *unc-30* or *unc-3* giving rise to glutamatergic-, GABAergic-, or cholinergic-like neurons, respectively. These effects

Table 14.1 Advances in cell transdifferentiation in vitro.

Germ layer	Cell type conversion	Cell type of origin	Species	Reprogramming factors	Reference
ECTODERM	Neurons (glutamatergic)	Fibroblast	Mouse	Ascl1, Brn2, Myt1L	[25]
	Neurons (glutamatergic)	Astrocyte	Mouse	Ngn2	[31]
	Neurons (glutamatergic)	Fibroblast	Human	Ascl1, Brn2, Myt1L, NeuroD1	[29]
	Neurons (glutamatergic)	Fibroblast	Human	Brn2, Myt1L, miR-124	[30]
	Neurons (glutamatergic)	Fibroblast	Human	Ascl1, Myt1L, NeuroD2, miR-124, miR-9/9	[28]
	Neurons (dopaminergic)	Fibroblast	Mouse/Human	Ascl1, Lmx1a, Nurr1	[26]
	Neurons (dopaminergic)	Fibroblast	Human	Ascl1, Lmx1a, Brn2, FoxA2, Myt1L	[27]
	Neurons (dopaminergic)	Astrocyte/Fibroblast	Mouse	Ascl1, Lmx1B, and Nurr1	[32]
	Spinal cord motoneurons	Fibroblast	Mouse/Human	Ascl1, Brn2, Myt1L, Ngn2, Hb9, Isl1, Lhx3/NeuroD1	[33]
	Neurons	Fibroblast	Human	Ascl1, Brn2, Myt1L, Zic1, Olig2	[34]
	Neurons	Hepatocyte	Mouse	Ascl1, Brn2, Myt1L	[35]
	Neural progenitor cells	Fibroblast	Mouse	Oct4, Sox2, Klf4, c-Myc	[45]
MESODERM	Cardiomyocytes	Fibroblast	Mouse	Gata4, Tbx5, Mef2c	[37]
	Cardiomyocytes	Fibroblast	Mouse	Oct4, Sox2, Klf4, (c-Myc)	[44]
	Hematopoietic progenitors	Fibroblast	Human	Oct4	[38]
ENDODERM	Hepatocytes	Fibroblast	Mouse	Hnf1α, FoxA3, Gata4, p19^{Arf} inact.	[41]
	Hepatocytes	Fibroblast	Mouse	FoxA1, FoxA2, FoxA3 and Hnf4α	[42]

were much more dramatic in larvae treated with valproic acid and trichostatin-A, highlighting the importance of epigenetic regulation of gene expression in the process of cell transdifferentiation. In addition, this work highlights the role of specific master genes that control cell fate changes during transdifferentiation in vivo.

Following on the steps of studies analyzing cell transdifferentiation in vivo, many successful attempts at transdifferentiating cells in vitro have been recently described (summarized in Table 14.1). The transcription factor *Ascl1* (achaete-scute homolog 1) has been demonstrated to be one of the master controllers of fibroblast transdifferentiation to neuronal fates, in the mouse [25,26] and also in human cells [26–29]. In addition to *Ascl1*, other factors play important roles in neuron-specific cell transdifferentiation. Thus, direct conversion of adult human fibroblasts to functional neurons has been achieved using a combination of micro-RNA (*miR-124*) and two transcription factors (*Myt1L* and *Brn2*) under defined conditions [30]. *Brn2* (also known as *Pou3f2*) and *Myt1L*, either alone [25] or in combination with *NeuroD1* [29], or *NeuroD2* with *miR-9/9* and *miR-124* [28], all induce glutamatergic transdifferentiation.

Glutamatergic neuron transdifferentiation also has been accomplished by ectopic expression of *Ngn2* in mouse cortical astrocytes [31], confirming that the particular hierarchical overexpression of defined neural-related genes induces cell-specific transdifferentiation from different cell sources. In addition, the instructive role of micro-RNAs on chromatin-remodeling complexes contributing to neural fate was shown in this context [28], underscoring the importance of epigenetic remodelers in cell transdifferentiation. Similar results have been obtained in GABAergic transdifferentiation approaches from human fibroblasts [28] or mouse cortical astrocytes [31]. Dopaminergic neuron conversions have been described from both human and mouse fibroblasts by the combination of *Ascl1*, *Lmx1a*, and *NurR1* [26]. Also, the combination of *Ascl1*, *Lmx1a*, *Brn2*, *FoxA2*, and *Myt1L* has been shown to work effectively in converting human fibroblasts into mature dopaminergic neurons [27]. In addition, a cocktail of *Ascl1*, *Lmx1B*, and *Nurr1* expressed from a single polycistronic lentiviral vector has been demonstrated to convert astrocytes into dopaminergic neurons [32]. A recent report has demonstrated that functional spinal cord motoneurons could be obtained by direct conversion of mouse fibroblasts using the factors *Ascl1*, *Brn2*, *Myt1l*, *Ngn2*, *Hb9*, *Isl1*, and *Lhx3*, and in addition to *NeuroD1* in their human counterparts as well [33]. Taken together, these reports highlight the importance of gene regulators of neural development, not only during in vivo or in vitro differentiation, but also during transdifferentiation events. Taking advantage of the possibilities created by such directed trans-differentiation approaches, human induced-neuronal (hiN) cells have recently been generated from adult skin fibroblasts of Alzheimer's disease patients, using key neural regulators (*Brn2*, *Myt1L*, *Zic1*, *Olig2*, and *Ascl1*) and extrinsic support factors (brain-derived neurotrophic factor, neurotrophin-3, and glial-conditioned media) [34]. This recent study highlights the notion that transdifferentiation approaches may become useful strategies for obtaining functional human differentiated cells, not only for cell replacement therapies, but also for disease modeling.

It is important to note that the phenomenon of direct lineage conversion does not appear to be restricted to cell types belonging to the same embryo germ layer, but that transdifferentiation of somatic cells across germ layers has also been accomplished. Thus, induced neurons have been obtained through transdifferentiation of somatic cells from ectoderm origin [31,32], but also from mesoderm derivatives [25–30,33,34], as well as from derivatives of definitive endoderm [35] (see Table 14.1). In the latter study, homogeneous populations of hepatocytes were trans-difffrentiated into neurons using essentially the same conditions used to transdifferentiate mouse embryonic fibroblasts, demonstrating that the same core of reprogramming factors is able to reset different epigenetic backgrounds to a neural fate, and further confirming the plasticity of the cell's developmental potency.

Direct cell fate conversion into mesoderm derivatives, while less explored than transdifferentiation into neuronal cells, has also been reported. In the context of mouse embryo development, ectopic expression of transcripts encoding the cardiac transcription factors Gata4 and Tbx5, together with *Baf60c*, encoding a cardiac-specific subunit of the BAF chromatin-remodeling complex, generated beating cardiomyocytes from non-cardiogenic mesoderm [36]. In addition, the action of these reprogramming factors induced the appearance of ectopic cardiomyocytes in extra-embryonic amniotic tissue, suggesting that their cardiogenic potential was also effective in other

cellular contexts, at least during early embryo development. In this context, Gata4 acts as a key factor in initiating the cardiac program in co-operation with Baf60c, whereas Tbx5 is required for full differentiation into contracting cardiomyocytes. However, this transdifferentiation phenomenon was not observed in cultured embryonic fibroblasts, suggesting that cell fate transitions in this case depend on the combination of specific permissive global transcriptional and epigenetic landscapes.

A further refinement of this approach included the use of Mef2c instead of Baf60c, along with Gata4 and Tbx5 to reprogram mouse cardiac and dermal fibroblasts into cardiomyocyte-like cells, termed induced cardiomyocytes (iCM) [37] (see Table 14.1). In this study, the combined overexpression of the three factors was sufficient to induce the activation of silent cardiac markers in fibroblasts. Moreover, it was shown that dermal fibroblasts were much more difficult to reprogram into iCMs than cardiac fibroblasts, indicating that while both cell types were amenable to direct conversion, epigenetic barriers, depending on the cellular origin, could influence chromatin remodeling. Importantly, this study also showed that markers of cardiac progenitors, such as *Islet1*, were not re-expressed during the process of lineage conversion, providing support for a mechanism of transdifferentiation, rather than dedifferentiation, toward multipotent progenitors, followed by cardiac differentiation. Taken together, the evidence from these studies reinforces the notion that transcription factors and specific chromatin-remodeling complexes that play important roles during cardiac differentiation, can also induce transdifferentiation of permissive cell types into cardiomyocytes. It should be interesting to investigate if the same or a different combination of factors can generate iCM from distantly related cell types such as endoderm or ectoderm derivatives.

Another recent example of mesoderm transdifferentiation has been achieved after forced expression of *Oct4* in human fibroblasts, which under culture conditions known to support hematopoietic progenitor cells, resulted in their transdifferentiation into cells expressing the pan-leukocyte marker CD45 [38]. The blood-cell progenitors obtained in this way were able to generate granulocytes, monocytes, erythrocytes, and megakaryocytes, confirming their hematopoietic multipotency. These results were somewhat unexpected since, unlike the case of trans-differentiation into cardiomyocytes discussed above,

Oct4 is not expressed during hematopoietic differentiation. Moreover, *Oct4* is well known as a master gene of pluripotency and is the only indispensable factor for correct and full reprogramming to pluripotency, being sufficient for generating iPSCs from neural progenitor cells [39]. In the light of this evidence, an alternative scenario to transdifferentiation in this case could be envisioned, with *Oct4* inducing fibroblast dedifferentiation (partial or total reprogramming to pluripotency) and the appropriate culture conditions subsequently promoting hematopoietic differentiation. Even though the authors did not detect re-expression of other pluripotency-associated factors, such as Nanog or Sox2 [38], conclusive evidence for either scenario will probably require further investigation and independent validation of these results.

Transdifferentiation of cells within the definitive endoderm lineage was first demonstrated in pioneering work in the Melton laboratory [40]. In this study, forced expression of *Pdx1*, *MafA*, and *Ngn3* was shown to reprogram differentiated pancreatic exocrine cells of adult mice into β-like cells. From a core of nine genes, the mutation of which resulted in defects in β-cell specification or differentiation in mice, a set of three (*Pdx1*, *MafA*, and *Ngn3*) was shown to be sufficient to reprogram exocrine pancreatic cells into functional insulin-producing cells in streptomycin-treated animals. However, this combination of factors failed to transdifferentiate embryonic fibroblasts into β-cells, indicating that the reprogramming ability of these factors was restricted to closely related, endoderm-derived cell lineages. This finding also suggests that cell fate transitions across cell types more distantly related, such as fibroblasts and β-cells, may require a core of selector genes that allows an appropriate chromatin context to establish a functional β-cell phenotype. The direct conversion of mesoderm-derived somatic cells into definitive endoderm cell lineages is very much the current focus of stem-cell research, with the ultimate goal of generating functional fully differentiated insulin-producing cells. In addition to this, two independent groups have recently demonstrated direct conversion of mouse fibroblasts to hepatocyte-like cells using two different approaches (see Table 14.1). In one study, forced expression of *Hnf1α*, *FoxA3*, and *Gata4*, in combination with inactivation of *p19^{Arf}*, induced transdifferentiation of mouse fibroblasts into mature hepatocyte-like cells [41]. In a second approach, ectopic expression of *FoxA1*, *FoxA2*, *FoxA3*, and *Hnf4α* induced a cell fate conversion in mouse fibroblasts to cells that expressed mature hepatocyte markers and were able to engraft in livers of genetic models of liver failure [42]. It is interesting to note that the same factors that have been shown to play pivotal roles in the transdifferentiation of fibroblasts into cardiac (*Gata4*) [37] or neural (*FoxA2*) [27] phenotypes could induce cell fate conversion into definitive endoderm lineages in specific contexts. This finding reinforces the notion that genes that are known to regulate cell fate during embryo development could promote specific lineage conversions, independent of the chromatin state in the cell of origin, therefore acting as "pioneer" factors [43].

Experimentally, most attempts thus far to induce cell fate conversions have relied on forced expression of transcriptional factors and epigenetic modulators that play important roles during normal development. However, alternative strategies for generating the desired target cell types from different donor sources have also been reported. Pioneering work in the laboratory of Sheng Ding has established a new paradigm for direct cell conversions without transition to full pluripotency. In this case, the reprogramming factors generally used to generate iPSCs (the "Yamanaka cocktail", including *Oct4*, *Sox2*, *Klf4*, and *c-Myc*) are overexpressed in fibroblasts and, upon specific cell selection conditions, cells of cardiac (mesoderm) [44] and neural (ectoderm) [45] phenotypes can be obtained. In this way, mouse embryonic fibroblasts can be directly reprogrammed to spontaneously contracting patches of differentiated cardiomyocytes over a period of 11–12 days, after forced expression of the Yamanaka factors, in LIF-free medium containing decreasing concentrations of fetal bovine serum (FBS), BMP4, and JAK-STAT inhibition [44]. Under these differentiating conditions, robust expression of cardiac markers appeared as soon as 9 days, and contracting colonies after 11 days of differentiation. This study also showed that three-factor-induced reprogramming (without *c-Myc*) is sufficient to activate the early cardiac program without transiting through a full pluripotent state, as *Nanog* is not re-expressed during the process. Using a conceptually similar approach, this group has also reprogrammed fibroblasts into neural progenitor cells by means of doxycycline-inducible expression of OSKM factors [45]. In this case, after 3 days of doxycycline treatment, and subsequent maturation in neural reprogramming media (containing FGF2, EGF, and FGF4, without LIF), colonies of neural progenitor cells appeared in only

9–13 days. Taken together, these data suggest that forced expression of the Yamanaka factors may generate various developmentally plastic intermediate cells that, when appropriately instructed by specific extrinsic signaling inputs, give rise to their transdifferentiating cellular counterparts. Moreover, these results offer an alternative use of general reprogramming factors, rather than lineage-specific transcription factors, to facilitate cell fate conversions.

Epigenetic memory

The dilemma of whether cells retain some type of memory of their origin during cell potency transitions dates to the very beginning of this research field. However, as modern genetic and molecular techniques have enabled robust cell-type-specific lineage-tracing experiments, this issue has begun to be addressed directly in the past few years. During limb regeneration in amphibians, blastema cells comprise a heterogeneous pool of progenitor cells derived from different cell types that dedifferentiate, but which retain a memory of the cell of origin [9]. This conclusion was obtained thanks to elegant experiments combining genetic cell-lineage tracing and transplantation, which showed that Schwann cells only regenerated Schwann cells, muscle cells gave rise to muscle, and blood vessels formed new blood vessels [9]. Similarly, it has also been shown that frog embryos generated by SCNT from *MyoD*-expressing somite cells show expression of this gene in cells where it is not normally expressed [46]. Moreover, the high frequency of developmental abnormalities in animals cloned by nuclear transfer has been proposed to depend on incomplete or less-than-perfect nuclear reprogramming. A more detailed understanding of the mechanisms at work during reprogramming, particularly of those responsible for resetting the epigenetic profile of reprogrammed cells, is clearly necessary to ascertain whether retention of memory of cell origin is consubstantial with this process, or a consequence of faulty or incomplete reprogramming.

The advent of iPSC technology has provided a powerful experimental platform for dissecting the mechanisms underlying cell fate transitions, and for addressing the issue of cell-of-origin memory erasure in reprogrammed cells. Early comparative analyses of genome-wide transcriptional and histone modification patterns of ESCs and iPSCs showed that they overlapped with each other to a large extent. However, more recent and detailed analyses have uncovered specific differences between ESCs and iPSCs at the molecular level, the significance of which is still debated. For instance, mouse ESCs and iPSCs have been shown to differ only in the levels of expression of transcripts encoded by the imprinted *Dlk1-Dio3* cluster [47]. Thus, most iPSC lines failed to erase imprinting in this region, so that maternally expressed genes in this cluster were aberrantly silenced. This study also showed that, while all iPSC lines were able to form chimeras (although with varying degrees of iPSC contribution), only those with a *Dlk1-Dio3* expression pattern equivalent to ESCs were able to generate "all-iPS"-derived adult mice after tetraploid complementation assays. In addition, SCNT-derived ESCs obtained from different cell types all show high levels of *Dlk1-Dio3* expression, indicating that SCNT is more efficient at generating fully reprogrammed cells than induced reprogramming with defined factors. These results open the question of which are the factors present in SCNT reprogramming that control the full erasure of chromatin/DNA epigenetic modifications. In addition, these findings reinforce the concept that certain epigenetic marks in the starting cell population predispose reprogrammed cells to different potency states after cell fate transition. Directly addressing this issue in human cells is currently limited by our ability to thoroughly test their pluripotent capacity. The stringency of pluripotency tests used for mouse cells (such as germline contribution of iPSC-derived chimeras or tetraploid complementation assays) far exceeds, for obvious ethical reasons, that of analyses employed for human cells. It follows that our inability to distinguish subtle differences in the degree of pluripotency in human stem cells may impede telling fully reprogrammed iPSCs apart from cells that have not undergone complete reprogramming, and therefore to ascribe residual epigenetic memory to the latter. Unambiguously addressing this critical issue will require the implementation of novel testing platforms and assays to accurately quantify the degree of potency of human stem cells.

Based on the principle that full reprogramming to pluripotency should involve completely resetting the chromatin architecture from a somatic state to a pluripotent one, equivalent to the ESC state, one would expect the absence of epigenetic memory after a round of efficient reprogramming. However, recent data show that depending on the cell type of origin, iPSCs retain some degree of epigenetic memory after induced reprogramming with defined factors, which is not apparent when adult somatic cells are reprogrammed to pluripotency by SCNT [48]. Residual DNA methylation signatures characteristic of the somatic tissue of origin could be reset by serial passaging [49], or by treating iPSCs with chromatin-modifying drugs [48]. These results suggest that low-passage iPSCs retain transient epigenetic marks of their cell type of origin, which can then influence their differentiation capacity. The mechanism by which passaging eliminates the molecular and functional differences between iPSCs of different origins remains to be determined. The analysis of genes that change their profile of expression during early-to-late iPSC transition could provide valuable information in this respect [50].

Numerous independent studies have recently identified retention of some sort of cell-of-origin memory in iPSCs. For example, iPSCs generated from a variety of cell types, including retinal pigmented epithelial cells, pancreatic β-cells, hepatocytes, skin fibroblasts, and melanocytes, show increased tendency to differentiate to the particular cell type from which they were obtained. However, as mentioned above, distinguishing between memory of cell of origin and incomplete reprogramming may be difficult due to current technical limitations, so these findings should be interpreted with care.

Concluding remarks

Extraordinary scientific and technological advances over the past 60 years have contributed to our current view of how cells regulate the genetic information encoded in the genome to give rise to the many cell types that make up an organism. Most of these processes take place during embryo development and are controlled by a remarkably complex, yet robust, plethora of high-order mechanisms that are essentially supracellular in nature, but whose ultimate effector are changes in individual cell phenotypes or behaviors. The derivation of pluripotent cells from embryos provided a revolutionary new approach for investigating the mechanisms that underlie the acquisition and maintenance of pluripotency and the differentiation of specific cell types. The combined knowledge gained in both these areas of research, in turn, created unique opportunities for developing cell reprogramming technologies, as well as methods for directed

cell differentiation in vitro. It comes, therefore, as no surprise that many genes that control the pluripotent state in embryonic stem cells have become critical and efficient reprogramming factors. Similarly, key genes controlling cell differentiation during embryo development are now used in the laboratory to direct the fate of pluripotent stem cells toward specific cell types, and even to transdifferentiate the fate of cells that were distantly related within the embryo.

The study of organ regeneration in certain animal models has also provided invaluable information as to the cellular and molecular mechanisms that underlie processes such as dedifferentiation and transdifferentiation. Comparing how natural instances of cell reprogramming and their experimental counterparts are regulated will surely identify commonalities, but also context-specific differences. In addition to bettering our understanding of fascinating biological phenomena, research on induced reprogramming to pluripotency and direct cell fate conversion is likely to have profound biomedical implications. These novel technologies offer unprecedented opportunities for the generation of unlimited amounts of tailored, functional, and specific cell types for autologous cell-therapy applications, as well as for creating genuinely human models of disease.

References

1. Yamanaka, S., Blau, H.M. Nuclear reprogramming to a pluripotent state by three approaches. *Nature*. 2010; 465: 704–712.

2. Takahashi, K., Yamanaka, S. Induction of pluripotent stem cells from mouse embryonic and adult fibroblast cultures by defined factors. *Cell*. 2006; 126: 663–676.

3. Park, I.H., Zhao, R., West, J.A. *et al*. Reprogramming of human somatic cells to pluripotency with defined factors. *Nature*. 2008; 451: 141–146.

4. Takahashi, K., Tanabe, K., Ohnuki, M. *et al*. Induction of pluripotent stem cells from adult human fibroblasts by defined factors. *Cell*. 2007; 131: 861–872.

5. Yu, J., Vodyanik, M.A., Smuga-Otto, K. *et al*. Induced pluripotent stem cell lines derived from human somatic cells. *Science*. 2007; 318: 1917–1920.

6. Jopling, C., Sleep, E., Raya, M. *et al*. Zebrafish heart regeneration occurs by cardiomyocyte dedifferentiation and proliferation. *Nature*. 2010; 464: 606–609.

7. Kikuchi, K., Holdway, J.E., Werdich, A.A. *et al*. Primary contribution to zebrafish heart regeneration

by gata4(+) cardiomyocytes. *Nature*. 2010; 464: 601–605.

8. Porrello, E.R., Mahmoud, A.I., Simpson, E. *et al.* Transient regenerative potential of the neonatal mouse heart. *Science*. 2011; 331: 1078–1080.

9. Kragl, M., Knapp, D., Nacu, E. *et al.* Cells keep a memory of their tissue origin during axolotl limb regeneration. *Nature*. 2009; 460: 60–65.

10. Chen, Z.L., Yu, W.M., Strickland, S. Peripheral regeneration. *Annual Review of Neuroscience*. 2007; 30: 209–233.

11. Thorel, F., Nepote, V., Avril, I. *et al.* Conversion of adult pancreatic alpha-cells to beta-cells after extreme beta-cell loss. *Nature*. 2010; 464: 1149–1154.

12. Wilmut, I., Schnieke, A.E., McWhir, J., Kind, A.J., Campbell, K.H. Viable offspring derived from fetal and adult mammalian cells. *Nature*. 1997; 385: 810–813.

13. Blau, H.M., Chiu, C.P., Webster, C. Cytoplasmic activation of human nuclear genes in stable heterocaryons. *Cell*. 1983; 32: 1171–1180.

14. Schneuwly, S., Klemenz, R., Gehring, W.J. Redesigning the body plan of Drosophila by ectopic expression of the homoeotic gene Antennapedia. *Nature*. 1987; 325: 816–818.

15. Davis, R.L., Weintraub, H., Lassar, A.B. Expression of a single transfected cDNA converts fibroblasts to myoblasts. *Cell*. 1987; 51: 987–1000.

16. Xie, H., Ye, M., Feng, R., Graf, T. Stepwise reprogramming of B cells into macrophages. *Cell*. 2004; 117: 663–676.

17. Cobaleda, C., Jochum, W., Busslinger, M. Conversion of mature B cells into T cells by dedifferentiation to uncommitted progenitors. *Nature*. 2007; 449: 473–477.

18. Waddington, C.H. *The Strategy of the Genes*. London: Geo Allen and Unwin. 1957.

19. Sleep, E., Boue, S., Jopling, C. *et al.* Transcriptomics approach to investigate zebrafish heart regeneration. *Journal of Cardiovascular Medicine (Hagerstown)*. 2010; 11: 369–380.

20. McGann, C.J., Odelberg, S.J., Keating, M.T. Mammalian myotube dedifferentiation induced by newt regeneration extract. *Proceedings of the National Academy of Sciences of the United States of America*. 2001; 98: 13699–13704.

21. Nutt, S.L., Heavey, B., Rolink, A.G., Busslinger, M. Commitment to the B-lymphoid lineage depends on the transcription factor Pax5. *Nature*. 1999; 401: 556–562.

22. Hanna, J., Markoulaki, S., Schorderet, P. *et al.* Direct reprogramming of terminally differentiated mature B lymphocytes to pluripotency. *Cell*. 2008; 133: 250–264.

23. Li, R., Liang, J., Ni, S. *et al.* A mesenchymal-to-epithelial transition initiates and is required for the nuclear reprogramming of mouse fibroblasts. *Cell Stem Cell*. 2010; 7: 51–63.

24. Tursun, B., Patel, T., Kratsios, P., Hobert, O. Direct conversion of C. elegans germ cells into specific neuron types. *Science*. 2011; 331: 304–308.

25. Vierbuchen, T., Ostermeier, A., Pang, Z.P. *et al.* Direct conversion of fibroblasts to functional neurons by defined factors. *Nature*. 2010; 463: 1035–1041.

26. Caiazzo, M., Dell'Anno, M.T., Dvoretskova, E. *et al.* Direct generation of functional dopaminergic neurons from mouse and human fibroblasts. *Nature*. 2011; 476: 224–227.

27. Pfisterer, U., Kirkeby, A., Torper, O. *et al.* Direct conversion of human fibroblasts to dopaminergic neurons. *Proceedings of the National Academy of Sciences of the United States of America*. 2011; 108: 10343–10348.

28. Yoo, A.S., Sun, A.X., Li, L. *et al.* MicroRNA-mediated conversion of human fibroblasts to neurons. *Nature*. 2011; 476: 228–231.

29. Pang, Z.P., Yang, N., Vierbuchen, T. *et al.* Induction of human neuronal cells by defined transcription factors. *Nature*. 2011; 476: 220–223.

30. Ambasudhan, R., Talantova, M., Coleman, R. *et al.* Direct reprogramming of adult human fibroblasts to functional neurons under defined conditions. *Cell Stem Cell*. 2011; 9: 113–118.

31. Heinrich, C., Blum, R., Gascon, S. *et al.* Directing astroglia from the cerebral cortex into subtype specific functional neurons. *PLoS Biology*. 2010; 8: e1000373.

32. Addis, R.C., Hsu, F.C., Wright, R.L. *et al.* Efficient conversion of astrocytes to functional midbrain dopaminergic neurons using a single polycistronic vector. *PLoS One*. 2011; 6: e28719.

33. Son, E.Y., Ichida, J.K., Wainger, B.J. *et al.* Conversion of mouse and human fibroblasts into functional spinal motor neurons. *Cell Stem Cell*. 2011; 9: 205–218.

34. Qiang, L., Fujita, R., Yamashita, T. *et al.* Directed conversion of Alzheimer's disease patient skin fibroblasts into functional neurons. *Cell*. 2011; 146: 359–371.

35. Marro, S., Pang, Z.P., Yang, N. *et al.* Direct lineage conversion of terminally differentiated hepatocytes to functional neurons. *Cell Stem Cell*. 2011; 9: 374–382.

36. Takeuchi, J.K., Bruneau, B.G. Directed transdifferentiation of mouse mesoderm to heart tissue by defined factors. *Nature*. 2009; 459: 708–711.

37. Ieda, M., Fu, J.D., Delgado-Olguin, P. *et al.* Direct reprogramming of fibroblasts into functional

cardiomyocytes by defined factors. *Cell*. 2010; 142: 375–386.

38. Szabo, E., Rampalli, S., Risueno, R.M. *et al.* Direct conversion of human fibroblasts to multilineage blood progenitors. *Nature*. 2010; 468: 521–526.

39. Kim, J.B., Greber, B., Arauzo-Bravo, M.J. *et al.* Direct reprogramming of human neural stem cells by OCT4. *Nature*. 2009; 461: 649–653.

40. Zhou, Q., Brown, J., Kanarek, A., Rajagopal, J., Melton, D.A. In vivo reprogramming of adult pancreatic exocrine cells to beta-cells. *Nature*. 2008; 455: 627–632.

41. Huang, P., He, Z., Ji, S. *et al.* Induction of functional hepatocyte-like cells from mouse fibroblasts by defined factors. *Nature*. 2011; 475: 386–389.

42. Sekiya, S., Suzuki, A. Direct conversion of mouse fibroblasts to hepatocyte-like cells by defined factors. *Nature*. 2011; 475: 390–393.

43. Smale, S.T. Pioneer factors in embryonic stem cells and differentiation. *Current Opinion in Genetic Development*. 2010; 20: 519–526.

44. Efe, J.A., Hilcove, S., Kim, J. *et al.* Conversion of mouse fibroblasts into cardiomyocytes using a direct reprogramming strategy. *Nature Cell Biology*. 2011; 13: 215–222.

45. Kim, J., Efe, J.A., Zhu, S. *et al.* Direct reprogramming of mouse fibroblasts to neural progenitors. *Proceedings of the National Academy of Sciences of the United States of America*. 2011; 108: 7838–7843.

46. Ng, R.K., Gurdon, J.B. Epigenetic memory of an active gene state depends on histone H3.3 incorporation into chromatin in the absence of transcription. *Nature Cell Biology*. 2008; 10: 102–109.

47. Stadtfeld, M., Apostolou, E., Akutsu, H. *et al.* Aberrant silencing of imprinted genes on chromosome 12qF1 in mouse induced pluripotent stem cells. *Nature*. 2010; 465: 175–181.

48. Kim, K., Doi, A., Wen, B. *et al.* Epigenetic memory in induced pluripotent stem cells. *Nature*. 2010; 467: 285–290.

49. Polo, J.M., Liu, S., Figueroa, M.E. *et al.* Cell type of origin influences the molecular and functional properties of mouse induced pluripotent stem cells. *Nature Biotechnology*. 2010; 28: 848–855.

50. Chin, M.H., Mason, M.J., Xie, W. *et al.* Induced pluripotent stem cells and embryonic stem cells are distinguished by gene expression signatures. *Cell Stem Cell*. 2009; 5: 111–123.

The metabolic framework of pluripotent stem cells and potential mechanisms of regulation

Alexandra J. Harvey, Joy Rathjen, and David K. Gardner

Introduction

It is becoming increasingly clear that standard measures of embryonic stem cell pluripotency do not necessarily reflect underlying differences in cell physiology. There is an immediate need to expand our knowledge of the basic physiology of pluripotent stem cells and to understand the impact of factors that regulate pluripotent stem-cell expansion, maintenance, and controlled differentiation on cell metabolism. Importantly, the responses of pluripotent stem cells to alterations in culture environment have not been extensively elucidated; this is especially relevant with the recent growth in specialized media formulations available. Coincident with the development and selection of media for pluripotent stem-cell culture, it is imperative to understand the impact each formulation has on the metabolism and physiology of the cells. This is particularly pertinent as cells are being considered for clinical and commercial applications. Consequently, medium selection needs to be made on both functional and physiological grounds.

Pluripotent stem cells are characterized by their differentiation potential (pluripotency), defined as their ability to differentiate into cell populations of the three primary lineages, ectoderm, mesoderm, and endoderm, and by their immortality. It is immortality, or the capacity for unlimited self-renewal, which enables continued proliferation of pluripotent stem cells without cellular senescence. Pluripotency is regulated by a complex transcription factor network, centred on *OCT4 (POU5F1)*, *NANOG*, and *SOX2*. In addition to these defining features it is becoming apparent that pluripotent stem cells are characterized by a unique physiology. This chapter will focus on the metabolic framework that sustains pluripotent stem cells in culture, potential mechanisms that regulate the physiology of these cells, and the effect of environmental factors on homeostasis in these cells.

Metabolism and the maintenance of pluripotency

Metabolism provides the energy (adenosine triphosphate; ATP) needed to sustain cell function and replication, and relies on the provision of appropriate nutrients in the surrounding environment. In culture this environment comprises the medium composition, gaseous atmosphere, extracellular matrix, and interactions between cells. The extracellular environment surrounding a cell in vitro constantly changes due to the activity of the cells themselves. Cells need to be able to respond to signals and interact actively with their environment, and to regulate metabolism accordingly in order to maintain cellular homeostasis. Maintenance of homeostasis is required to minimize cell stress and facilitates a cell's interaction with the environment. In this chapter we will focus on the effect of medium composition and gaseous atmosphere on pluripotent cells in culture as these areas have, to date, been the best characterized in terms of their ability to modulate pluripotent metabolism.

Studies examining mitochondrial (oxidative) and glycolytic metabolism in pluripotent stem cells have generally compared their metabolic activities with those of somatic cells. Human embryonic stem (ES) cells contain low levels of intracellular ATP when compared with somatic cells. The level of ATP in human ES cells has been reported to be approximately a quarter to a third of levels in human fibroblasts [1–3]. Human and mouse ES cells rely heavily on glycolysis for ATP production, despite culture conditions maintaining the cells in atmospheric (20%)

Stem Cells in Reproductive Medicine 3rd edition, ed. Carlos Simón, Antonio Pellicer and Renee Reijo Pera.
Published by Cambridge University Press. © Cambridge University Press 2013.

oxygen [1,2,4,5,6] (Figure 15.1), with an estimated 50–70% of glucose metabolized to lactate (Harvey, Rathjen, unpublished results). High rates of aerobic glycolysis are typical of rapidly dividing cells such as lymphocytes and tumour cells [7]. A high glycolytic flux is correlated with ES cell proliferation, and the inhibition of glycolysis with non-metabolizable 2-deoxyglucose significantly reduces mouse ES cell self-renewal [4]. Of significance, the inner cell mass cells of the pre-implantation blastocyst, from which ES cells are derived, similarly generate a large proportion of ATP from glycolysis [8,9], reflecting the origin of such characteristic metabolism. This contrasts with somatic cells, which typically rely heavily on oxidative phosphorylation (OXPHOS), coupling metabolism of pyruvate through the tricarboxylic acid (TCA) cycle and the electron transport chain (ETC), although most cultured cells rely on both mitochondrial metabolism and glycolysis to generate ATP under aerobic conditions [10] (Figure 15.1). When compared with mouse embryonic fibroblasts, mouse ES cells also contain higher levels of glycolytic enzymes, including phosphoglycerate kinase (PGK) and phosphoglyceromutase (PGM), and consume less oxygen [4]. A high level of aerobic glycolysis is a common characteristic of rapidly dividing cells and tumors [11–13]. High levels of glucose utilization are required for the synthesis of triacylglycerols and phospholipids, and as a precursor for complex sugars and glycoproteins. Glucose metabolized by the pentose phosphate pathway (PPP) generates ribose moieties required for nucleic acid synthesis and the NADPH required for the biosynthesis of lipids and other complex molecules [13,14]. NADPH is also required for the reduction of intracellular glutathione. Interestingly, the percentage of the total glucose consumed which is metabolized through this pathway in ES cells is not known.

Pluripotent stem cells are generally cultured in medium containing in excess of 10 mM glucose and have been shown to metabolize glucose for energy. In addition, mouse ES cells have been shown to have an absolute requirement for threonine, in the presence of glucose, where inhibition of threonine dehydrogenase results in loss of proliferative capacity and induction of autophagy [15,16]. Threonine may function to provide acetyl-CoA for TCA activity or produce glycine for the glycine cleavage system with a concomitant reduction of NAD^+. Fernandes *et al.* [5] reported the dependence of mouse ES cells on glutamine consumption shortly after seeding, when cell density is at its lowest, with

metabolism of glucose through glycolysis becoming more important as cell density increased [5].

While these studies have established some basic metabolic characteristics of ES cells, the majority of studies are limited to the analysis of one or two lines, failing to explore interline variability, and use a variety of culture conditions, making comparison between studies difficult. Furthermore, glycolytic activity is often inferred from lactate production alone [1,2,5], and few studies have investigated OXPHOS in parallel to establish the relative contribution of each pathway to ATP production.

Mitochondria not only provide the energy required to maintain cellular activity through OXPHOS, act as a site for amino-acid metabolism, and supply intermediates for glycolysis, they also function in a number of other pathways including ion homeostasis, signal transduction, and apoptosis. ES cells are reported to contain a low number of mitochondria, inferred by approximately 5–10-fold lower mitochondrial DNA copy numbers when compared with day 6 or older ES-cell-derived fibroblasts or with somatic cells [1,17,18]. ES cell mitochondria have a distinct morphology. The overwhelming majority of ES cell mitochondria are small, spherical, have a low electron density, contain few cristae, and cluster perinuclearly [19–21]; this compares to elongated, reticular, electron-dense, and cristae-rich mitochondria of somatic cells. Despite their distinct morphology, pluripotent stem cell mitochondria are functional and can consume oxygen at rates similar to differentiated cells [6]. The low numbers of mitochondria within these cells, however, may limit generation of ATP through OXPHOS [22]. Reprogramming of somatic cells to pluripotent stem cells is associated with restructuring of cristae-rich mitochondria to a more cristae-poor morphology [1,2,23], suggesting that mitochondrial architecture is important in pluripotent cells.

The proton pump across the inner mitochondrial membrane establishes a proton gradient (mitochondrial membrane potential; MMP) correlated to levels of oxidative metabolism. MMP can be studied through the use of fluorescent probes. Like other cultured cell lines [24], ES cells within a population vary considerably in MMP [25], and differences in mitochondrial activity have been seen between ES cell lines [26]. Sorting and comparing the 5% of mouse ES cells with the lowest MMP and the corresponding 5% of the ES cell population with the highest MMP showed cells with higher MMP were

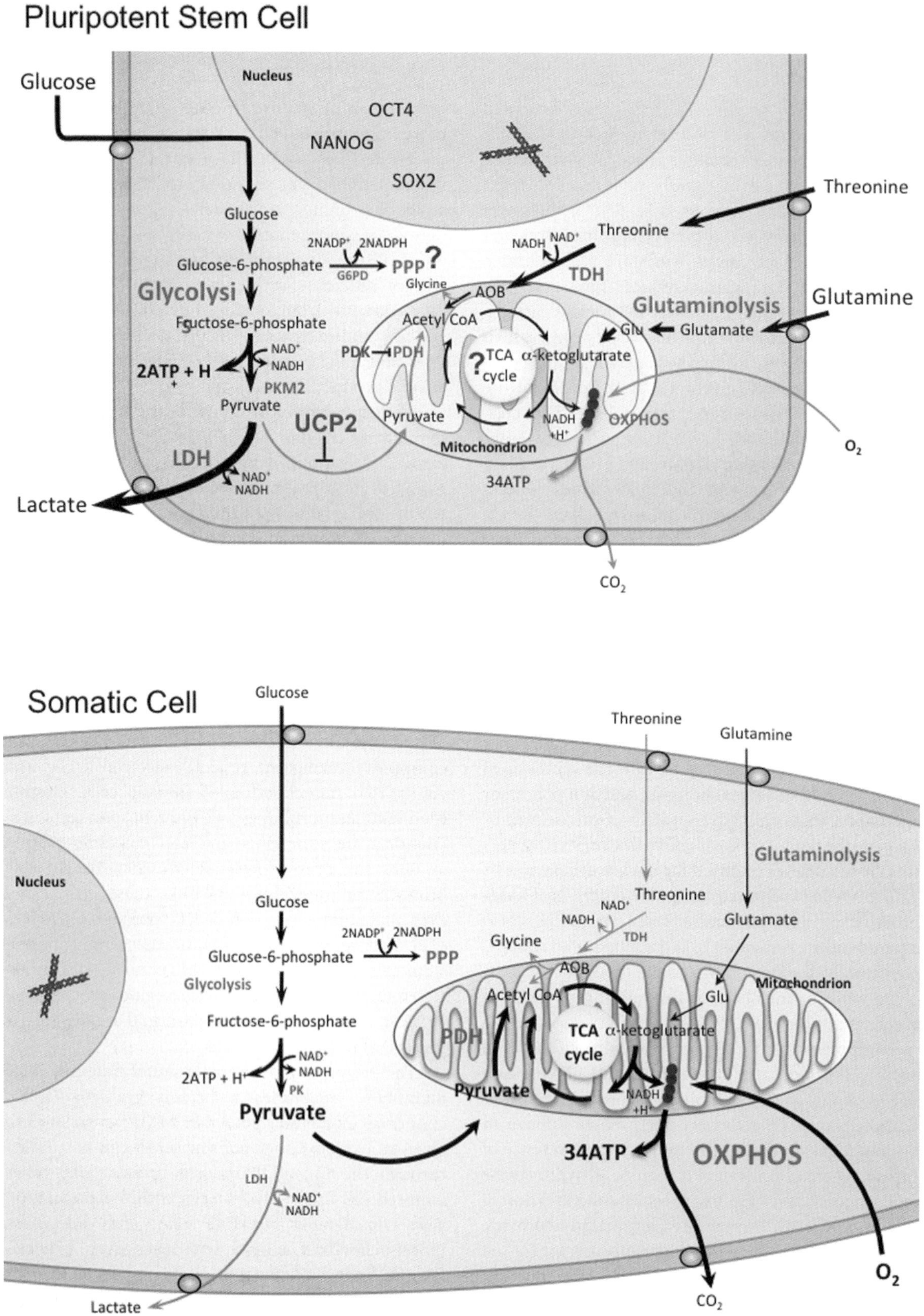

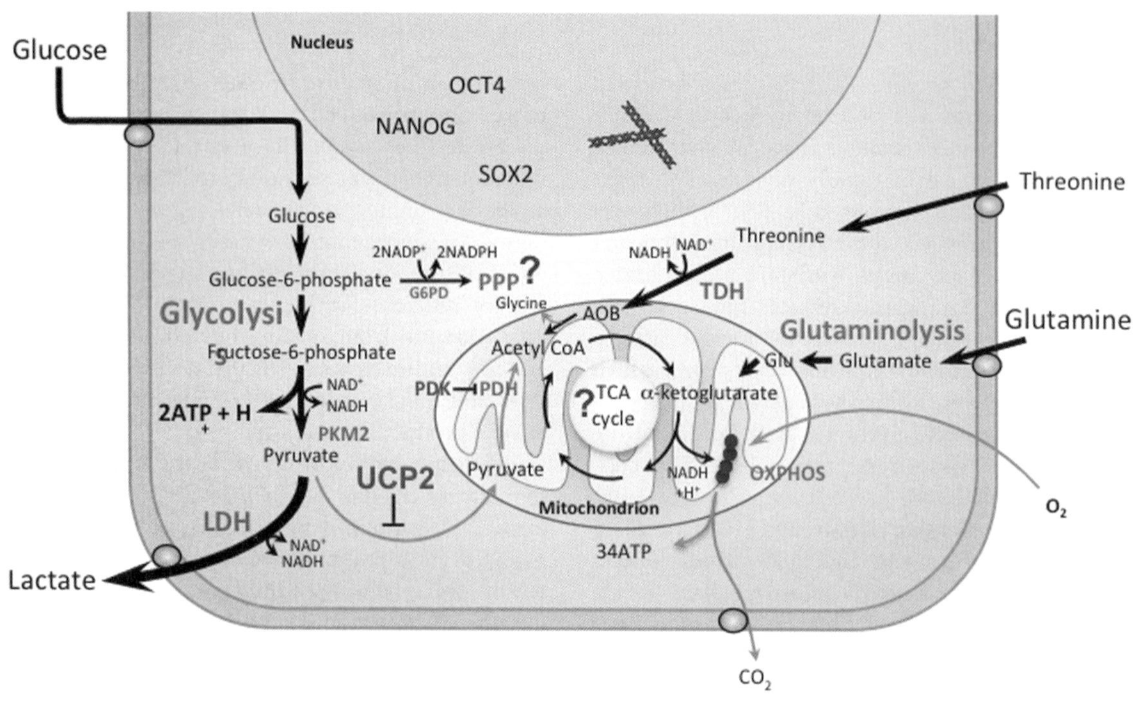

Figure 15.1 Schematic representation of differences between pluripotent stem cell and somatic cell metabolism. Pluripotent stem cells (PSCs) are characterized by spherical, electron-poor mitochondria which contain few cristae and rely heavily on glycolysis for ATP generation

metabolically more active without exhibiting a detectable difference in intracellular ATP concentrations or pluripotent marker expression [25]. These observations suggest that within a population ES cells vary in energetic activity, but balance energy consumption and production to maintain equivalent intracellular ATP concentrations. Glycolysis plays a role in maintaining MMP in pluripotent stem cells as addition of sodium oxamate, which dissipates the glycolysis-dependent component of MMP, resulted in a partial reduction in MMP in human ES cells. Sodium oxamate had no effect on MMP in fibroblast mitochondria [6]. Assessment of the differentiation potential of MMP-sorted ES cell populations showed differences in their propensity to form mesoderm and teratomas, suggesting that cellular metabolism at the time of differentiation impacts on outcome, and provides evidence for a link between mitochondrial activity and the regulation of differentiation. MMP characteristics were not maintained with continued culture, and sorted populations reverted to a normal distribution within 48 hours [25]. This is not unlike other markers that detect ES cell heterogeneity and which, when used to subdivide ES cell populations, are not maintained on further culture; purified populations revert to a normal distribution, suggesting that heterogeneity within an ES cell population represents a number of interchangeable cell states [27,28].

Mitochondrial function is dependent upon regulation of biogenesis and dynamics, involving the coordinated regulation of nuclear and mitochondrial genomes [29]. The importance of mitochondria in maintaining pluripotency has been demonstrated in experiments that modulate the number and function of mitochondria in ES cells. Reducing levels of mitochondrial polymerase PolG (polymerase gamma), which regulates mitochondrial DNA (mtDNA) replication, with siRNA results in loss of pluripotency of mouse ES cells [22]. Similarly, ES cells deficient in growth factor *erv-1*-like (*Gfer*) show a loss of mitochondrial integrity, evidenced by fragmentation and mitophagy, which is associated with decreased pluripotency marker expression, impaired embryoid body (EB) formation, and reduced cell survival [30]. Expression of dynamin-related protein 1 (Drp1), a protein that mediates mitochondrial fission, was increased in these cells; pharmacological inhibition of Drp1 rescued the defects of mitochondrial function and cell viability that resulted from depletion of *Gfer* [30]. Overexpression of *Gfer* in ES cells resulted in elongation of mitochondria, increased expression of *Oct4* and *Nanog*, and down-regulation of Drp1. Together these data support a requirement for mitochondria in ES cells and define a key role for *Gfer* in maintaining organelle integrity.

Despite a clear requirement for mitochondria by ES cells, inhibition of mitochondrial metabolism in human ES cells enhances pluripotency [31,32]. The addition of antimycin, a complex III inhibitor, or carbonyl cyanide *m*-chlorophenyl hydrazone (CCCP), an uncoupler of the proton gradient, to ES cells increased glycolytic flux and expression of pluripotent markers [31]. Antimycin also maintained pluripotency of human ES cells in the absence of bFGF [32]. These data suggest that the role of mitochondria in pluripotent cells is complex, with the paradox that there is an absolute requirement for the organelle, but that pluripotency is enhanced when organelle function is inhibited, suggesting a novel relationship between the stem cell and its unusual mitochondria that underpins cell functionality. Understanding this relationship and manipulating mitochondrial metabolism may provide useful strategies for regulating pluripotency in culture.

Metabolism and the differentiation of pluripotent cells

ES cells differ metabolically from somatic cells (Figure 15.1), implying that metabolic changes occur

---

(black arrows), resulting in significant lactate production through the conversion of pyruvate to lactate by lactate dehydrogenase (LDH). Consequently, oxidative phosphorylation (OXPHOS) contributes minimally to total ATP in PSCs. In PSCs, uncoupling protein 2 (UCP2) functions to shunt pyruvate away from the tricarboxylic acid (TCA) cycle, facilitating lactate production [81]. Pyruvate dehydrogenase kinase (PDK) activity also prevents the conversion of pyruvate to acetyl coenzyme A (acetyl CoA) [6]. PSCs also use both glutamine [2] and threonine [5] metabolism in culture, while the role of the pentose phosphate pathway (PPP) in PSCs is less clear. Most somatic cells in culture rely primarily on mitochondrial metabolism to generate ATP under aerobic conditions, with limited lactate production. In contrast, somatic cells are characterized by long, electron-dense mitochondria that contain numerous cristae, producing ATP largely through OXPHOS (black arrows); glycolysis provides pyruvate for TCA activity, while lactate production is minimal (grey arrows). Abbreviations: ATP, adenosine triphosphate; CO_2, carbon dioxide; O_2, oxygen; NAD^+, nicotinamide adenine dinucleotide; NADH, reduced form of NAD+; TCA, tricarboxylic acid cycle; PKM2, pyruvate kinase M2; LDH, lactate dehydrogenase. (See also color plate.)

as cells differentiate. The timing and regulation of these metabolic changes, however, have been largely unexplored. Removal of LIF from mouse ES cells for 6–8 days is associated with reductions in cell proliferation and glycolytic flux [4]. Differentiation of mouse ES cells towards a neural fate is similarly associated with reductions in glucose and glutamine consumption 4 days after the initiation of differentiation [33]. Examination of human ES cells induced to differentiate in the presence of retinoic acid over four consecutive days showed a gradual decrease in glycolysis, as determined by the extracellular acidification rate (ECAR) and lactate production, with a significant but modest reduction first seen on day 2 [6]. The level of glycolysis after four days of differentiation, however, was still higher than in fibroblasts. These reports suggest that changes in energy generation occur gradually after the initiation of pluripotent stem-cell differentiation. Consistent with this, we have found that differentiating human ES cells exhibited a slow acquisition of metabolic change (Rathjen *et al.* unpublished). This may be a function of the cell population formed or of the chemically defined and feeder-independent culture conditions used (mTeSR) [34]. A reduction in glycolysis with differentiation is likely accompanied by an increase in OXPHOS. Disruption of the mitochondrial ETC with antimycin or rotenone compromises the differentiation of ES cells within EBs, or towards the cardiac lineage [20], suggesting a requirement for increased oxidative metabolism as differentiation of pluripotent stem cells progresses.

The analysis of other metabolites has shown few changes accompanying cell differentiation. In our hands, the turnover of the majority of individual amino acids remained unchanged with human ES cell differentiation (Rathjen *et al.* unpublished data). Exceptions to this included proline, an imino acid which has been shown to play a role in regulating differentiation in mouse ES cells [35,36]. In mouse ES cells a similar stability in amino-acid profiles was seen with differentiation [16]. Analyzing intracellular metabolites showed that the levels of the amino acids monitored were unchanged, with the exception of threonine, which was increased with differentiation. Threonine has been shown to be required by mouse ES cells [16]. In this analysis few changes in other metabolites were detected, although folic acid and 5-aminoimidazolecarboxamine-R (AICAR), an intermediate of purine biosynthesis, decreased in abundance with differentiation.

It is surprising that so few metabolites have been shown to change between ES cells and their differentiated progeny. The metabolite changes that do occur, however, appear to be indicators of pathways that control or regulate stem-cell maintenance or differentiation. It will be valuable to expand on the approaches outlined above to include the analysis of metabolites in cells as they differentiate to detect early and potentially transient metabolic events that accompany the initial stages of differentiation and which may provide insight into the pathways involved in the loss of pluripotency and commitment to differentiation.

A comparative analysis of metabolite abundance in ES cells and their differentiated progeny has suggested that changes in redox status occur with ES cell differentiation [37]. When compared to differentiated progeny, ES cells have a metabolome rich in unsaturated structures [37]. Changes in redox regulators were detected with differentiation, with a significant but transient decrease in GSH/GSSG ratio after 4 days of differentiation and a concomitant increase in ascorbic acid [37]. GSH plays a significant antioxidant role within the cell and a reduction in the GSH/GSSG ratio suggests that differentiation is associated with an increase in oxidative stress; this may explain the increases in molecular saturation and the up-regulation of other antioxidants, such as ascorbic acid. Inhibition of select oxidative pathways promoted pluripotency of mouse ES cells, delaying the loss of pluripotency markers in conditions that would otherwise induce neuronal differentiation [37]. Conversely, the addition of fatty acids to both mouse and human ES cells enhanced neuronal differentiation [37]. Redox changes associated with differentiation were also seen following differentiation of reprogrammed cells; intracellular peroxide concentrations increased following induced pluripotent stem-cell differentiation [17], and reactive oxygen species (ROS) levels increase with differentiation in human ES cells [20]. These data imply that ES cells are characterized by low levels of oxygen radicals, potentially as a result of their reliance on glycolysis for ATP generation, and that the formation of ROS increases with differentiation, potentially as a result of increasing OXPHOS and ETC activity within the cell.

Low mitochondrial copy number and distinctive mitochondrial architecture persist as pluripotent cells differentiate. In the pre-implantation embryo, mitochondrial restructuring occurs gradually in the trophectoderm after lineage segregation [38]. Expansion of mitochondria from the perinuclear space to a dispersed distribution occurs within 3–7 days of the initiation of ES cell differentiation [21,22,31]. Induction of differentiation of human ES cells is accompanied by an increase in mtDNA copy number [19], with mitochondrial elongation occurring within the first week of differentiation [31]. Retinoic-acid (RA)-induced differentiation results in an up-regulation of mtDNA copy number on day 1 and day 6 of differentiation only; these changes were not accompanied by significant changes in the expression of three genes involved in mtDNA replication [22]. Yet another study documents no significant change in mitochondrial mass over a 4-week period of differentiation [17]. This data suggests an apparent absence of coupling between mitochondrial biogenesis and changes in metabolism to a more oxidative phenotype with differentiation, although changes in metabolism were not assessed in parallel in these studies. Differentiated ES cells also display a decrease in the expression of genes regulating mitochondrial fission and fusion [1,17,20], suggesting that these processes are more important for the maintenance of pluripotency prior to lineage commitment and not the early stages of differentiation. Examination of enzyme activity, ultrastructural changes, and post-translation regulation of mitochondrial biogenesis and dynamics as ES cells differentiate would greatly enhance our understanding of the role of mitochondria during differentiation.

Although many of the studies discussed above have generated data suggesting that differentiation of pluripotent stem cells is linked to a switch to oxidative metabolism, or changes in mitochondrial properties, comparisons are often made with pluripotent cells maintained using different basal medium formulations or conditions, and differentiation is induced using different protocols (EB formation vs. directed by exogenous growth factors). Data may also be biased by the selection of differentiation pathway and differentiated cell population used in the comparison, as different cell populations differ significantly in mitochondrial activity; cardiomyocytes and neurons, for example, depend heavily on mitochondrial activity. The data collected to date suggest that metabolism changes progressively after the initiation of differentiation. The focus on the metabolism of fully differentiated cells has meant that the events that occur within hours of a differentiation stimulus remain unknown.

Reprogramming energy metabolism

Induced pluripotent stem (iPS) cells promise enormous potential for the generation of cells for regenerative medicine, drug discovery, and understanding disease etiology. iPS cells result from the reprogramming of a somatic cell to a pluripotent cell-like state, a process effected by the modulation of transcription factors in the somatic cell [39]. A number of methods have been developed to establish pluripotency, including viral transduction of various combinations of transcription factors and the use of chemical inducers of pluripotency (reviewed in [40]).

Characterization of iPS cells has, until recently, focused largely on pluripotency, epigenetic characteristics, and differentiation potential, with little emphasis placed on the characterization of metabolism. Like ES cells, iPS cells rely heavily on glycolysis for ATP production, with significantly higher glucose consumption and lactate production than fibroblasts or their somatic parental cells [1,2,41]. Total cellular ATP [2,23,41,42], mitochondrial mass [23], and mtDNA copy number [42], are all reduced to more ES-cell-like levels in iPS cells, while the genes regulating glycolysis, the pentose phosphate pathway (PPP), the TCA cycle, and mitochondrial complex activity are increased to levels analogous with ES cells [2,41,43]. Oxygen consumption changes with reprogramming, with iPS cells consuming significantly less oxygen than differentiated cells [41,44], which is consistent with an increased reliance on glycolysis. By NMR, iPS cells can be distinguished from MEFs, and clustered with ES cells, on acetate, lactate, fumarate, and taurine concentrations [41], suggesting that other modifications to metabolism occur as a somatic cell is reprogrammed into an iPS cell. Finally, reprogramming of human adult dermal fibroblasts resulted in a reduction in the expression of antioxidant genes to levels similar to those observed in human ES cells [17]. These data indicate that iPS cells acquire not only functional characteristics of pluripotent cells but also a metabolism that is characteristic of ES cells.

The modification of metabolism may not be merely a consequence of reprogramming, but a required component of the process. Stimulating glycolysis with D-fructose-6-phosphate enhances reprogramming, while inhibiting glycolysis with 2-deoxy-D-glucose inhibits reprogramming [41,43]. Together these data illustrate the importance of intact glycolytic machinery in reprogramming. As with ES cells, however, there is a lack of comparative metabolic data collected from multiple lines that allow a comprehensive appreciation of the importance of metabolic reprogramming and which provide a solid baseline of metabolic activity against which to compare new lines. iPS cell lines generated by different methods can differ in their metabolic activity, such that reprogramming with three transcription factors resulted in cells that produced less lactate when compared to cells formed in response to exogenous expression of four factors; the lower lactate production was more similar to ES cells [41]. These observations, however, are limited to two cell lines and may reflect inherent variability in the metabolism of iPS cell lines rather than a consequence of different methodology.

Although several changes in metabolism occur in iPS cell formation that make these cell more ES-cell-like, a number of metabolic characteristics are not equivalent between ES and iPS cells [2,42,45], and iPS cell lines retain some characteristics of their somatic history. Microarray analysis has highlighted differences in the expression of genes controlling mitochondrial regulation between ES and iPS cells [45,46], suggesting incomplete reprogramming of the nuclear and mtDNA compartments regulating mitochondrial function and metabolism. Transmission electron micrographs show that a proportion of mitochondria in iPS cells retain a cristae-rich, elongated architecture [1,2,23], although the extent of this retention has not been quantified. It has been concluded, however, that reprogramming leads to the complete remodeling of mitochondria to a pluripotent state in iPS cells. How these elongated, cristae-rich mitochondria contribute to iPS cell physiology and integrity has not been investigated. Mouse ES cells are characterized by high levels of unsaturated fatty acid metabolites, the levels of which decrease upon differentiation [37]. In contrast, iPS cells have reduced levels of unsaturated fatty acid metabolites when compared with ES cells [43]; this potentially reflects their somatic cell history. Finally, in comparison to ES cells, iPS cells have higher levels of metabolites involved in the *S*-adenosyl methionine (SAM) cycle [43]. The SAM cycle links metabolism to epigenetic modifications [47], and suggests a link between metabolic activity and epigenetic stability. These data, which represent an incomplete comparative survey of metabolism between iPS cells and pluripotent cells, suggest that although iPS cells are functionally pluripotent, they are potentially incompletely programmed with respect to metabolism and retain features reflecting the metabolism of their parental lineage. It is simply too early to assess the extent of the metabolic misprogramming or the implications of this on the differentiation and use of these cells.

More seriously, Prigione *et al.* report the occurrence of mutations in the mtDNA of iPS cells that were not present in the parental cells [3]. While these mutations did not appear to impact on the reprogramming of the majority of metabolic parameters measured, the affected lines had an increased ATP reserve, similar to the reserves seen in fibroblasts. Potentially these mutations may impact the ability of cells to respond to changes in energy requirements and supply, and to differentiate into functional somatic cells. Regardless of the ramifications of these mutations, it is unlikely that cells harboring mtDNA mutations and aberrant metabolism will be suitable for commercial and clinical uses.

Differences between iPS cells and ES cells highlight the need for more exhaustive evaluations of both pluripotent stem-cell sources, at the genetic, epigenetic, functional, and physiological level, before the utility of these cells in research, disease models, and drug testing can be realized.

Regulation of ES cell metabolism by the culture environment

A lack of optimized and standardized conditions for the derivation and culture of pluripotent stem cells will limit their use in research, and in commercial and clinical applications, and may increase heterogeneity between lines. The development of the preimplantation embryo in vitro has been shown to be impacted by a number of culture variables, including oxygen concentration, medium formulation, and supplementation strategies [48]. Optimization of embryo culture conditions, and translation of these conditions into the clinic, has had a significant and measurable impact on pregnancy rates following in vitro fertilization; advances in embryo culture conditions have been cited as one of the most important developments in the field of assisted human conception [49]. There is a growing realization among stem-cell biologists of the importance of understanding of how culture variables affect the growth and function of ES cells, and of the need for optimization of culture conditions to promote functional and physiologically normal cells in culture. Culture variables include the composition of the gaseous phase, predominantly the concentration of oxygen, the medium formulation, and the presence of culture additives such as serum.

In the past decade a number of laboratories have investigated the role of oxygen concentration on ES cell culture. The oxygen concentration in the reproductive tract has been measured to be between 2 and 8% [50], however pluripotent stem cells are most often cultured under an atmospheric (~20%) oxygen concentration, reflecting the disconnect between in vivo and in vitro conditions. There have been reports demonstrating that reduced oxygen concentrations are correlated with increased pluripotency marker expression [51,52], improved chromosomal stability [53], decreased differentiation [52,54,55], enhanced derivation of mouse [56] and human [57] ES cells, and improved generation of iPS cells from mouse embryonic fibroblasts [58]. There are, however, reports that have failed to demonstrate enhanced ES cell pluripotency marker expression [52,53,55] or proliferation [52,54] in cells cultured in lower oxygen concentrations. The lack of compelling experimental data on the effect of oxygen on ES cells probably reflects the subtle effects elicited in the cells, the use of a limited range of cellular characteristics, and, potentially, characteristics that are insensitive to the ambient oxygen levels, to detect these differences and the confounding effect of different cell lines and different experimental approaches used to culture ES cells and modify ambient oxygen. The lack of concordant data on the detrimental effects of atmospheric oxygen concentrations on ES cells, coupled with the ability to maintain pluripotency in a high proportion of cells within an ES cell population cultured in atmospheric oxygen, and the cost and inconvenience of maintaining culture incubators at low oxygen concentrations, probably underlies the reluctance of the field to adopt physiological oxygen concentrations for pluripotent stem cell culture and maintenance.

Approaches to characterize the effect of oxygen concentration on ES cells in culture have focused on monitoring the molecular and biochemical manifestations of pluripotency, and have largely neglected the effect of oxygen on ES cell metabolism. Recent research by our laboratory has found changes in carbohydrate and amino acid use by human ES cells cultured in mTeSR, defined and feeder-free culture system (mTeSR) [34], under 5% oxygen compared to 20% oxygen; these changes occurred without significant changes in colony morphology, proliferation, or pluripotent and differentiation marker expression (Harvey *et al.* unpublished). The effect of oxygen concentration on oxygen consumption and the oxygen uptake rate (OUR) of human ES cells and iPS cells in culture has also been investigated [44]. Reductions in oxygen concentration, to physiological and hypoxic levels, did not change oxygen consumption, but the OURs of both cell populations were less in lower oxygen concentrations. Similarly, glycolysis can be enhanced when mouse ES cells are cultured in a more physiological oxygen concentration (3%) [4]. These data suggest that pluripotent cells have mechanisms that promote adaptation to lower oxygen concentrations within the environment. The response of human ES cells and iPS cells to oxygen concentration was similar, although in atmospheric oxygen the OUR of iPS cells was significantly higher; this may reflect the different origin of these cells or an underlying variability in this parameter in pluripotent cells when cultured in 20% oxygen.

A number of observations, including the heterogeneity of mouse ES cell cultures [27,28], the ability of distinct pluripotent cell populations to be enriched in manipulated culture conditions [59,60], and the differences that have been documented between mouse and human ES cells [61], have led to the definition of a number of pluripotent cell states in culture. Preliminary analysis of the metabolism of different cell states indicates that culture conditions that modulate cell state can alter the metabolic response to environmental perturbations. Mouse ES cells maintained in serum-containing medium with LIF are considered to be a mixed population comprising several cell states and have been defined as primed for differentiation [59,60]. When cultured in 2% oxygen this population has a lower uptake of glucose, increased flux of glucose through glycolysis, and a decreased proliferation rate than equivalently cultured populations in atmospheric oxygen [33]. In serum-free medium with inhibitors of intracellular signaling, culture conditions that promote the ground-state pluripotent cell, proliferation is not reduced in 2% oxygen, and both glucose uptake and lactate production appear increased when compared with 20% oxygen conditions [33]. Glycolytic flux is not significantly different between the two oxygen conditions. It is not clear from these approaches if the differences in metabolic responses to oxygen concentration reflect the response of the different cell states or differences in the culture medium used affecting cell behavior.

A comparison of mouse ES and EpiSC cells, and human ES cells, also demonstrated differences in metabolism between pluripotent cell states, specifically between ICM-like cells, represented by mouse ES cells, and epiblast-like populations, represented by EpiSC and human ES cells [62]. Mouse ES cells were shown to be characterized by the generation of ATP through glycolysis and mitochondrial metabolism, which was flexible enough to support the cell when glycolysis was inhibited. In contrast, mouse EpiSC and human ES cells were more glycolytic and less capable of generating ATP from OXPHOS; inhibition of glycolysis in these cells led to a loss of cell viability as a result of their impaired ability to increase mitochondrial respiration [62]. Likewise, others have also reported that, despite containing functional mitochondria, human ES cells generate very little ATP by OXPHOS [62]. The differences in metabolism between cell states were reflected in lower ATP levels, lower expression levels of genes required for mitochondrial metabolism, a 40% reduction in COX protein activity and a lower mitochondrial membrane potential in EpiSC and human ES cells when compared to mouse ES cells. Paradoxically, despite having reduced mitochondrial function, EpiSC and human ES cells had more mtDNA and mitochondria that appeared, in comparison, to be more elongated, electron dense, and which contained more developed cristae. This suggests that although the mitochondria are essential for pluripotent cells, this reliance is not a requirement for mitochondrial respiration, but suggests a more complex relationship between mitochondria and pluripotency. Although a reduction in COX gene expression was demonstrated in freshly isolated epiblast when compared to ICM, it is still difficult to interpret the differences in metabolism as resulting exclusively from differences in cell state, as the media used to culture mouse ES cells or EpiSC and human ES cells were different, most notably in the use of serum for the former and Knockout™ Serum Replacement (Knockout™ SR) for the latter.

The development of xeno-free systems for the derivation and maintenance of pluripotent stem cells has become a priority to ensure the safety of cells for use in regenerative medicine, paralleling the development of defined conditions for pre-implantation embryo culture. The inclusion of serum or feeders to support stem cells introduces undefined components to the system, and impairs the clinical and pharmaceutical applications of pluripotent stem cells. In embryo culture, serum has been shown to damage embryonic cell ultrastructure, specifically affecting mitochondrial state and function, thereby compromising embryo metabolism and oxidative function, culminating in impaired embryo development, and abnormal gene expression and imprinting [48,63]. In cultured human ES cells addition of animal-derived components to the medium leads to metabolic incorporation of metabolites, including N-glycolylneuramine (Neu5Gc). Subsequent exposure of these cells to human sera containing antibodies directed against Neu5Gc suggested that the incorporation of the xeno-antigen could elicit an immune response on transplantation [64].

Knockout™ SR, a defined supplement specifically formulated to support mouse ES cell self-renewal, has been used extensively in the development of xeno-free culture media for human ES cells. The use of Knockout™ SR, and specifically the ascorbate within this medium supplement, has been reported to cause DNA demethylation in human ES cells leading to increased expression of CD30 [65]. Findings by our laboratory suggest that human ES cells interact with their surrounding medium. In response to supplementation with serum or Knockout™ SR, human ES cells changed carbohydrate use and amino-acid turnover without significantly impacting on pluripotency (Rathjen *et al.*, unpublished). In mouse ES cells, glucose consumption and lactate production were also sensitive to medium supplementation, with higher carbohydrate use in cells cultured in serum-supplemented medium when compared with medium containing Knockout™ SR [5]. The development of xeno-free culture systems to date has relied on defining conditions that maximize pluripotent cell numbers and inhibit differentiation almost exclusively; these data stress the importance of understanding optimal metabolic characteristics and including evaluation of cell metabolic parameters during medium development.

Adaptation of ES cells to different culture conditions, using a comparative system that can monitor metabolic response to culture conditions, has been used to assess mitochondrial properties in human ES cells cultured in two feeder-conditioned culture media [26]. Cells cultured without feeders in a mesenchymal stem-cell-conditioned medium showed higher MMP, mtDNA content and mitochondrial gene expression, correlated with higher expression levels of the pluripotent markers, when compared to cells cultured in human fibroblast-cell-conditioned medium [26]. Mitochondrial characteristics were not fixed in each population, as adaptation of a human ES cell line from one condition into the other was accompanied by co-ordinated changes in mtDNA levels, mitochondrial gene expression, and pluripotency marker expression [26]. Mitochondrial changes have been detected with time in culture. Human ES cells propagated for 120 passages displayed reduced oxygen consumption, significantly higher MMP, enlarged mitochondrial volume, and higher levels of ROS when compared to cells from the same line at a lower passage number [26]. High and low passage number cells were both able to differentiate into derivatives of all three germ lineages in teratomas. Gene-expression analysis revealed a modest reduction in the expression of endoderm-associated markers and increased expression in one of two ectodermal markers tested in teratomas derived from higher passage-number cells, perhaps indicating that time in culture can affect differentiation outcome [66].

These studies provide evidence that long-term culture and exposure to different culture conditions can impact ES cell physiology and differentiation capacity without necessarily influencing markers of pluripotency. It is important to consider that while pre-implantation embryos are able to adapt to their environment in vitro, this adaptation results in perturbations in metabolite use, leading to a loss of subsequent developmental capacity and viability [48]. Perturbed metabolism may also alter the epigenome [47]. The question remains as to whether this is also the case for stem cells; does adaptation of ES cells to in vitro culture, with the concomitant changes in metabolite use, compromise viability and function?

Molecular regulation of metabolic pathways in pluripotent stem cells

Cellular responses to changes in oxygen involve the regulation of hypoxia-inducible factors (HIFs). HIFs are activated in cells in low oxygen concentrations; in a range of cell types, HIF activation has been shown to increase exponentially once oxygen concentrations drop below 7% oxygen, with maximal activation at 0.5%. HIFs reprogram metabolism to ensure continued energy production at low oxygen concentrations via the regulation of transcription, including the up-regulation of genes involved in glycolytic metabolism (reviewed in [67]). Long-term adaptation of human ES cells to physiological oxygen conditions has recently been attributed to HIF2α (reviewed in [51]), the only HIFα protein shown to be detectable at the blastocyst stage to date [68]. HIF2α has been shown to regulate Oct4 [69] and chemical inhibition of HIFα proteins reduces transcriptional and protein expression of Oct4, Nanog, and Sox2 in mouse and rat ES cells [70]. More recently, activation of HIF1α has been shown to switch ES cell metabolism from a reliance on both OXPHOS and glycolysis, to predominantly glycolysis, rendering ES cell morphologically and metabolically similar to EpiSC [71]. The regulation of a number of pathways shown to be involved in ES cell maintenance and the continued expression of the core pluripotent stem-cell regulator by HIFs suggests that oxygen concentration plays a role in regulating pluripotency (Figure 15.2).

Recognition and response by cells to changes in energy availability are regulated by interactions between the AMP-activated protein-kinase (AMPK), the mammalian target of rapamycin (mTOR), and the sirtuin-1 (SIRT1) pathways. These pathways act to maintain energy homeostasis within the cell and ensure consistency of ATP concentration. AMPK positively regulates ATP generation and negatively regulates ATP consumption and has been shown to be up-regulated in cells cultured in low oxygen concentrations. Up-regulation of ATP generation by AMPK is largely mediated through increased glucose uptake and the activation of glycolysis, as well as through the regulation of mitochondrial biogenesis (reviewed in [72]). The activation of AMPK in pluripotent stem cells has not provided a clear understanding of the role of this protein in pluripotency. Adamo *et al.* demonstrated improved maintenance of mouse ES cell pluripotency and inhibition of RA-induced differentiation in the presence of 1 mM AICAR, an AMPK activator [73]. The addition of 0.5 mM AICAR to mouse ES cells, however, inhibited proliferation and induced differentiation [74]. The activation of AMPK with alternative compounds, such as metformin, prior to or during reprogramming decreased the generation of mouse and human iPS cells [75]. These data

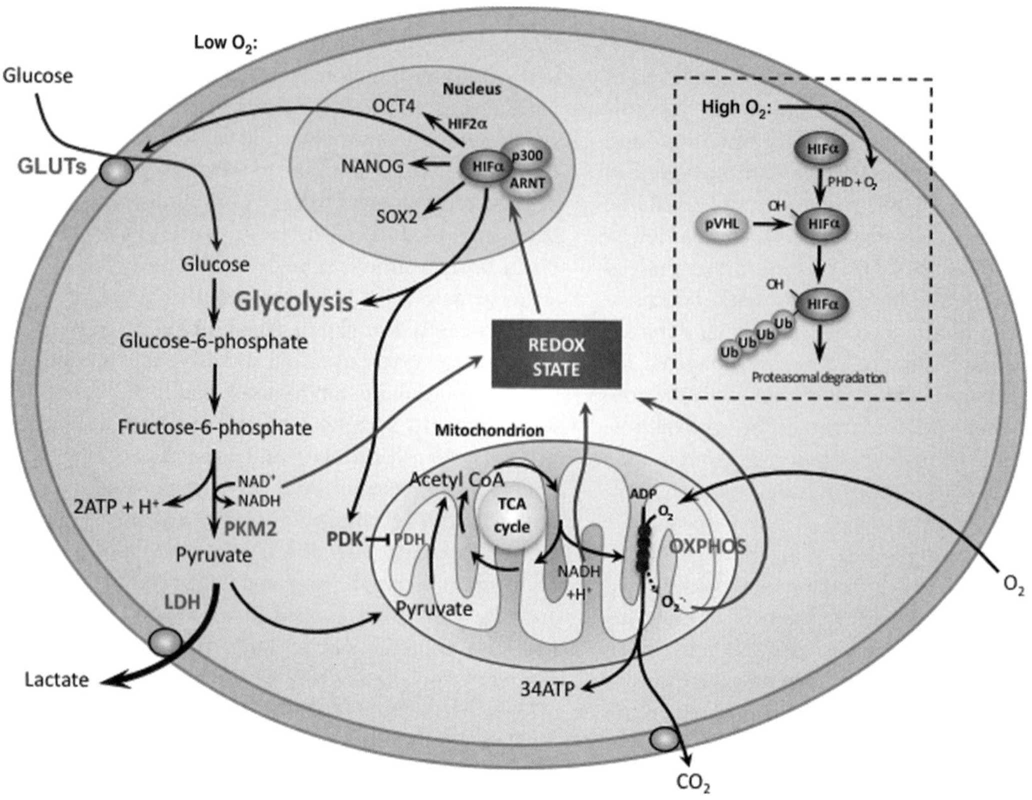

Figure 15.2 Schematic representation of oxygen and redox-regulated HIF modulation of ES cell metabolism. Under conditions of high oxygen concentrations (dashed box), HIFα proteins are targeted for proteasomal degradation through hydroxylation by proline hydroxylases (PHD) and recognition by pVHL (von Hippel Lindau tumor suppressor protein), leading to tagging of HIFα with polyubiquitin. In response to low oxygen concentrations, proline hydroxylation is inhibited, leading to stabilization and accumulation of HIFα protein, and translocation to the nucleus. This enables dimerization of HIFα with HIF1β (ARNT) and p300, and subsequent binding to hypoxia response elements within target genes. HIF targets include glucose transporters (GLUTs), glycolytic enzymes, and the pyruvate dehydrogenase kinase (PDK), resulting in increased glycolytic activity to maintain ATP [16]. Chemical inhibition of HIFα proteins reduces transcriptional and protein expression of *Oct4*, *Nanog*, and *Sox2* in mouse and rat ES cells [66], supporting a role for HIF in regulating pluripotency markers; HIF2α is known to activate *Oct4* directly in mouse ES cells [69], while HIF2α silencing results in reduced *OCT4*, *NANOG*, and *SOX2* protein expression in human ES cells [68]. More recently, activation of HIF1α has been shown to switch mouse ES cell metabolism from a reliance on both oxidative and glycolytic metabolism, to predominantly glycolytic, rendering ES cells morphologically and metabolically similar to EpiSCs [51]. Changes in redox state have also been shown to stabilize HIF1α. The cellular redox state relies on the rates of production and elimination of reactive oxygen species, and the production and oxidation of reducing equivalents from cytoplasmic and mitochondrial metabolism (blue arrows), and functions to modulate cellular signalling and homeostasis. Abbreviations: HIF, hypoxia-inducible factor; Ub, ubiquitin; ATP, adenosine triphosphate; O_2, oxygen; $O_2^{\cdot-}$, hydroxyl radical; NAD^+, nicotinamide adenine dinucleotide; NADH, reduced form of NAD^+; TCA, tricarboxylic acid cycle; PKM2, pyruvate kinase M2; LDH, lactate dehydrogenase. (See also color plate.)

suggest a role for AMPK in regulating ATP levels within pluripotent cells, where perturbation of AMPK regulation can affect cell function and/or pluripotency. However, the effect of activating AMPK is variable, potentially reflecting the influence of different culture conditions on ES cell processes required to maintain homeostasis.

Downstream targets of AMPK – SIRT1, UCP2, and mTOR – have been shown to regulate ES cell biology in culture with effects on pluripotency and cell differentiation. SIRT1, a NAD^+-dependent histone deacetylase, has been shown to modulate the translocation of p53 and regulate apoptosis in mouse ES cells in response to oxidative stress, preserving pluripotency by maintaining p53-dependent *Nanog* expression [76]. SIRT1 is also up-regulated during the reprogramming of mouse fibroblasts to iPS cells [77]. In contrast, human ES cells may not require SIRT1 to maintain pluripotency, as treatment of human ES cells for 2 days with SIRT1 siRNA leads to a greater change in the percentage of differentiation markers altered by SIRT1 inhibition than in the percentage of pluripotency markers [78]. Down-regulation of SIRT1 is observed 15 days after the induction of differentiation of human ES cells to EBs [78], although it is unclear whether SIRT1 decreases at earlier stages of differentiation. Notably, there are seven mammalian Sirtuins, many of which are currently poorly characterized. Whether other Sirtuins are capable of compensating for the loss of SIRT1 remains to be determined. In addition to their roles in epigenetic silencing, Sirtuins require NAD^+ as a co-factor, linking SIRT1 activity to cellular redox state and metabolism. As histone signatures are central to ES cell pluripotency, and differentiation, SIRT1 may play a role in modulating epigenetic silencing in ES cells, as well as during the reprogramming process.

Expression of uncoupling protein 2 (UCP2) has been correlated with pluripotency, and down-regulation of the protein has been shown to be required for ES cell differentiation [6]. UCP2 has been hypothesized to regulate the relative contributions of glycolysis and OXPHOS to energy production, reducing glucose flux through mitochondrial oxidation, and facilitating glycolysis through a substrate-shunting mechanism [6]. Decreased expression of UCP2 in human ES cells reduced metabolic activity but did not affect the expression of pluripotency markers, suggesting that it is not required for pluripotency [6]. Differentiation of human ES cells was shown to be accompanied by down-regulation of UCP2 and a slow transition from glycolysis to OXPHOS over successive days. Ectopic expression of UCP2 in human ES cells prevented this transition and inhibited up-regulation of differentiation markers during retinoic-acid-induced differentiation; these data suggest that the regulation of UCP2 and metabolism is a key step in human ES cell differentiation and that UCP2 is functioning to enforce glycolytic metabolism in human ES cells. It is also tempting to speculate that UCP2 may function in the transition of pluripotent cells from a metabolism reliant on both OXPHOS and glycolysis in ICM-like cells to the predominantly glycolytic metabolism of epiblast-like stem cells.

mTOR is a conserved serine/threonine kinase that plays a central role in regulating cell growth and metabolism, and functions as a sensor of cellular nutrient and energy levels, and redox status. mTOR comprises two complexes, the rapamycin-sensitive mTOR complex 1 (mTORC1; mTOR-Raptor), and the rapamycin-insensitive complex mTORC2 (mTOR-Rictor). Mice with disruption of the kinase domain of mTOR die shortly after implantation with defects in embryonic and extra-embryonic cell proliferation; ES cells carrying this mutation failed to proliferate [79]. Inhibition of mTORC1 with rapamycin in mouse ES cells that exhibit a high MMP led to decreased MMP, oxygen consumption, and lactate production, features characteristic of ES cells sorted for low MMP, suggesting a role for mTOR in the interconversion of these two cell populations and potentially in the regulation of mitochondrial activity in ES cells [25]. Similarly, inhibition of mTOR appears to prevent EPL cell formation from ES cells, a conversion representative of the formation of later epiblasts from ICM in the embryo [36]. In human ES cells the effect of rapamycin treatment is not consistent. Loss of human ES cell pluripotency and proliferative capacity following mTOR inhibition by rapamycin has been demonstrated; these defects could be rescued by activation of mTOR [80]. In contrast, others have shown that inhibition of mTOR with rapamycin did not affect pluripotency, although constitutive activation of p70 S6K, downstream of mTORC1, was associated with loss of human ES cell morphology and *OCT4* expression [81]. Activation of mTOR, through deletion of the mTOR suppressor tuberous sclerosis complex 2 (TSC2), prevents reprogramming of mouse embryonic fibroblasts; inhibition of mTOR activation with rapamycin in these $Tsc2^{-/-}$ cells leads to the formation of alkaline phosphatase-positive cells [82].

These data suggest a role for energy-sensing in modulating pluripotent stem-cell physiology. As modulation of these pathways alters ES cell function, this implies a critical relationship between the maintenance of homeostasis and ATP levels, and the maintenance of pluripotency. Significantly, the variability in experimental results suggests a diverse physiological profile across ES cell lines, a diversity that has not been detected by the analysis of gene expression, epigenetics, or differentiation potential alone. This variability likely reflects the multiplicity of culture conditions used in the isolation and maintenance of these cells, and amplifies diversity attributable to inherent inter-line variation.

Conclusions

Metabolic features are a recent addition to the portfolio of characteristics that can be used to describe and define pluripotent stem cells in culture. In comparison to somatic cells, pluripotent stem cells are metabolically distinct, relying largely on glycolysis for the generation of ATP, containing morphologically diverse mitochondria and maintaining low levels of intracellular ATP. Several lines of evidence imply that the pluripotent cell metabolism is not only a characteristic of these cells, but may act to maintain and regulate pluripotency, proliferation, and differentiation. The acquisition of pluripotency during the formation of iPS cells requires metabolic reprogramming to a pluripotent stem-cell metabolism [41,43,82]. Approaches to understanding the role of pluripotent stem-cell mitochondria are uncovering a complex relationship between the cell and its mitochondria, predicting a role for the organelle in regulating cell function. Transcriptome analyses have begun to show links between core transcriptional circuitry and metabolic gene regulation within pluripotent stem cells [83]. Unlike other cell systems, however, there is as yet no direct demonstration of a nexus between specific metabolic pathways in pluripotent stem cells and the regulation of other pluripotent cell functions. Finding these will provide new avenues for regulating pluripotency and differentiation in culture.

The unique metabolism of pluripotent stem cells predicates that they may not respond to medium formulations and supplements like somatic cells. The proliferation of specialized and optimized media to support these cells in culture recognizes this, but medium formulation still appears to be largely empirical and not informed by metabolic processes. It is clear that pluripotent stem cells react and adapt to suboptimal culture conditions by altering their metabolism, particularly changing metabolism to ensure ATP levels are maintained. A result of working in a cell-based system, however, is that the consequences of these metabolic alterations on cell function are difficult to appreciate. Despite this, unravelling the effects of the culture environment on pluripotent stem cells and defining an optimal metabolism to be achieved in culture needs to be a priority, particularly for cells destined for medical applications. These aims should be coupled with approaches to understand the underlying variability in metabolism in these cells in culture to provide a baseline metabolism against which all new cell isolates and culture conditions can be appraised. Approaches to optimizing the culture environment will need to recognize and incorporate the differences in metabolism

that have been detected between pluripotent cell states, developing conditions that maintain each population in a metabolically appropriate configuration. Lastly, in the view of the authors, optimal culture conditions need to strive to achieve metabolic states that mirror the physiology of embryonic cell states in vivo.

References

1. Prigione, A., Fauler, B., Lurz, R. *et al.* The senescence-related mitochondrial/oxidative stress pathway is repressed in human induced pluripotent stem cells. *Stem Cells.* 2010; 28(4): 721–733.

2. Varum, S., Rodrigues, A.S., Moura, M.B. *et al.* Energy metabolism in human pluripotent stem cells and their differentiated counterparts. *PLoS One.* 2011; 6(6): e20914.

3. Prigione, A., Lichtner, B., Kuhl, H. *et al.* Human induced pluripotent stem cells harbor homoplasmic and heteroplasmic mitochondrial DNA mutations while maintaining human embryonic stem cell-like metabolic reprogramming. *Stem Cells.* 2011; 29(9): 1338–1348.

4. Kondoh, H., Lleonart, M.E., Nakashima, Y. *et al.* A high glycolytic flux supports the proliferative potential of murine embryonic stem cells. *Antioxid ants and Redox Signaling.* 2007; 9(3): 293–299.

5. Fernandes, T.G., Fernandes-Platzgummer, A.M., da Silva, C.L. *et al.* Kinetic and metabolic analysis of mouse embryonic stem cell expansion under serum-free conditions. *Biotechnology Letters.* 2010; 32(1): 171–179.

6. Zhang, J., Khvorostov, I., Hong, J.S. *et al.* UCP2 regulates energy metabolism and differentiation potential of human pluripotent stem cells. *EMBO Journal.* 2011; 30(24): 4860–4873.

7. Newsholme, E.A., Crabtree, B., Ardawi, M.S. The role of high rates of glycolysis and glutamine utilization in rapidly dividing cells. *Bioscience Reports.* 1985; 5(5): 393–400.

8. Gopichandran, N., Leese, H.J. Metabolic characterization of the bovine blastocyst, inner cell mass, trophectoderm and blastocoel fluid. *Reproduction.* 2003; 126(3): 299–308.

9. Hewitson, L.C., Leese, H.J. Energy metabolism of the trophectoderm and inner cell mass of the mouse blastocyst. *Journal of Experimental Zoology.* 1993; 267(3): 337–343.

10. Sariban-Sohraby, S., Magrath, I.T., Balaban, R.S. Comparison of energy metabolism in human normal and neoplastic (Burkitt's lymphoma) lymphoid cells. *Cancer Research.* 1983; 43(10): 4662–4664.

11. Hume, D.A., Weidemann, M.J. Role and regulation of glucose metabolism in proliferating cells. *Journal of the National Cancer Institute.* 1979; 62(1): 3–8.

12. Mandel, L.J. Energy metabolism of cellular activation, growth and transformation. *Current Topics in Membrane and Transport.* 1986; 27: 261–291.

13. Morgan, M.J., Faik, P. Carbohydrate metabolism in cultured animal cells. *Bioscience Reports.* 1981; 1(9): 669–686.

14. Reitzer, L.J., Wice, B.M., Kennell, D. The pentose cycle. Control and essential function in HeLa cell nucleic acid synthesis. *Journal of Biological Chemistry.* 1980; 255(12): 5616–5626.

15. Alexander, P.B., Wang, J., McKnight, S.L. Targeted killing of a mammalian cell based upon its specialized metabolic state. *Proceedings of the National Academy of Sciences of the United States of America.* 2011; 108(38): 15828–15833.

16. Wang, J., Alexander, P., Wu, L. *et al.* Dependence of mouse embryonic stem cells on threonine catabolism. *Science.* 2009; 325(5939): 435–439.

17. Armstrong, L., Tilgner, K., Saretzki, G. *et al.* Human induced pluripotent stem cell lines show stress defense mechanisms and mitochondrial regulation similar to those of human embryonic stem cells. *Stem Cells.* 2010; 28(4): 661–673.

18. Kelly, R.D., Sumer, H., McKenzie, M. *et al.* The effects of nuclear reprogramming on mitochondrial DNA replication. *Stem Cell Reviews.* 2011 Oct 13. [Epub ahead of print.]

19. Cho, Y.M., Kwon, S., Pak, Y.K. *et al.* Dynamic changes in mitochondrial biogenesis and antioxidant enzymes during the spontaneous differentiation of human embryonic stem cells. *Biochemistry and Biophysics Research Communications.* 2006; 348(4): 1472–1478.

20. Chung, S., Dzeja, P.P., Faustino, R.S. *et al.* Mitochondrial oxidative metabolism is required for the cardiac differentiation of stem cells. *Nature Clinical Practice Cardiovascular Medicine.* 2007; 4 Suppl 1: S60–S67.

21. St John, J.C., Ramalho-Santos, J., Gray, H.L. *et al.* The expression of mitochondrial DNA transcription factors during early cardiomyocyte *in vitro* differentiation from human embryonic stem cells. *Cloning and Stem Cells.* 2005; 7(3): 141–153.

22. Facucho-Oliveira, J.M., Alderson, J., Spikings, E.C. *et al.* Mitochondrial DNA replication during differentiation of murine embryonic stem cells. *Journal of Cell Science.* 2007; 120 (Pt 22): 4025–4034.

23. Suhr, S.T., Chang, E.A., Tjong, J. *et al.* Mitochondrial rejuvenation after induced pluripotency. *PLoS One.* 2010; 5(11): e14095.

24. Smiley, S.T., Reers, M., Mottola-Hartshorn, C. *et al.* Intracellular heterogeneity in mitochondrial membrane potentials revealed by a J-aggregate-forming lipophilic cation JC-1. *Proceedings of the National Academy of Sciences of the United States of America.* 1991; 88(9): 3671–3675.

25. Schieke, S.M., Ma, M., Cao, L. *et al.* Mitochondrial metabolism modulates differentiation and teratoma formation capacity in mouse embryonic stem cells. *Journal of Biological Chemistry.* 2008; 283(42): 28506–28512.

26. Ramos-Mejia, V., Bueno, C., Roldan, M. *et al.* The adaptation of human embryonic stem cells to different feeder-free culture conditions is accompanied by a mitochondrial response. *Stem Cells and Development.* 2012; 21: 1145–1155.

27. Hayashi, K., Lopes, S.M., Tang, F. *et al.* Dynamic equilibrium and heterogeneity of mouse pluripotent stem cells with distinct functional and epigenetic states. *Cell Stem Cell.* 2008; 3(4): 391–401.

28. Toyooka, Y., Shimosato, D., Murakami, K. *et al.* Identification and characterization of subpopulations in undifferentiated ES cell culture. *Development.* 2008; 135(5): 909–918.

29. Harvey, A., Gibson, T., Lonergan, T. *et al.* Dynamic regulation of mitochondrial function in preimplantation embryos and embryonic stem cells. *Mitochondrion.* 2011; 11(5): 829–838.

30. Todd, L.R., Damin, M.N., Gomathinayagam, R. *et al.* Growth factor erv1-like modulates Drp1 to preserve mitochondrial dynamics and function in mouse embryonic stem cells. *Molecular Biology of the Cell.* 2010; 21(7): 1225–1236.

31. Mandal, S., Lindgren, A.G., Srivatava, A.S. *et al.* Mitochondrial function controls proliferation and early differentiation potential of embryonic stem cells. *Stem Cells.* 2010; 29: 486–495.

32. Varum, S., Momcilovic, O., Castro, C. *et al.* Enhancement of human embryonic stem cell pluripotency through inhibition of the mitochondrial respiratory chain. *Stem Cell Research.* 2009; 3(2–3): 142–156.

33. Fernandes, T.G., Diogo, M.M., Fernandes-Platzgummer, A. *et al.* Different stages of pluripotency determine distinct patterns of proliferation, metabolism, and lineage commitment of embryonic stem cells under hypoxia. *Stem Cell Research.* 2010; 5(1): 76–89.

34. Ludwig, T.E., Levenstein, M.E., Jones, J.M. *et al.* Derivation of human embryonic stem cells in defined conditions. *Nature Biotechnology.* 2006; 24(2): 185–187.

35. Tan, B.S., Lonic, A., Morris, M.B. *et al.* The amino acid transporter SNAT2 mediates L-proline-induced differentiation of ES cells. *American Journal of Physiology, Cell Physiology.* 2011; 300(6): C1270–C1279.

36. Washington, J.M., Rathjen, J., Felquer, F. *et al.* L-Proline induces differentiation of ES cells: a novel role for an amino acid in the regulation of pluripotent cells in culture. *American Journal of Physiology, Cell Physiology.* 2010; 298(5): C982–C992.

37. Yanes, O., Clark, J., Wong, D.M. *et al.* Metabolic oxidation regulates embryonic stem cell differentiation. *Nature Chemical Biology.* 2010; 6(6): 411–417.

38. Sathananthan, A.H., Trounson, A.O. Mitochondrial morphology during preimplantational human embryogenesis. *Human Reproduction.* 2000; 15 Suppl 2: 148–159.

39. Takahashi, K., Yamanaka, S. Induction of pluripotent stem cells from mouse embryonic and adult fibroblast cultures by defined factors. *Cell.* 2006; 126(4): 663–676.

40. Wang, P., Na, J. Mechanism and methods to induce pluripotency. *Protein and Cell.* 2011; 2(10): 792–799.

41. Folmes, C.D., Nelson, T.J., Martinez-Fernandez, A. *et al.* Somatic oxidative bioenergetics transitions into pluripotency-dependent glycolysis to facilitate nuclear reprogramming. *Cell Metabolism.* 2011; 14(2): 264–271.

42. Prigione, A., Adjaye, J. Modulation of mitochondrial biogenesis and bioenergetic metabolism upon *in vitro* and *in vivo* differentiation of human ES and iPS cells. *International Journal of Developmental Biology.* 2010; 54(11–12): 1729–1741.

43. Panopoulos, A.D., Yanes, O., Ruiz, S. *et al.* The metabolome of induced pluripotent stem cells reveals metabolic changes occurring in somatic cell reprogramming. *Cell Research.* 2012; 22(1): 168–177.

44. Abaci, H.E., Truitt, R., Luong, E. *et al.* Adaptation to oxygen deprivation in cultures of human pluripotent stem cells, endothelial progenitor cells, and umbilical vein endothelial cells. *American Journal of Physiology, Cell Physiology.* 2010; 298(6): C1527–C1537.

45. Chin, M.H., Mason, M.J., Xie, W. *et al.* Induced pluripotent stem cells and embryonic stem cells are distinguished by gene expression signatures. *Cell Stem Cell.* 2009; 5(1): 111–123.

46. Lowry, W.E., Richter, L., Yachechko, R. *et al.* Generation of human induced pluripotent stem cells from dermal fibroblasts. *Proceedings of the National Academy of Sciences of the United States of America.* 2008; 105(8): 2883–2888.

47. Donohoe, D.R., Bultman, S.J. Metaboloepigenetics: interrelationships between energy metabolism and epigenetic control of gene expression. *Journal of Cell Physiology.* 2012; 227: 169–177.

48. Gardner, D.K., Lane, M. *Ex vivo* early embryo development and effects on gene expression and imprinting. *Reproduction, Fertility and Development.* 2005; 17(3): 361–370.

49. Oddens, B., Ledger, B. (eds.) *A Decade of Success in ART: The Most-cited Research Articles on Assisted Reproduction Treatments From the Last 10 Years.* Amsterdam: Excerpta Medica; 2006.

50. Fischer, B., Bavister, B.D. Oxygen tension in the oviduct and uterus of rhesus monkeys, hamsters and rabbits. *Journal of Reproduction and Fertility.* 1993; 99(2): 673–679.

51. Forristal, C.E., Wright, K.L., Hanley, N.A. *et al.* Hypoxia inducible factors regulate pluripotency and proliferation in human embryonic stem cells cultured at reduced oxygen tensions. *Reproduction.* 2010; 139(1): 85–97.

52. Prasad, S.M., Czepiel, M., Cetinkaya, C. *et al.* Continuous hypoxic culturing maintains activation of Notch and allows long-term propagation of human embryonic stem cells without spontaneous differentiation. *Cell Proliferation.* 2009; 42(1): 63–74.

53. Forsyth, N.R., Musio, A., Vezzoni, P. *et al.* Physiologic oxygen enhances human embryonic stem cell clonal recovery and reduces chromosomal abnormalities. *Cloning and Stem Cells.* 2006; 8(1): 16–23.

54. Ezashi, T., Das, P., Roberts, R.M. Low O2 tensions and the prevention of differentiation of hES cells. *Proceedings of the National Academy of Sciences of the United States of America.* 2005; 102(13): 4783–4788.

55. Zachar, V., Prasad, S.M., Weli, S.C. *et al.* The effect of human embryonic stem cells (hESCs) long-term normoxic and hypoxic cultures on the maintenance of pluripotency. *In Vitro Cellular and Developmental Biology, Animal.* 2010; 46(3–4): 276–283.

56. Gibbons, J., Hewitt, E., Gardner, D.K. Effects of oxygen tension on the establishment and lactate dehydrogenase activity of murine embryonic stem cells. *Cloning and Stem Cells.* 2006; 8(2): 117–122.

57. Peura, T.T., Bosman, A., Stojanov, T. Derivation of human embryonic stem cell lines. *Theriogenology.* 2007; 67(1): 32–42.

58. Yoshida, Y., Takahashi, K., Okita, K. *et al.* Hypoxia enhances the generation of induced pluripotent stem cells. *Cell Stem Cell.* 2009; 5(3): 237–241.

59. Rathjen, J., Lake, J.A., Bettess, M.D. *et al.* Formation of a primitive ectoderm like cell population, EPL cells, from ES cells in response to biologically derived factors. *Journal of Cell Science.* 1999; 112 (Pt 5): 601–612.

60. Ying, Q.L., Wray, J., Nichols, J. *et al.* The ground state of embryonic stem cell self-renewal. *Nature.* 2008; 453(7194): 519–523.

61. Pera, M.F., Tam, P.P. Extrinsic regulation of pluripotent stem cells. *Nature.* 2010; 465(7299): 713–720.

62. Zhou, W., Choi, M., Margineantu, D. *et al.* HIF1alpha induced switch from bivalent to exclusively glycolytic metabolism during ESC-to-EpiSC/hESC transition. *EMBO Journal.* 2012; 31: 2103–2116.

63. Khosla, S., Dean, W., Brown, D. *et al.* Culture of preimplantation mouse embryos affects fetal development and the expression of imprinted genes. *Biology of Reproduction.* 2001; 64(3): 918–926.

64. Martin, M.J., Muotri, A., Gage, F., Varki, A. Human embryonic stem cells express an immunogenic nonhuman sialic acid. *Nature Medicine.* 2005; 11(2): 228–232.

65. Chung, T.L., Turner, J.P., Thaker, N.Y. *et al.* Ascorbate promotes epigenetic activation of CD30 in human embryonic stem cells. *Stem Cells.* 2010; 28(10): 1782–1793.

66. Xie, X., Hiona, A., Lee, A.S. *et al.* Effects of long-term culture on human embryonic stem cell aging. *Stem Cells and Development.* 2011; 20(1): 127–138.

67. Semenza, G.L. Regulation of oxygen homeostasis by hypoxia-inducible factor 1. *Physiology (Bethesda).* 2009; 24: 97–106.

68. Harvey, A.J., Kind, K.L., Pantaleon, M. *et al.* Oxygen-regulated gene expression in bovine blastocysts. *Biology of Reproduction.* 2004; 71(4): 1108–1119.

69. Covello, K.L., Kehler, J., Yu, H. *et al.* HIF-2alpha regulates Oct-4: effects of hypoxia on stem cell function, embryonic development, and tumor growth. *Genes and Development.* 2006; 20(5): 557–570.

70. Moreno-Manzano, V., Rodriguez-Jimenez, F.J., Acena-Bonilla, J.L. *et al.* FM19G11, a new hypoxia-inducible factor (HIF) modulator, affects stem cell differentiation status. *Journal of Biological Chemistry.* 2010; 285(2): 1333–1342.

71. Mazumdar, J., O'Brien, W.T., Johnson, R.S. *et al.* O2 regulates stem cells through Wnt/beta-catenin signalling. *Nature Cell Biology.* 2010; 12(10): 1007–1013.

72. Finley, L.W., Haigis, M.C. The coordination of nuclear and mitochondrial communication during aging and calorie restriction. *Ageing Research Reviews.* 2009; 8(3): 173–188.

73. Adamo, L., Zhang, Y., Garcia-Cardena, G. AICAR activates the pluripotency transcriptional network in embryonic stem cells and induces KLF4 and KLF2 expression in fibroblasts. *BMC Pharmacology.* 2009; 9: 2.

74. Chae, H.D., Lee, M.R., Broxmeyer, H.E. 5-Aminoimidazole-4-carboxyamide ribonucleoside induces G(1)/S arrest and Nanog downregulation via p53 and enhances erythroid differentiation. *Stem Cells.* 2012; 30(2): 140–149.

75. Chen, T., Shen, L., Yu, J. *et al.* Rapamycin and other longevity-promoting compounds enhance the generation of mouse induced pluripotent stem cells. *Aging Cell.* 2011; 10(5): 908–911.

76. Han, M.K., Song, E.K., Guo, Y. *et al.* SIRT1 regulates apoptosis and Nanog expression in mouse embryonic stem cells by controlling p53 subcellular localization. *Cell Stem Cell.* 2008; 2(3): 241–251.

77. Saunders, L.R., Sharma, A.D., Tawney, J. *et al.* miRNAs regulate SIRT1 expression during mouse embryonic stem cell differentiation and in adult mouse tissues. *Aging (Albany NY).* 2010; 2(7): 415–431.

78. Calvanese, V., Lara, E., Suarez-Alvarez, B. *et al.* Sirtuin 1 regulation of developmental genes during differentiation of stem cells. *Proceedings of the National Academy of Sciences of the United States of America.* 2010; 107(31): 13736–13741.

79. Murakami, M., Ichisaka, T., Maeda, M. *et al.* mTOR is essential for growth and proliferation in early mouse embryos and embryonic stem cells. *Molecular and Cellular Biology.* 2004; 24(15): 6710–6718.

80. Zhou, J., Su, P., Wang, L. *et al.* mTOR supports long-term self-renewal and suppresses mesoderm and endoderm activities of human embryonic stem cells. *Proceedings of the National Academy of Sciences of the United States of America.* 2009; 106(19): 7840–7845.

81. Easley, C.A., Ben-Yehudah, A., Redinger, C.J. *et al.* mTOR-mediated activation of p70 S6K induces differentiation of pluripotent human embryonic stem cells. *Cellular Reprogramming.* 2010; 12(3): 263–273.

82. He, J., Kang, L., Wu, T. *et al.* An elaborate regulation of mammalian target of rapamycin activity is required for somatic cell reprogramming induced by defined transcription factors. *Stem Cells and Development.* 2012; 21: 2630–2641.

83. Chen X, Xu, H., Yuan, P. *et al.* Integration of external signaling pathways with the core transcriptional network in embryonic stem cells. *Cell.* 2008; 133(6): 1106–1117.

Index

Locators in *italic* refer to figures and tables